ATLAS
OF
CARDIOVASCULAR
PATHOLOGY

ATLASES IN
DIAGNOSTIC SURGICAL PATHOLOGY

Consulting Editor
Gerald M. Bordin, M.D.
Department of Pathology
Scripps Clinic and Research Foundation

Published:

WOLD, McCLEOD, SIM, AND UNNI:
ATLAS OF ORTHOPEDIC PATHOLOGY

COLBY, LOMBARD, YOUSEM, AND KITAICHI:
ATLAS OF PULMONARY SURGICAL PATHOLOGY

KANEL AND KORULA:
ATLAS OF LIVER PATHOLOGY

OWEN AND KELLY:
ATLAS OF GASTROINTESTINAL PATHOLOGY

WENIG:
ATLAS OF HEAD AND NECK PATHOLOGY

Forthcoming Titles:

RO, AMIN, GRIGNON, AYALA:
ATLAS OF SURGICAL PATHOLOGY OF THE MALE REPRODUCTIVE TRACT

ATLAS OF CARDIOVASCULAR PATHOLOGY

Renu Virmani, M.D.
Chairman
Department of Cardiovascular Pathology
Armed Forces Institute of Pathology
Washington, D.C.

Allen Burke, M.D.
Associate Chairman
Department of Cardiovascular Pathology
Armed Forces Institute of Pathology
Washington, D.C.

Andrew Farb, M.D.
Chief, Division of Cardiovascular Research
Department of Cardiovascular Pathology
Armed Forces Institute of Pathology
Washington, D.C.

W.B. SAUNDERS COMPANY
A Division of Harcourt Brace & Company
Philadelphia London Toronto Montreal Sydney Tokyo

W.B. SAUNDERS COMPANY
A Division of Harcourt Brace & Company

The Curtis Center
Independence Square West
Philadelphia, Pennsylvania 19106

Library of Congress Cataloging-in-Publication Data

Virmani, Renu.
    Atlas of cardiovascular pathology / Renu Virmani, Allen Burke,
Andrew Farb.

        p.   cm.   —   (Atlases in diagnostic surgical pathology)

    ISBN 0-7216-4476-7

    1. Cardiovascular system—Diseases—Atlases.   2. Pathology,
Surgical—Atlases.   I. Burke, Allen.   II. Farb, Andrew.
III. Title.   IV. Series.
    [DNLM: 1. Cardiovascular Diseases—pathology—atlases.
WG 17 V819a   1996]
RC669.9.V57   1996   616.1′07—dc20

DNLM/DLC   95-9479

Atlas of Cardiovascular Pathology   ISBN 0-7216-4476-7

Printed in the United States of America.

Last digit is the print number: 9   8   7   6   5   4   3   2   1

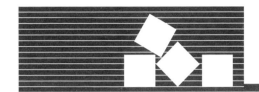

AUTHORS and CONTRIBUTORS

Authors:

Allen Burke, M.D.
Associate Chairman
Department of Cardiovascular Pathology
Armed Forces Institute of Pathology
Washington, D.C.

Andrew Farb, M.D.
Chief, Division of Cardiovascular Research
Department of Cardiovascular Pathology
Armed Forces Institute of Pathology
Washington, D.C.

Renu Virmani, M.D.
Chairman
Department of Cardiovascular Pathology
Armed Forces Institute of Pathology
Washington, D.C.

Contributor:

James B. Atkinson, M.D.
Associate Professor of Pathology
Vanderbilt University Medical Center
Nashville, Tennessee
Endomyocardial Biopsy of Cardiac Allografts and Transplant Atherosclerosis

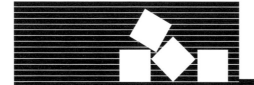

PREFACE

Surgical pathology of the cardiovascular system is a relatively new field. Textbooks of surgical pathology have, in the past, provided only a superficial discussion of the heart and blood vessels or ignored them altogether. Since the advent of cardiac bypass and newer techniques in vascular surgery, pathologists now commonly encounter biopsies of the heart and great vessels. What was once the realm of the autopsy pathologist has now entered the surgical pathologist's world, and there is an increasing need for cardiovascular pathology texts with a bias toward surgical specimens.

This atlas is specifically aimed, therefore, to meet what we see as a void in the current medical literature: a useful reference book with ample illustrations of the common and rare surgical diseases of both the heart *and* blood vessels. Although the emphasis in this volume is clearly on surgical specimens, autopsy specimens are occasionally included, especially for the illustration of aortic diseases, the gross appearance of which are important to the understanding of the underlying pathologic processes.

This book is structured for ease of use; pathologic entities are discussed essentially by organ. The first section on endomyocardial biopsy is arranged by indications for biopsy and outlines the technical and histologic evaluation of biopsy specimens. It stresses common pitfalls in diagnosis and illustrates the majority of conditions that the pathologist will encounter, as well as typical biopsy sign-out for the evaluation of dilated cardiomyopathy and other common diseases.

The second section, on valvular disease, is organized within the context of clinical indications for surgical excision. Each cardiac valve is discussed separately. This organization results in duplicate discussions of certain entities, such as rheumatic valvular disease, but it allows easy reference for the pathologist who must make a diagnosis on a specimen. A discussion of prosthetic valves illustrates the more common valves that will be encountered and various etiologies for prosthetic valve failure.

Although cardiac tumors are rare, it is becoming more common to see them as surgical specimens because they are increasingly encountered with new imaging techniques. The third section extensively illustrates the diagnostic criteria for myxoma, the most common cardiac neoplasm, and discusses the various differential diagnoses and pitfalls in diagnosis. Malignant primary and metastatic lesions of the heart are illustrated. The fourth section, on diseases of the pericardium, illustrates common and unusual neoplasms and focuses on the differential diagnoses, especially between reactive mesothelial hyperplasia, malignant mesothelioma, and metastatic carcinoma.

This Atlas addresses a broad spectrum of vascular diseases that may be diagnosed by surgical biopsy, including those involving the aorta and pulmonary vessels. The pathologic examination of specimens obtained by newer techniques, such as endarterectomy and atherectomy, are amply covered in the fifth section. A simplified classification and approach to vasculitis will prove helpful to the practicing pathologist in the differential diagnosis of inflammatory vascular disease. The more common peripheral vascular tumors are illustrated in the sixth section, with a recent classification of hemangiomas that will, we hope, elucidate this complex area.

An all-inclusive textbook on a subject as vast as this would require several thousand pages. This Atlas is not intended to be an exhaustive reference work. Rather, we hope that it will readily guide the pathologist to the proper interpretation of cardiovascular surgical material and provide a springboard for further investigation. As the designation "atlas" indicates, the emphasis is on illustrations, often multiple, of the different disease processes. We hope that areas of cardiovascular pathology that were previously difficult or obscure to the practicing surgical pathologist will hereby become clarified. If the interpretation of cardiac biopsies, of valve specimens, and of blood vessels is made any easier by access to this volume, then our major goals will have been met.

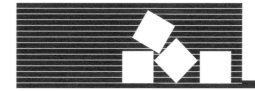

CONTENTS

Section 3
SURGICAL PATHOLOGY OF CARDIAC MASSES

Section 4
DISEASES OF THE PERICARDIUM

Section 5
DISEASES OF THE GREAT VESSELS
AND PULMONARY CIRCULATION

Section 6

DISEASES OF PERIPHERAL VESSELS

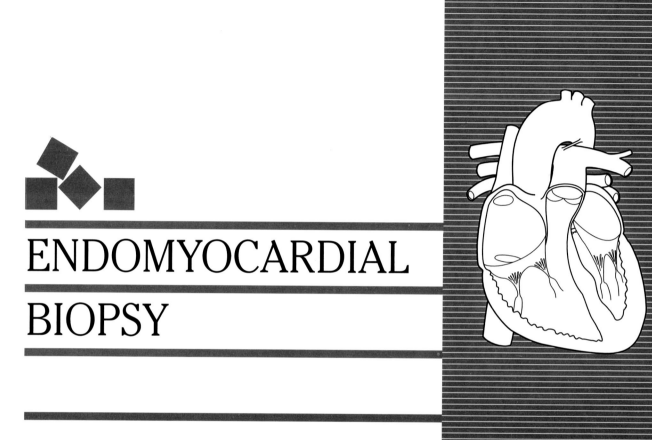

ENDOMYOCARDIAL

BIOPSY

CHAPTER 1

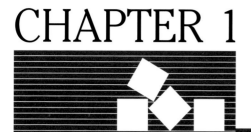

Approach to Endomyocardial Biopsy

TECHNIQUE

Bioptomes

- Stanford bioptome
- Konno bioptome (commonly used in Japan)
- King's College bioptome (modified Olympus bronchoscopic forceps), popular in Europe
- Cordis disposable bioptome (yields smaller myocardial fragments)
- Myocardial tissue obtained via catheterization of the right side of the heart through a sheath in the right internal jugular vein under fluoroscopic guidance

INDICATIONS FOR BIOPSY

Cardiac Transplant Rejection

- For diagnosis, grading, and follow-up

Anthracycline Cardiotoxicity

- For diagnosis, grading, and follow-up

Myocarditis

- For diagnosis and follow-up

Dilated Cardiomyopathy

- To exclude specific diseases (e.g., amyloidosis, hemochromatosis, myocarditis, storage diseases)

Restrictive Cardiomyopathy

- For diagnosis of specific entities (amyloidosis, endocardial fibrosis)
- To distinguish between fibrosing pericarditis and infiltrative myocardial diseases

Idiopathic Arrhythmias

- Myocarditis and infiltrative disease occasionally present as arrhythmias.

Neoplasms

- For diagnosis of cardiac tumors (including primary sarcomas and metastatic tumors); specific diagnosis often cannot be rendered because there is insufficient material

Indications for Left Ventricular Biopsy

- Endomyocardial fibrosis
- Scleroderma involving the heart
- Left-sided heart irradiation
- Left-sided failure greater than right-sided failure

COMPLICATIONS

Incidence

- The rate of serious complications of endomyocardial biopsy is very low, less than 0.1%.

Types

- Cardiac perforation and hemopericardium
- Pneumothorax
- Tricuspid valve biopsy
- Air embolism
- Atrial fibrillation, ventricular ectopy
- Transient nerve palsies (right Horner's syndrome, right recurrent laryngeal nerve paralysis, right phrenic nerve palsy)
- Cervical soft-tissue hematoma

SPECIMEN PROCESSING

Diagnostic Biopsies (Cardiomyopathy, Myocarditis Evaluation)

- Light microscopy: four or more pieces are needed.
- Electron microscopy: one piece is needed.
- One piece each of frozen tissue for special studies (in situ hybridization) and culture medium for viral culture is optional and not recommended for routine diagnosis.

Cardiac Transplant Rejection

▪ All biopsy fragments should be submitted for light microscopy; one fragment may be submitted for frozen section and immunofluorescence for the evaluation of vascular rejection (see Chap. 3).

Anthracycline Toxicity

▪ All biopsy fragments should be submitted for electron microscopy.
▪ At least 10 thick sections should be examined and 4 should be submitted for thin section examination.

ARTIFACTS AND NONSPECIFIC FINDINGS

Due to Sampling

▪ The greatest limiting factor of endomyocardial biopsy may be the small amount of tissue obtained; focal processes, especially myocarditis, cannot be excluded on the basis of a negative biopsy.
▪ Myofiber disarray is normally present in the right ventricle near the septum; for this reason, the diagnosis of hypertrophic cardiomyopathy generally cannot be made by endomyocardial biopsy.

Due to Biopsy Procedure

▪ Acute fibrin platelet thrombi may occur on the endocardial surface; these are usually secondary to the procedure and not indicative of mural thrombus.
▪ In subsequent biopsies, especially in transplants, the bioptome is often guided by the anatomic configuration to the same location; areas of scarring and granulation tissue should not be diagnosed as rejection.
▪ Mesothelial cells may be present and indicate focal perforation of the pericardium; these perforations are often minute and do not generally result in hemopericardium.
▪ Pinching artifact is often the result of postbiopsy handling by forceps, which may result in crush artifact.

Histologic Artifacts and Caveats

▪ Contraction bands are common and are especially marked when cold fixative has been used; these are not indicative of contraction band necrosis as is seen with reperfusion or catecholamine injury.
▪ Contraction bands often result in artifactual loss of contractile elements in adjacent areas of the myocyte; this change should not be mistaken for myocytolysis or myofibrillar loss.
▪ Telescoping of vessels is common and indicates the herniation or intussusception of the outer walls within the lumen; this change should not be mistaken for vascular disease.
▪ Endothelial and other mesenchymal cells cut tangentially may mimic lymphocytes; for this reason, immunohistochemical staining for common leukocyte or T-cell antigens may be helpful.
▪ Tangential orientation of the endocardium may mimic

endocardial thickening; the presence of multiple, layered endocardial elastic lamellae is required for the diagnosis of endocardial fibroelastosis.

GENERAL APPROACH TO BIOPSY DIAGNOSIS

Sections

▪ Serial sectioning of endomyocardial biopsy fragments enhances the diagnostic sensitivity for myocarditis and other inflammatory diseases.
▪ At least one thick section (8–10 μm) is recommended for Congo red stains for amyloidosis.

Stains

▪ Hematoxylin and eosin stains are routine and adequate for the diagnosis of myocarditis.
▪ Congo red or sulfated alcian blue stains for amyloid and iron stains are sometimes recommended as a routine procedure.
▪ Masson trichrome stain is helpful in the diagnosis of increased interstitial collagen, which may be indicative of cardiomyopathy. It may also be helpful in identifying myocyte necrosis when screening for myocarditis; necrotic cells lose red staining and appear gray-blue with Masson trichrome stain.
▪ Elastic stains may be helpful for the evaluation of endocardial fibroelastosis and pseudoxanthoma elasticum.
▪ A periodic acid–Schiff (PAS) stain highlights basophilic degeneration, a nonspecific finding that is especially prevalent in the myocytes of patients with thyroid disease and cardiomyopathies.
▪ Special stains for organisms (especially fungi) are important to rule out infections in transplant patients.
▪ Immunohistochemical markers for T-cell subsets may be helpful in the diagnosis of transplant rejection; immunohistochemical stains for light chains and transthyretin are helpful in establishing the chemical nature of amyloid.

Myocytes

▪ Nuclear enlargement with irregular outlines is characteristic of myocyte hypertrophy. In hearts without dilatation, there is an increase in myocyte cytoplasm; in hearts with cardiac dilatation, myocyte size is normal, but nuclear enlargement persists.
▪ Increased lipofuscin in a perinuclear location is especially prominent in elderly patients and in patients with catabolic disorders; it can be distinguished from iron by Prussian blue stain. Iron pigment indicates a pathologic process and may be missed without iron stains.
▪ Basophilic degeneration is a nonspecific accumulation of glycoprotein that is amphophilic on hematoxylin and eosin stains but stains bright pink with PAS stain.
▪ Myofibrillar loss is difficult to assess by light microscopy and may be an artifact of contraction bands.
▪ Contraction bands are generally a biopsy artifact.

- Myocyte necrosis is generally associated with lymphocytic infiltrates and is characterized by fluffy, eosinophilic cytoplasm.
- Ischemic myocyte necrosis may be accompanied by neutrophils; healing lesions may be accompanied by interstitial hemosiderin or hemosiderin-laden macrophages.
- Vacuolated cytoplasm may indicate Fabry's disease or Pompe's disease (see Chap. 2).
- Cysts of toxoplasmosis may be present in immunocompromised patients.
- Irregular, enlarged nuclei suggest myocyte hypertrophy; nuclear inclusions of cytomegalovirus should be sought, especially in transplant cases.

Endocardium

- Increased (>3–5) layers of elastic fibers are indicative of endocardial fibroelastosis, which may be secondary to cardiomyopathy; irregular, thickened fibers may be suggestive of pseudoxanthoma elasticum.
- Tangential orientation may result in endocardial thickening.
- In patients undergoing immunosuppressive therapy, especially cyclosporine therapy, endocardial aggregates of lymphocytes, predominantly T cells, may occur (Quilty effect); these aggregates are not indicative of rejection.

Interstitium

- Aggregates of lymphocytes with associated myocyte necrosis indicate myocarditis. Scattered lymphocytes are not indicative of a pathologic process, and quantitative criteria for normal numbers of lymphocytes are not particularly helpful. Aggregates of lymphocytes may be found in cases of dilated cardiomyopathy.
- Lymphocytes may be difficult to discern from mesenchymal cells cut on end; immunohistochemical stains for lymphoid markers may be helpful.
- Eosinophils are present in hypersensitivity myocarditis; they may also be present in giant cell myocarditis or hypereosinophilic syndrome.
- Anitschkow's cells are nonspecific and may be present in hypersensitivity myocarditis, infectious myocarditis, or acute rheumatic fever.
- Histiocytes may be found in hypersensitivity myocarditis and healing ischemic lesions (hemosiderin is often present). Aggregates of histiocytes may represent Whipple's disease, and aggregates of oncocytic myocytes, resembling histiocytes, may indicate histiocytoid (oncocytic) cardiomyopathy (Purkinje cell hamartoma; see Chaps. 2 and 11).
- Mast cells are found in small numbers in the normal interstitium; these may be increased in hypersensitivity myocarditis.

- Amyloid may be interstitial, perivascular, or nodular in distribution.
- A diffuse interstitial fibrosis is suggestive of cardiomyopathy.
- Rarely, foreign material (e.g., talc crystals in drug addicts) or endogenous crystals (e.g., oxalosis) may be present within the interstitium and are identified when viewed under polarized light.

Ultrastructure

- In choosing thin sections, those with longitudinally oriented myocytes should be used if possible.
- In noting the myocyte size, if the cell fills a 3000× field, it is probably hypertrophic.
- Irregular myocyte nuclear contours are suggestive of cardiac hypertrophy.
- In evaluation of myofibrillar loss, contractile elements may be sparse in many myocytes if there is end-stage cardiomyopathy or Adriamycin toxicity.
- In ascertaining the morphology of mitochondria, rare forms of infantile cardiomyopathies, often with skeletal involvement, are associated with numerous enlarged, abnormal mitochondria. Mitochondria are sensitive to hypoxia, and, if tissue is not immediately fixed, flocculent densities and mitochondrial swelling with clearing of the mitochondrial matrix occur.
- The interstitium and pericapillary areas should be evaluated for the presence of amyloid fibrils (100-angstrom nonbranching filaments).
- The presence of lamellated electron-dense bodies (or "myelin figures") and curvilinear bodies should be sought. These may be seen in isolated cells in patients with cardiomyopathy. If they are numerous, chloroquine toxicity, amiodarone toxicity, or Fabry's disease should be considered.
- Lipofuscin is often present in a perinuclear location and is a nonspecific degenerative change, especially in the elderly; if lipofuscin is unusually prominent, catabolic disorders and anorexia should be considered.
- An increase in membrane-bound lipid is nonspecific and is seen in various cardiomyopathies and ischemic states.

References

Billingham ME. Role of endomyocardial biopsy in diagnosis and treatment of heart disease. In Silver MD (ed). *Cardiovascular Pathology.* New York, Churchill Livingstone, 1991, pp 1465–1486.

Edwards WD. Pathology of endomyocardial biopsy. In Waller BF (ed). *Pathology of the Heart and Great Vessels.* New York, Churchill Livingstone, 1988, p 191.

Mason J, O'Connell JB. Clinical merit of endomyocardial biopsy. Circulation 79:971, 1989.

Yoshizato T, Edwards WD, Alboliras ET, Hagler DJ, Driscoll DJ. Safety and utility of endomyocardial biopsy in infants, children and adolescents: a review of 66 procedures in 53 patients. J Am Coll Cardiol 15:436–442, 1990.

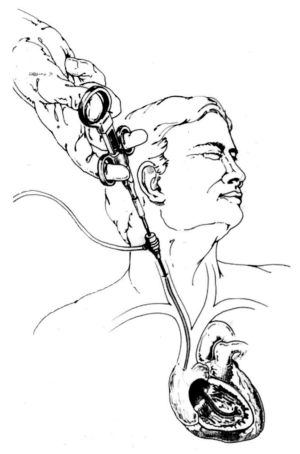

Figure 1–1. Schematic of right ventricular endomyocardial biopsy, right internal jugular vein approach. The bioptome is advanced past the tricuspid valve, and the hemispherical cutting jaws are positioned against the apical portion of the septum. (From Atkinson JB, Virmani R. The endomyocardial biopsy: techniques, indications, and limitations. In Virmani R, Atkinson JB, Fenoglio JJ, Jr [eds]. *Cardiovascular Pathology.* Philadelphia, WB Saunders, 1991, pp 203–219.)

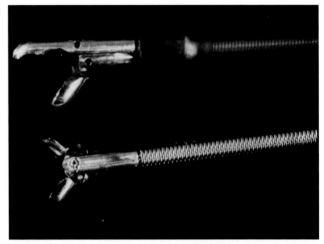

Figure 1–2. Cordis bioptome *(bottom).* Note both jaws open at the hinge. The Stanford bioptome *(top)* is larger, and only one jaw is moveable.

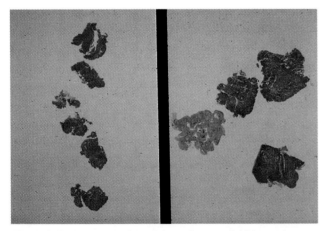

Figure 1–3. Low-power view of the endomyocardial biopsy pieces removed by the Cordis *(left)* and the Stanford *(right)* bioptomes. The Stanford bioptome removes larger pieces of the heart than does the Cordis. Therefore, to avoid sampling errors, more myocardial fragments must be examined with the Cordis bioptome.

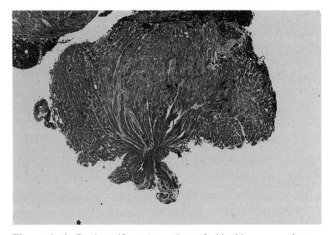

Figure 1–4. Crush artifact. A portion of this biopsy sample was squeezed by forceps before fixation, rendering interpretation difficult.

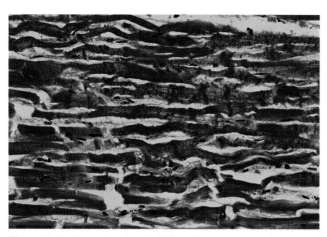

Figure 1–5. Contraction bands. This artifact occurs at the time of biopsy and can be reduced by maintaining the fixative at room or body temperature and by adding potassium to the fixative. Contraction bands are recognized as hypereosinophilic transverse bands with intervening light zones. Contraction bands should not be interpreted as ischemic areas.

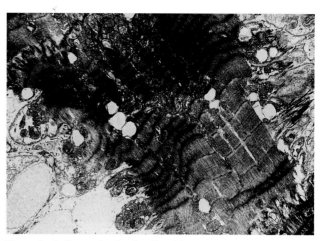

Figure 1–6. Contraction band artifact. Ultrastructurally, there is approximation of Z bands in the myocyte in the center of the photomicrograph.

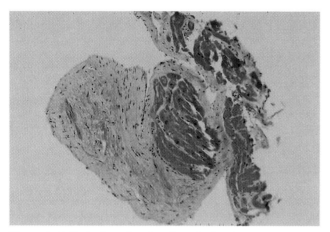

Figure 1–7. Evaluation of endocardium. Endocardium should be assessed only in areas that are sectioned at right angles. In this figure, there is tangential orientation resulting from an oblique cut.

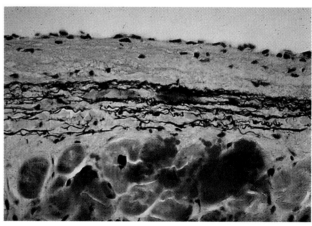

Figure 1–8. Normal endocardium, cut at right angles. A Movat pentachrome stain demonstrates elastic lamellae.

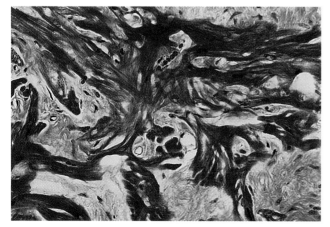

Figure 1–9. Myofiber disarray. This is a normal finding in the right ventricle at sites of insertion of the trabeculae carneae into the free wall or septum. In hypertrophic cardiomyopathy, myofiber disarray occurs in the middle third of the septum and is too deep to access by biopsy bioptome. The myofiber disarray of hypertrophic cardiomyopathy, unlike normal right ventricle, is accompanied by a marked increase in cell size.

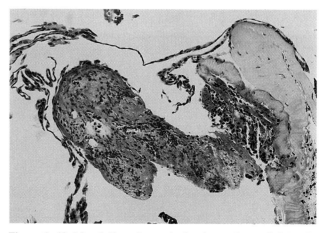

Figure 1–10. Mesothelium. Removal of a layer of mesothelial cells does not necessarily indicate clinically significant perforation. Although mesothelial cells are frequently present in endomyocardial biopsies, it is prudent to report their presence in the surgical pathology diagnosis. Note the thrombus associated with the mesothelial cells.

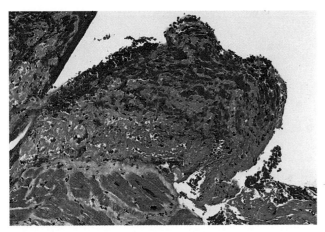

Figure 1–11. Acute thrombus adherent to endocardium is a common finding in endomyocardial biopsy and is secondary to the procedure.

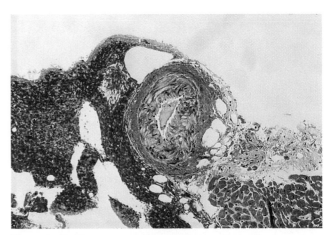

Figure 1–12. The presence of a muscular artery in the biopsy specimen does not indicate risk for pericardial hemorrhage; muscular arteries are normally found in the myocardium.

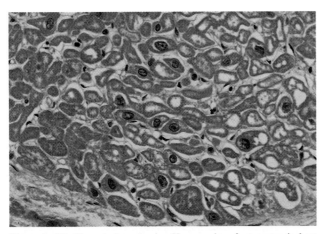

Figure 1–13. Myocyte hypertrophy. Hypertrophy of myocytes is best diagnosed by nuclear changes; myocyte cytoplasm may appear decreased in size subsequent to the development of hypertrophy if there is cardiac dilatation. Nuclear changes of hypertrophy include nuclear enlargement, irregular shapes, hyperchromatism, and often binucleation.

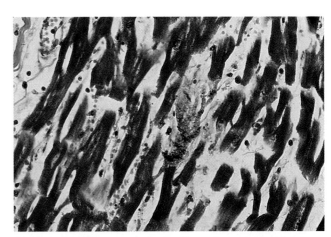

Figure 1–14. Myocyte necrosis. In this section stained with Masson trichrome, note the necrotic myocyte in the center of the field. The cytoplasm is bluish gray, unlike the dark red of the normal surrounding myocytes.

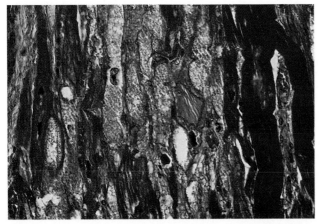

Figure 1–15. Myofibrillar loss. Intracellular absence of myofilaments is best assessed by ultrastructure. However, in extreme examples, such as this of cardiomyopathy due to cobalt toxicity, a large number of myocytes are nearly devoid of muscle and are filled with mitochondria.

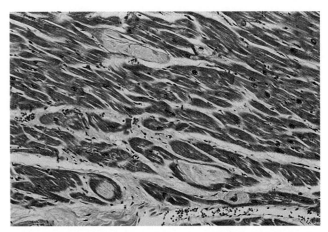

Figure 1–16. Basophilic degeneration. A nonspecific finding in most biopsies, basophilic degeneration may be associated with thyroid disease and cardiomyopathies. It is recognizable by amphophilic intracytoplasmic material in scattered myocytes.

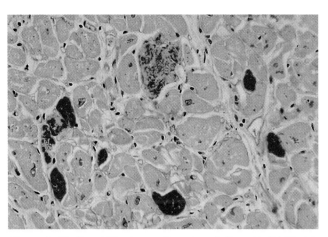

Figure 1–17. Basophilic degeneration. A periodic acid–Schiff stain highlights the material, which is a glycoprotein of uncertain origin.

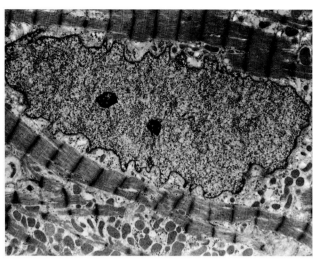

Figure 1–18. Myocyte ultrastructure. There is mild nuclear irregularity, which may occur with contraction of the cell, or, if more marked, myocyte hypertrophy. The presence of multiple nucleoli generally indicates a degree of hypertrophy. In this longitudinally oriented section, the thick, dark lines are Z bands. In the center of the sarcomere, bound by Z bands on each side, are less distinct M bands, which are formed by interfilamentous cross links between myosin filaments. Mitochondria are normally plentiful.

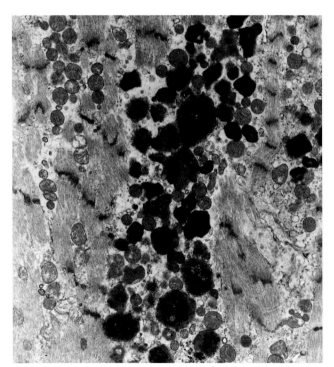

Figure 1–19. Lipofuscin. In this electron micrograph, lipofuscin is identified as electron-dense bodies. Also present are myofilaments, mitochondria, and portions of the Golgi complex.

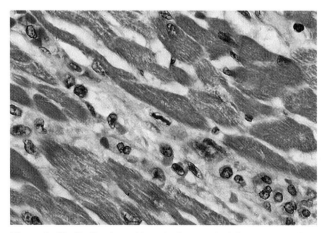

Figure 1–20. Cardiac interstitium. An increase in inflammatory cells in the cardiac interstitium may be a reflection of hypersensitivity or infection, or it may be of uncertain significance. Note Anitschkow's cell with condensed, wavy chromatin. These cells are found only in the heart and are modified connective tissue cells that may be found in a variety of inflammatory conditions, including hypersensitivity myocarditis, bacterial infections, and acute rheumatic fever.

CHAPTER 2

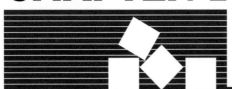

Endomyocardial Biopsy in the Nontransplant Setting

Table 2-1 lists diseases that can be diagnosed by endomyocardial biopsy.

Table 2-1
DISEASES DIAGNOSABLE BY
ENDOMYOCARDIAL BIOPSY

Allograft rejection
Myocarditis
    Lymphocytic myocarditis[1]
    Giant cell myocarditis
    Hypersensitivity myocarditis/hypereosinophilic syndrome
    Acute rheumatic fever
    Sarcoidosis
    Specific infections
Cardiomyopathies
    Dilated cardiomyopathy[2]
    Drug-induced cardiomyopathy
        Anthracycline cardiomyopathy
        Chloroquine toxicity
        Amiodarone toxicity
    Amyloidosis
    Hemochromatosis
    Endomyocardial disease
    Fabry's disaease
    Right ventricular dysplasia[3]
    Hypertrophic cardiomyopathy[4]
Tumors
Ischemia

[1]There is, in general, poor correlation between the clinical diagnosis of myocarditis and the histologic diagnosis made by endomyocardial biopsy. This discrepancy may, in part, be due to sampling error.
[2]The diagnosis of dilated cardiomyopathy by endomyocardial biopsy is primarily one of exclusion.
[3]The usefulness of endomyocardial biopsy in the diagnosis of right ventricular dysplasia is limited.
[4]Most authorities believe that hypertrophic cardiomyopathy cannot be diagnosed by endomyocardial biopsy.

MYOCARDITIS

Lymphocytic Myocarditis

Definition

Lymphocytic myocarditis is an inflammatory process resulting in lymphocytic infiltration and myocyte necrosis. It is thought to be the result of enteroviral (often coxsackievirus B) infection. The necrosis involves single cells or a cluster of cells, unlike the zonal coagulative necrosis present in ischemic necrosis.

Clinical Findings

- Approximately 9% of patients with unexplained congestive heart failure of less than 2 years' duration are shown to have myocarditis or borderline myocarditis on biopsy.
- Cardiac arrhythmias are common.
- A history of viral syndrome is variable.
- The value of immunosuppressive therapy is not substantiated in double-blind studies.
- The histologic diagnosis by endomyocardial biopsy correlates poorly with the clinical diagnosis.
- Patients with connective tissue disease, especially systemic lupus erythematosus, may develop lymphocytic myocarditis, presumably by an autoimmune mechanism.

Histologic Findings

- Histologic findings are generally focal and may, therefore, be missed by biopsy (a negative biopsy does not rule out the diagnosis).
- Serial sectioning of biopsies may enhance the yield of a positive diagnosis.

- The following Dallas criteria were developed to standardize reporting of myocardial biopsies performed to rule out myocarditis:

> First biopsy
>> Myocarditis, with or without fibrosis
>> Borderline myocarditis (suggest subsequent biopsy)
>> No myocarditis
> Subsequent biopsy
>> Ongoing (persistent) myocarditis, with or without fibrosis
>> Healing (resolving) myocarditis, with or without fibrosis
>> Healed (resolved) myocarditis, with or without fibrosis

Additional Facts

- The role of in situ hybridization and polymerase chain reaction (PCR) for the detection of viral RNA in myocardial tissues in patients with myocarditis is under investigation.
- Enteroviral-specific RNA sequences may be found in noninflammatory diseases, and their presence by PCR is not considered specific for the diagnosis of viral myocarditis.
- In situ hybridization for enteroviral RNA is not a routine diagnostic method and has low sensitivity.
- Small vessel vasculitis may coexist in patients with connective tissue disease and lymphocytic myocarditis.

Giant Cell Myocarditis

Definition

Giant cell myocarditis is an idiopathic inflammatory process resulting in myocyte necrosis associated with an inflammatory infiltrate composed of histiocytic giant cells, lymphocytes, and scattered eosinophils.

Clinical Findings

- Giant cell myocarditis occurs in young and middle-aged adults.
- Usually rapidly fatal, giant cell myocarditis may be an indication for cardiac transplantation.
- Although it is usually localized to the heart, there is rare association with skeletal muscle inflammation, thymoma, systemic lupus erythematosus, and thyrotoxicosis.

Histopathology

- There is myocardial necrosis.
- Chronic inflammation is composed of lymphocytes, plasma cells, macrophages, eosinophils, and multinucleated giant cells, most of which are histiocytic in origin. Multinucleated myocytes may also be present. The two types of giant cells are easily discerned by nuclear morphology.

Differential Diagnosis

- Sarcoidosis: There is a lack of myocyte necrosis, there are well-formed granulomas, and there are few or no eosinophils. Lymph node or lung involvement is almost always present in sarcoidosis.

Hypersensitivity Myocarditis

Definition

Hypersensitivity myocarditis is characterized by infiltrates of histiocytes, lymphocytes, and eosinophils along natural planes of dissection, with little myocyte necrosis; it is often associated with hypersensitivity to medications.

Clinical Findings

- Patients are often elderly, taking multiple medications, and have known allergies.
- Mild peripheral eosinophilia is common.
- More than 20 drugs have been implicated in hypersensitivity myocarditis; classically, methyldopa, sulfonamide, and penicillin are cited.
- Symptoms include arrhythmias, sudden death, and, rarely, congestive heart failure.
- Hypersensitivity myocarditis is only rarely clinically suspected and, therefore, only rarely diagnosed by biopsy, except in transplant patients.

Histopathology

- There are perivascular, subendocardial, and interstitial infiltrates of macrophages, eosinophils, lymphocytes, and Anitschkow's cells.
- Collections of histiocytes may suggest poorly formed granulomas, but fibrinoid necrosis, epithelioid granulomas, and giant cells are uncommon.
- Myocyte necrosis is either absent or focal and sparse.

Active Rheumatic Carditis

Clinical Findings

- Rheumatic fever continues to be a major cardiovascular health problem in developing countries.
- Although rheumatic carditis is relatively rare in this country, there has been a recent resurgence in North America.
- Diagnosis is based on the finding of either two major or one major and two minor manifestations in the presence of antecedent group A streptococcal infection.
- Major criteria are carditis, polyarthritis, chorea, subcutaneous nodules, erythema marginatum; minor criteria are fever, arthralgias, increased sedimentation rate or other acute phase reactant, and prolonged P-R interval.

Endomyocardial Biopsy

- Aschoff's nodules are present in biopsy samples from one fourth of patients with acute rheumatic fever or with suspected carditis and preexisting rheumatic heart disease.
- Aschoff's nodules are not present in patients with

chronic rheumatic disease in the absence of acute carditis.

■ Histologically, the Aschoff's nodules are characterized by multinucleated giant cells (Aschoff's cells), histiocytes (Anitschkow's cells), and fibrin deposition in a nodular, interstitial pattern.

Hypereosinophilic Syndrome

Definition

Hypereosinophilic syndrome is a systemic illness characterized by persistent peripheral eosinophilia ($> 1500/mm^2$) for 6 months and multiorgan infiltration by eosinophils.

Clinical Findings

■ Patients are often men in their third to fifth decade of life.
■ A total of 75% of patients have cardiac involvement, which results in congestive heart failure, arrhythmias, and mural thrombi.
■ Scarring of the endocardium typically results in a restrictive cardiomyopathy.

Histopathology

■ Endocardial and myocardial infiltrates of eosinophils are found.
■ Mural thrombi with eosinophils are characteristic.
■ Granulomas with extracellular eosinophil granules may be present.
■ Although there is a histologic spectrum formed with hypersensitivity myocarditis, the presence of endomyocardial fibrosis, eosinophilic microabscesses, and granulomas suggest the diagnosis of hypereosinophilic syndrome.

Sarcoidosis

Clinical Findings

■ Cardiac involvement in patients with sarcoidosis is present in 20% to 30% of autopsied cases.
■ Less than 5% of patients with sarcoidosis have cardiac symptoms, including heart block, congestive heart failure, ventricular arrhythmias, and sudden death; both restrictive and congestive cardiomyopathy may occur.
■ Myocardial sarcoidosis is a disease of young or middle-aged adults of either sex.

Histopathology

■ Endomyocardial biopsy is positive in up to 50% of patients with myocardial sarcoidosis; a negative biopsy does not exclude the diagnosis.
■ Granulomas of sarcoidosis primarily affect the ventricular septum and left ventricular free wall, although any area may be involved.
■ Histologic features of myocardial sarcoidosis are similar to those of extracardiac sarcoidosis.
■ Granulomas typically heal as large scars, and areas of lymphocytic infiltrates may occur adjacent to granulomas.

■ Endomyocardial biopsy may be negative or demonstrate nonspecific changes of scarring or lymphocytic infiltrates, mimicking lymphocytic myocarditis.

Differential Diagnosis of Cardiac Granulomas

■ In sarcoidosis, lymph nodes and lungs are involved and there are well-formed granulomas; there is little myocyte necrosis or eosinophilic infiltrate.
■ The edge of a healing infarct may contain giant cells; these are myogenic, not histiocytic, and there are features of healed ischemic changes (hemosiderin-laden macrophages, granulation tissue).
■ Mycobacterial infections rarely involve the heart and may result in necrotizing granulomas with giant cells.
■ In hypersensitivity, poorly formed interstitial granulomas may be present, but multinucleated giant cells with myocyte necrosis do not occur.
■ Giant cell myocarditis generally does not demonstrate well-formed granulomas, but giant cells with myocyte necrosis are present.

Specific Infections

■ The etiologic agent of Lyme disease (Borrelia burgdorferi) has been identified in an endomyocardial biopsy; generally, the histology is nonspecific lymphocytic myocarditis; organisms are rarely identified by silver stains.
■ A variety of infectious agents may be encountered in immunosuppressed patients (see Chap. 3); infections that could possibly be diagnosed by biopsy in immunocompetent patients include Chagas' disease, rickettsial diseases, rare bacterial disease, and spirochetal diseases.
■ The heart is involved in more than half of patients dying of Whipple's disease. Whipple's lesions involve the valves, myocardium, and pericardium. Clinically, murmurs and friction rubs may occur; histologically, there are collections of foamy macrophages with fibrosis. Diagnosis depends on demonstration of organisms (Tropheryma whippelii) by periodic acid–Schiff stain or ultrastructural confirmation; rarely, the diagnosis of cardiac involvement is made by endomyocardial biopsy.

Toxic Myocarditis

■ Most toxic insults to the heart result in noninflammatory cardiomyopathy.
■ Lithium, emetine, cocaine, endogenous and exogenous catecholamines, and 5-fluorouracil have been associated with myocardial inflammation with or without cardiomyopathy.

References

Aretz H, Billingham ME, Edwards WD, et al. A histologic definition and classification. Am J Cardiovasc Pathol 1:3–14, 1987.
Mason JW, O'Connell JB. Clinical merit of endomyocardial biopsy. Circulation 79:971–973, 1989.
Narula J, Chopra P, Talwar K, et al. Does endomyocardial biopsy aid in the diagnosis of active rheumatic carditis? Circulation 88:2198–2205, 1993.
Reznick JW, Braunstein DB, Walsh RL, et al. Lyme carditis. Electrophysiologic and histopathologic study. Am J Med 81:923–927, 1986.

CARDIOMYOPATHIES

Clinical Definition

- The term "cardiomyopathy" is a general term referring to diseases of cardiac muscle resulting in cardiac failure. These include a variety of primary and secondary processes.
- Functionally, cardiomyopathies are divided into three groups: congestive (dilated), hypertrophic, and restrictive. Specific disease processes may result in either congestive or restrictive cardiomyopathy; biopsy may be most useful to separate restrictive cardiomyopathy from constrictive pericarditis.

Dilated (Congestive) Cardiomypathy

- Dilated cardiomyopathy occurs when there is increased left ventricular end diastolic volume, decreased ejection fraction, and diffuse hypokinesis of the ventricles. Secondary mitral or tricuspid regurgitation may occur.
- Dilated cardiomyopathy may be the result of 1 of more than 75 specific heart diseases, including the following:
  - Idiopathic dilated cardiomyopathy
  - Myocarditis
  - Storage diseases
  - Amyloidosis
  - Hemochromatosis
  - Toxic cardiomyopathies
  - Human immunodeficiency virus (HIV) infection
- Although the clinical picture of dilated cardiomyopathy may result from systemic hypertension, atherosclerotic coronary artery disease, and valvular heart disease, the term "dilated cardiomyopathy" should not be used in the presence of these diseases.

Hypertrophic Cardiomyopathy

- Hypertrophic cardiomyopathy occurs when there is decreased left ventricular end-diastolic volume, normal or increased ejection fraction, and myocardial hypertrophy, usually resulting in asymmetric thickening of the ventricular septum.
- Most patients with hypertrophic hemodynamic parameters suffer from idiopathic hypertrophic cardiomyopathy, but similar hemodynamic parameters may rarely occur in primary cardiac tumors that infiltrate primarily the ventricular septum and in other infiltrative diseases, such as Fabry's disease.
- Generally, hypertrophic cardiomyopathy cannot be diagnosed by endomyocardial biopsy because histologic changes are usually found in the middle third of the ventricular septum.
- Biopsy may be helpful in excluding rare causes of asymmetric hypertrophy.

Restrictive Cardiomyopathy

- Restrictive (infiltrative) cardiomyopathy occurs when there is decreased ventricular compliance resulting in impaired myocardial relaxation, often accompanied by reduced contractility; there is decreased cardiac output with normal systolic function.
- Restrictive cardiomyopathy may mimic constrictive pericarditis; endomyocardial biopsy may help in this distinction.
- Restrictive (infiltrative) cardiomyopathy may result from any of the following:
  - Amyloidosis
  - Hemochromatosis
  - Endocardial fibrosis
  - Sarcoidosis
  - Storage disease
  - Carcinoid heart disease
  - Radiation-induced myocardial fibrosis
  - Methysergide-induced endocardial fibrosis

Pathologic Definition

- The pathologic term "cardiomyopathy" is often restricted to idiopathic dilated cardiomyopathy, hypertrophic cardiomyopathy, and idiopathic endocardial fibrosis.
- Right ventricular dysplasia is sometimes termed "right ventricular cardiomyopathy," and may rarely be diagnosed by biopsy.

Idiopathic Dilated Cardiomyopathy

Clinical Findings

Clinical findings include the following:

- Progressive congestive heart failure
- Arrhythmias
- Family history occasionally positive, mostly autosomal dominant and less commonly autosomal recessive or X-linked
- Demonstration of four-chamber dilatation, decreased ejection fraction, and normal valve structure on echocardiogram; demonstration of normal coronary arteries on angiogram
- Absence of long-standing hypertension

Etiology

- The cause of idiopathic dilated cardiomyopathy is generally unknown. It may be a heterogeneous group of diseases. Approximately 5% to 10% of cases are familial.
- Five percent to 10% of cases of idiopathic dilated cardiomyopathy may represent the end stage of myocarditis.
- When dilated cardiomyopathy occurs during the last 3 months of pregnancy or within 6 months post partum, the term "peripartum cardiomyopathy" is used.
- Peripartum cardiomyopathy occurs in 1/1300 to 1/15,000 term pregnancies, and the incidence is greater in twin pregnancies, multiparous pregnancies, black patients, and patients older than 30 years of age.
- Immunologic abnormalities, including humoral and cytotoxic abnormalities, have been implicated as causes.
- There is an association between dilated cardiomyopathy

and alcohol use, diabetes mellitus, doxorubicin (Adri-amycin) toxicity, cocaine use, and HIV infection.

Histopathology

- Although a large percentage of endomyocardial biopsies are performed in patients with presumed idiopathic dilated cardiomyopathy, the histologic features are nonspecific.
- Hypertrophic myocytes are intermixed with atrophied myocytes, which show myofibrillar loss. Myocyte size and diameter vary.
- Interstitial fibrosis is variable and is appreciated primarily in the late stages of disease.
- Diagnosis is one of exclusion (i.e., absence of iron deposition, amyloidosis, sarcoidosis, and lymphocytic myocarditis on biopsy, and absence of valvular, hypertensive, and coronary disease clinically).
- Basophilic degeneration is occasionally present.
- Occasionally, the biopsy can be essentially normal, even in patients with clinically documented dilated cardiomyopathy.

Additional Facts

- Ultrastructural analysis may corroborate the findings of myofibrillar loss in some myocytes and of myocyte hypertrophy in others.
- Areas of contraction band necrosis should not be assessed.
- A typical diagnosis report may read "Myocyte hypertrophy, focal myofibrillar loss, mild interstitial fibrosis. In the absence of coronary, valvular, and hypertensive heart disease, the findings are consistent with dilated cardiomyopathy."
- A detailed history and catheterization report is necessary for the histologic diagnosis of dilated cardiomyopathy.

Drug-Induced Cardiomyopathy

Anthracycline Toxicity

- Anthracycline toxicity is usually a result of doxorubicin (Adriamycin) toxicity. The incidence of cardiotoxicity with doxorubicin is 1.7%, compared with 4.4% for daunorubicin.
- The maximal nontoxic dose is 550 mg/m^2 doxorubicin. Some patients develop toxicity at lower doses, especially if there is a history of heart disease, radiation therapy, advanced age, or systemic hypertension.
- The entire biopsy specimen should be submitted for ultrastructural examination.
- Ten plastic-embedded blocks should be reviewed.
- The grading scheme of toxic changes is as follows (pathologic changes may persist for months or years after initial damage):
  - Grade O: Normal myocardial ultrastructure
  - Grade 1: Isolated myocytes affected by distended sarcotubular system or early myofibrillar loss; damage to fewer than 5% of all cells in 10 plastic-embedded blocks of tissue
  - Grade 1.5: Changes similar to those in grade 1 but

with damage to 6% to 15% of all cells in 10 plastic-embedded blocks of tissue
  - Grade 2: Clusters of myocytes affected by myofibrillar loss or vacuolization, with damage to 16% to 25% of all cells in 10 plastic-embedded blocks of tissue
  - Grade 2.5: Many myocytes, 26% to 35% of all cells, in 10 plastic-embedded blocks affected by vacuolization or myofibrillar loss; at this stage, only one more dose of anthracycline should be given without further evaluation
  - Grade 3: Severe and diffuse myocyte damage (more than 35% of all cells affected); no more anthracycline should be given

Chloroquine Cardiomyopathy

- Patients may develop cardiac failure.
- Histologic features at biopsy are electron-dense concentric and parallel lamellae and curvilinear bodies within cardiac myocytes.
- Similar deposits are found in chloroquine-induced skeletal myopathy.

Amiodarone Toxicity

- Electron-dense lamellae similar to those seen in chloroquine toxicity have been reported.
- Curvilinear bodies associated with chloroquine toxicity have not been described in amiodarone toxicity.
- Electron-dense lamellae occur in pneumocytes, alveolar macrophages, liver cells, lymph nodes, and other cells.
- Lamellae are presumed to be lysosome-derived structures made of phospholipids.

Miscellaneous Toxic and Drug-Induced Cardiomyopathies

- Cobalt cardiomyopathy resulted from drinking beer with cobalt sulfate added for foam stabilization; no cases have been reported since the mid-1960s because cobalt is no longer used as an additive.
- Cardiomyopathy has been reported following treatment with 5-fluorouracil and lithium.

References

Arbustini E, Grasso M, Salerno JA, et al. Endomyocardial biopsy finding in two patients with idiopathic dilated cardiomyopathy receiving long-term treatment with amiodarone. Am J Cardiol 67:661–662, 1991.

McAllister HA Jr, Ferrans VJ, Hall RJ, Strickman NE, Bossart MI. Chloroquine-induced cardiomyopathy. Arch Pathol Lab Med 111:953–956, 1987.

Amyloidosis

Clinical Findings

- Amyloidosis accounts for up to 10% of all noncoronary cardiomyopathies.
- One third to one half of patients with amyloidosis associated with plasma cell dyscrasias (amyloid AL, derived from immunoglobulin light chains) develop cardiac symptoms.

- Cardiac amyloidosis in patients with secondary amyloidosis resulting from chronic inflammatory processes (nonimmunoglobulin amyloid AA) is uncommon, occurring in less than 10% of patients.
- Cardiac amyloidosis resulting from the deposition of amyloid AS (derived from transthyretin) is common in patients older than 80 years of age.
- Familial forms of cardiac amyloidosis (also amyloid AS) are also seen in older patients but may occur in patients as young as 35 years old.
- Although cardiac amyloidosis is classically considered to cause a restrictive type of cardiomyopathy, congestive heart failure and dilated cardiomyopathy develop in some patients.
- Mean survival of patients with primary amyloidosis (AL) is less than 6 months.
- Mean survival of patients with senile amyloidosis (AS) is more than 2 years.

Histopathology

- Regardless of the type of amyloid, histologic findings are similar.
- There are four patterns of amyloid deposition in the heart: interstitial, nodular, subendocardial, and vascular. There is often an overlap of patterns.
- Interstitial amyloid is seen in more than 95% of amyloid AS and amyloid AL cases.
- Nodular amyloid is more frequent in amyloid AS than in amyloid AL.
- Endocardial and vascular amyloid are more common in amyloid AL than in amyloid AS.
- The diagnosis of amyloid is confirmed by Congo red staining with apple green birefringence with polarized light on 10-μm sections, by metachromasia with methyl violet, by ultraviolet fluorescence with thioflavin T, and by green staining with sulfated alcian blue stain.
- AL and AS may be distinguished by immunohistochemical stains for light chains (AL) and for transthyretin (previously known as prealbumin, AS).

References

Crotty TB, Edwards WD, Li CY. Are immunohistochemical stains necessary to distinguish primary (AL) from senile (AS) amyloidosis in endomyocardial biopsy tissues? Mod Pathol 7:27A, 1994.

Pomerance A, Slavin G, McWatt J. Experience with the sodium sulphate-alcian blue stain for amyloid in cardiac pathology. J Clin Pathol 29:22–28, 1976.

Hemochromatosis

Clinical Findings

- Hemochromatosis is a congenital disorder of iron metabolism that causes a dilated or, less commonly, restrictive cardiomyopathy.
- Secondary forms of hemosiderosis may occur from excessive blood transfusion, hemolytic anemia, or increased iron intake.
- Diagnosis is aided by elevated plasma iron, low total iron binding capacity, and markedly elevated serum ferritin and transferrin saturation levels.
- Treatment consists of chelation and phlebotomy.

Histopathology

- There is iron in the perinuclear region (normal myocyte does not contain iron).
- Multiple biopsies may be required because epicardium is involved before the endocardium.

Endomyocardial Disease

Hypereosinophilic Syndrome

- Hypereosinophilic syndrome is also called Löffler's endocarditis.
- Cardiac involvement occurs in $>75\%$ of patients with hypereosinophilic syndrome.
- Echocardiography demonstrates thickening of the posterobasal left ventricular wall, limited motion of the posterior leaflet of the mitral valve, and apical mural thrombus.
- Restrictive cardiomyopathy is the most common hemodynamic abnormality.
- Pathologically, there is eosinophilic myocarditis, endocardial fibrosis up to several millimeters in thickness, and mural thrombi with eosinophils.

Idiopathic Endomyocardial Fibrosis (Davies Disease)

- Idiopathic endomyocardial fibrosis is the prototypic disease resulting in primary restrictive cardiomyopathy.
- It is rare in the United States and generally occurs in subtropical Africa, India, and South America.
- Pathologically, there is a thick collagen layer under the endocardium; myocardium is relatively spared.
- Endomyocardial biopsy may support the diagnosis; most reports of biopsy diagnosis of idiopathic endomyocardial fibrosis are from patients from Africa or India.
- Idiopathic endomyocardial fibrosis is believed to represent the end stage of Löffler's endocarditis.

Pseudoxanthoma Elasticum

- Idiopathic disease is characterized by fragmentation, thickening, and calcification of elastic fibers.
- Pseudoxanthoma elasticum involves the heart, skin, eye, and gastrointestinal tract.
- Although the endocardium demonstrates fibroelastosis, restrictive cardiomyopathy is rare because there is preferential atrial involvement.
- The major cardiac problem is accelerated atherosclerosis.
- Pseudoxanthoma elasticum may also clinically present as dilated cardiomyopathy.
- Diagnosis may be made by noting characteristic endocardial changes on endomyocardial biopsy.

Miscellaneous Diseases of the Endocardium

- Endocardial fibroelastosis is a common secondary finding in dilated cardiomyopathy, regardless of cause.
- Endocardial fibroelastosis is a disease of infants and children that may be idiopathic, related to intrauterine myocardial inflammation, or a form of infantile dilated cardiomyopathy; there may be coexistent structural congenital heart disease.

▪ Radiation therapy, carcinoid heart disease, and methysergide therapy may result in endocardial fibrosis and restrictive cardiomyopathy; histologic features are nonspecific.

▪ Endocardial fibrosis in patients with scleroderma is rarely clinically significant; more often, there is coronary artery spasm, intramural myocardial arterial sclerosis, and pericarditis.

Fabry's Disease

▪ Fabry's disease is also called angiokeratoma corporis diffusum universale.

▪ Fabry's disease is an X-linked disorder. Most men become symptomatic with cardiovascular disease by middle age, whereas women are often asymptomatic.

▪ Cardiac symptoms may mimic amyloidosis, mitral valve prolapse, hypertrophic cardiomyopathy, or restrictive cardiomyopathy.

▪ Biopsy demonstrates vacuolization of myocytes. Electron microscopy demonstrates electron-dense lamellated bodies (myelin figures), with alternating light and dark bands.

Histiocytoid Cardiomyopathy

▪ Histiocytoid cardiomyopathy is a rare entity that causes incessant ventricular tachycardia in infants.

▪ Synonyms include Purkinje cell hamartoma, infantile cardiomyopathy, and oncocytic cardiomyopathy.

▪ The proper classification of this entity is unclear; it may represent a hamartoma or developmental disorder.

▪ Because it shares some features with cardiac rhabdomyoma, histiocytoid cardiomyopathy is further discussed in Chapter 11.

Right Ventricular Dysplasia

Synonyms and Related Terms

▪ Right ventricular cardiomyopathy
▪ Arrhythmogenic right ventricular dysplasia
▪ Uhl's anomaly

Clinical Findings

▪ Ventricular tachyarrhythmias
▪ Young adults and adolescents
▪ Strong familial tendency
▪ Sudden death, often during exercise
▪ Right ventricular dysfunction

Pathology

▪ Fatty infiltration of right ventricular wall
▪ Focal scarring of right ventricular wall with occasional foci of inflammation
▪ Focal absence of right ventricular myocardium

Endomyocardial Biopsy Diagnosis

▪ Diagnosis of right ventricular dysplasia by endomyocardial biopsy is difficult because fat is normally present within the right ventricle.

▪ A presumed diagnosis is possible only if fat and fibrous tissue are found and there is a clinical suspicion based on clinical and familial findings.

Reference

Kirsch LR, Weinstock DJ, Magid MS, Levin AR, Gold JP. Treatment of presumed arrhythmogenic right ventricular dysplasia. Chest 104: 298–300, 1993.

CARDIAC TUMORS

▪ Primary and metastatic tumors of the heart have occasionally been diagnosed by endomyocardial biopsy.

▪ The classification of primary cardiac sarcomas may be hampered by limited tissue sampling; for a discussion of open biopsy of cardiac sarcoma, see Chapter 12.

References

Flipse TR, Tazelaar HD, Holmes DR Jr. Diagnosis of malignant cardiac disease by endomyocardial biopsy. Mayo Clin Proc 65:1415–1422, 1990.

Hausheer FH, Josephson RA, Grochow LB, Weissman D, Brinker JA, Weisman HF. Intracardiac sarcoma diagnosed by left ventricular endomyocardial biopsy. Chest 92:177–179, 1987.

ISCHEMIC HEART DISEASE

▪ The diagnosis of ischemic heart disease is not generally made on the basis of biopsy.

▪ However, failure of diagnosis of ischemic heart disease by conventional methods may lead to biopsy in patients with unexplained cardiac symptoms.

▪ The presence of necrosis with acute inflammation should suggest the diagnosis of acute ischemia.

▪ The presence of hemosiderin in an area of healing fibrosis is suggestive of an anginal lesion or edge of a healing infarct.

▪ Occasionally, the differential diagnosis between ischemia and myocarditis is difficult in small samples.

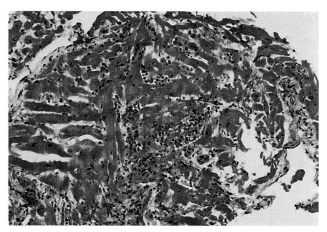

Figure 2–1. Myocarditis. Endomyocardial biopsy demonstrating a diffuse infiltration of lymphocytes. The patient was a young woman with sudden onset congestive heart failure.

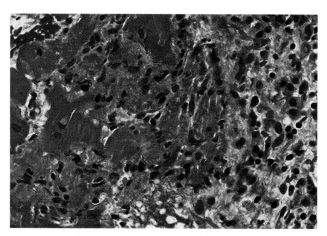

Figure 2–2. Myocarditis. Biopsy sample of the case illustrated in Figure 2–1 performed 2 years later. There is again a dense infiltrate of lymphocytes; myocyte necrosis is evident. The patient had responded well to treatment with steroids after her initial presentation but had discontinued them 2 weeks before rebiopsy, leading to recurrence of symptoms.

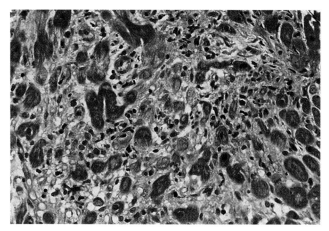

Figure 2–3. Healing myocarditis. Sparse lymphocytic infiltrate is combined with interstitial fibrosis. Note the scattered atrophic myocytes.

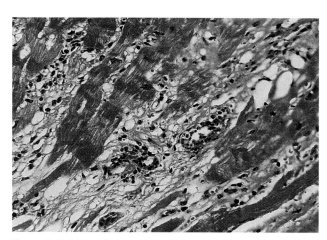

Figure 2–4. Myocarditis, systemic lupus erythematosus. In addition to lymphocytic myocarditis, a small vessel vasculitis is also present. The photomicrograph is from a different area of that illustrated in Figure 2–3.

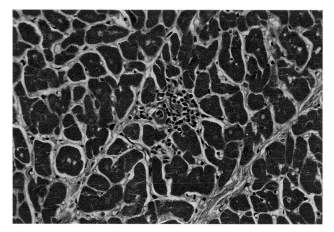

Figure 2–5. Focal myocarditis. Inflammation can be quite focal. Note the necrotic myocyte is infiltrated by lymphocytes.

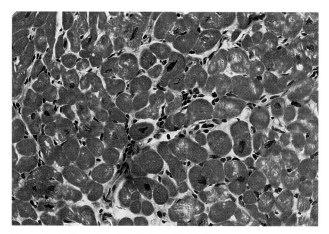

Figure 2–6. Focal lymphocytic interstitial infiltrate, myocardium. Occasional lymphocytes are normally present in the cardiac interstitium. The diagnosis of borderline myocarditis may be made if there are interstitial lymphocytes without myocyte necrosis in a biopsy from a patient with suspected myocarditis. A second biopsy is recommended for such patients.

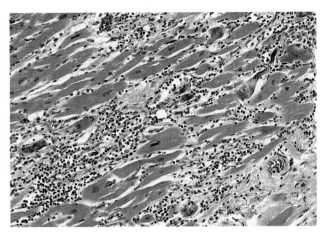

Figure 2–7. Giant cell myocarditis. There is a dense infiltrate of lymphocytes with prominent giant cells. Note the absence of well-formed granulomas.

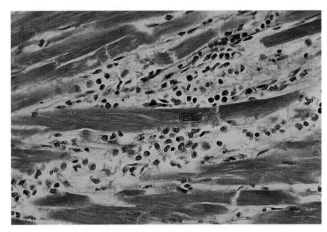

Figure 2–8. Hypersensitivity myocarditis. The inflammation is interstitial and composed of histiocytes, lymphocytes, and eosinophils.

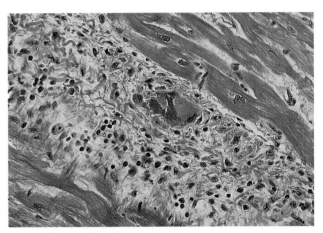

Figure 2–9. Hypereosinophilic syndrome. The interstitial infiltrate is reminiscent of hypersensitivity myocarditis. In addition, there is a granulomatous reaction to eosinophilic breakdown products, a feature not typical of hypersensitivity.

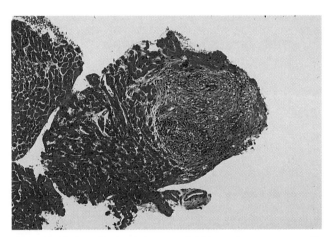

Figure 2–10. Sarcoidosis. Endomyocardial biopsy demonstrates a well-formed granuloma.

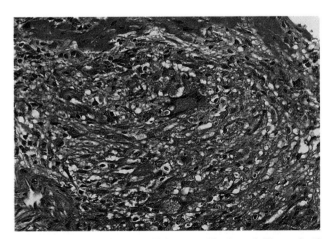

Figure 2–11. Sarcoidosis. A higher magnification of Figure 2–10 demonstrating a non-necrotizing, well-formed granuloma.

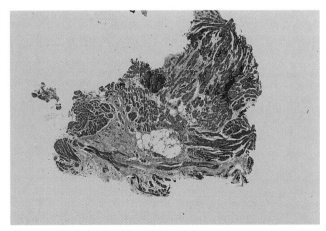

Figure 2–12. Dilated cardiomyopathy. A large percentage of endomyocardial biopsies are performed to rule out secondary causes of dilated cardiomyopathy. In this example of a patient with presumed dilated cardiomyopathy, there are nonspecific findings of interstitial fibrosis and myocyte hypertrophy. Fat is a normal finding in right ventricular biopsies.

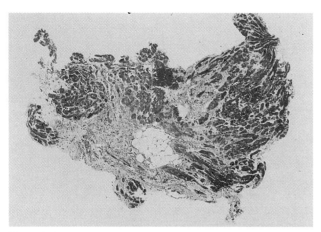

Figure 2–13. Dilated cardiomyopathy. A Masson trichrome stain highlights focal interstitial fibrosis.

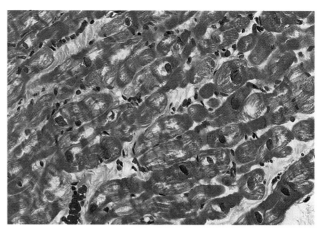

Figure 2–14. Dilated cardiomyopathy. Note the myocyte hypertrophy, which is a nonspecific finding that is present in dilated cardiomyopathy and cardiomegaly of diverse causes. There is a contraction band artifact, which imparts a false appearance of myofibrillar loss.

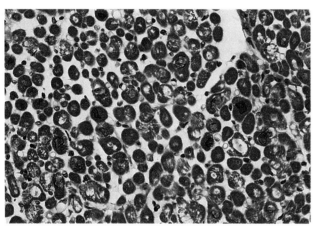

Figure 2–15. Dilated cardiomyopathy. A cross section of the biopsy sample shown in Figure 2–14 demonstrates myocyte hypertrophy characterized by enlarged, hyperchromatic nuclei. The myocyte diameter may be normal after cardiac dilatation occurs, or there may be variation in myocyte diameter, as seen in this illustration.

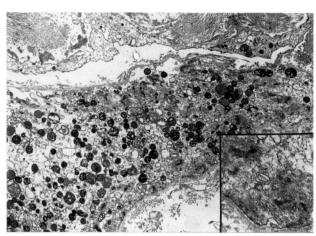

Figure 2–16. Dilated cardiomyopathy. The ultrastructural findings are nonspecific. In this particular example, there is marked myofibrillar loss. The myocyte contains largely mitochondria; note the remnants of Z bands at the periphery of the cell *(inset).*

Figure 2–17. Adriamycin toxicity, grade 1.5. The changes of Adriamycin toxicity are best appreciated by plastic sections and ultrastructure. In this 1-μm-thick toluidine blue–stained plastic section of a biopsy specimen from a patient with presumed Adriamycin cardiotoxicity, several cells demonstrate toxic effects, seen as cytoplasmic vacuolization (adria cells).

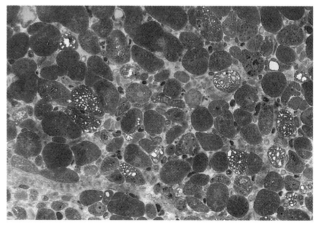

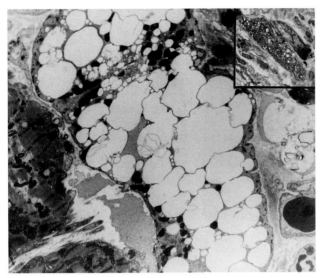

Figure 2–18. Adriamycin toxicity. There is marked coalescence of vacuoles. The inset shows a single myocyte with marked vacuolization as seen in the l-μm-thick toluidine blue–stained sections.

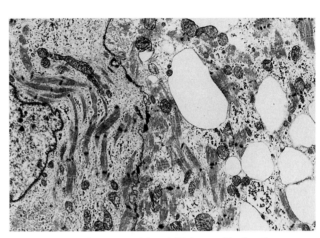

Figure 2–19. Adriamycin toxicity. A high magnification demonstrates dilated T tubules; unlike artifact, membranes line the vacuoles. (Courtesy of Dr. Victor Ferrans.)

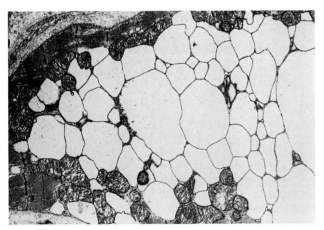

Figure 2–20. Adriamycin toxicity. A high magnification demonstrates severe sarcotubulur dilatation. Note the membranes lining individual vacuoles. (Courtesy of Dr. Victor Ferrans.)

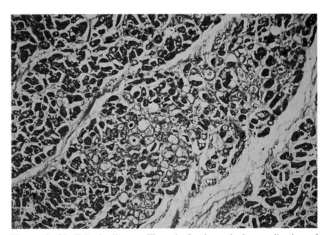

Figure 2–21. Fabry's disease. There is focal, marked vacuolization of cardiac myocytes.

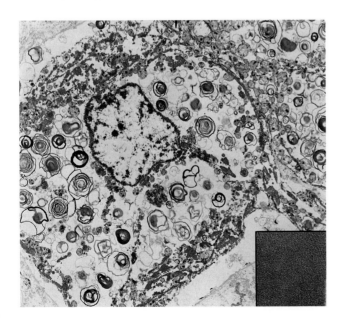

Figure 2–22. Fabry's disease. Lamellated electron-dense bodies, so-called myelin figures, are typical of Fabry's disease and may also be present in fewer numbers in chloroquine and amiodarone toxicity and in idiopathic dilated cardiomyopathy. The inset shows myelin figures at higher magnification; note the alternating light and dark bands.

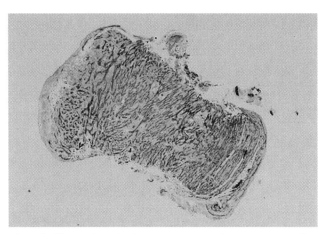

Figure 2–23. Amyloidosis. Cardiac biopsy sample demonstrates diffuse interstitial infiltrates.

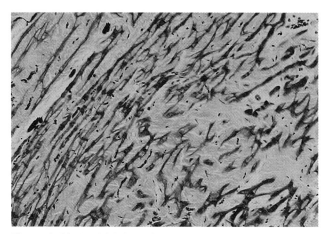

Figure 2–24. Amyloidosis. A higher magnification of Figure 2–23 demonstrates interstitial deposits of amorphous hyaline material.

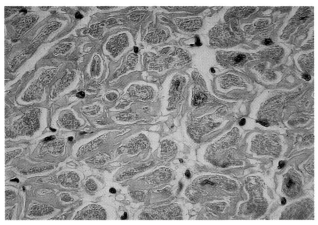

Figure 2–25. Amyloidosis. A characteristic feature of cardiac amyloidosis is circumferential interstitial distribution surrounding individual myocytes, seen here on cross section.

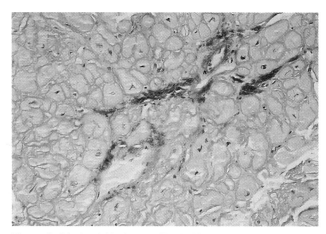

Figure 2–26. Amyloidosis. A sulfated alcian blue stain demonstrates amyloid (green) surrounding individual myocytes; there is focal interstitial fibrosis (red). In cases of cardiac amyloidosis, sulfated alcian blue has been shown to have greater sensitivity than Congo red stains.

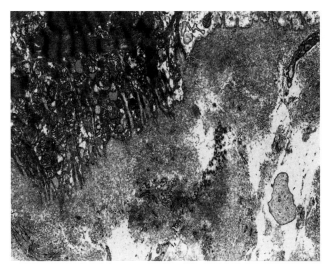

Figure 2–27. Amyloidosis, electron microscopy. A low magnification demonstrates interstitial expansion by fibrillar deposits.

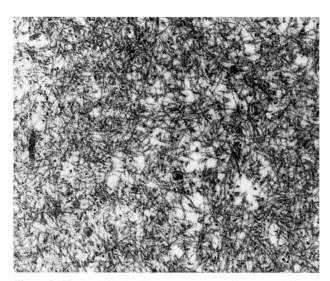

Figure 2–28. Amyloidosis, electron microscopy. The amyloid fibril is extracellular, nonbranching, and randomly oriented; it most often measures 10 nm in diameter.

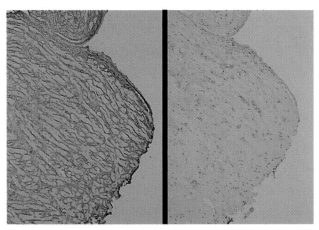

Figure 2–29. Primary amyloidosis, immunohistochemistry for light chains. Labeled antibodies to lambda light chains *(left)* demonstrate staining in contrast with kappa light chains *(right)*. In cases of senile amyloidosis, antibodies to transthyretin (prealbumin) bind the amyloid deposits.

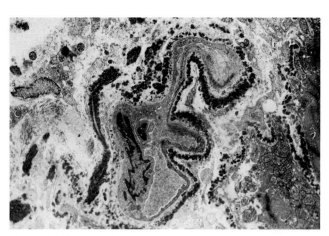

Figure 2–30. Light chain disease. In patients with plasma cell dyscrasias, light chains may rarely be deposited as electron-dense, perivascular deposits (not as amyloid). This section was prepared from a cardiac biopsy sample of an elderly man with Waldenström's macroglobulinemia and restrictive cardiomyopathy; the light chains were of kappa subtype.

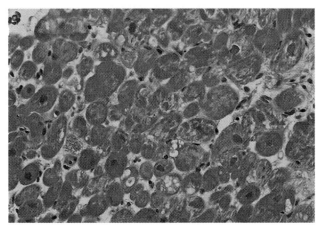

Figure 2–31. Hemochromatosis, endomyocardial biopsy. Note the brown intracellular pigment.

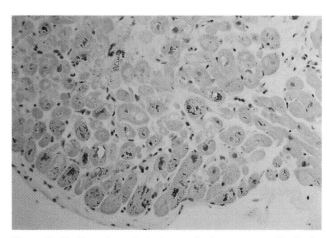

Figure 2–32. Hemochromatosis, iron stain. In contrast to lipofuscin, iron stains bright blue with Prussian blue reagent. Normal cardiac myocytes contain no stainable iron pigments.

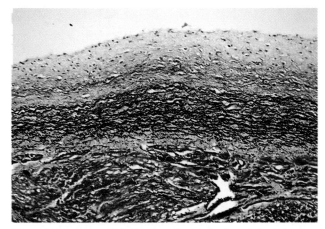

Figure 2–33. Endocardial fibroelastosis. Duplication of elastic laminae may occur in primary forms of the endocardial fibroelastosis, which is a congenital cardiomyopathy, and as a secondary finding in patients with dilated cardiomyopathy. The normal endocardium has fewer than five elastic layers.

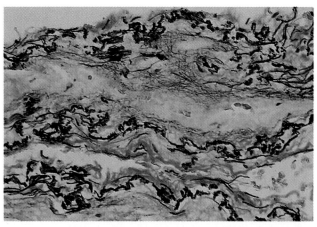

Figure 2–34. Pseudoxanthoma elasticum. This endomyocardial biopsy is from a 50-year-old woman with congestive heart failure and decreased ventricular compliance. Note the calcified, thickened, split elastic layers of the endocardium. Pseudoxanthoma elasticum is often asymptomatic in women and usually results in coronary artery disease, with clinically insignificant endocardial disease.

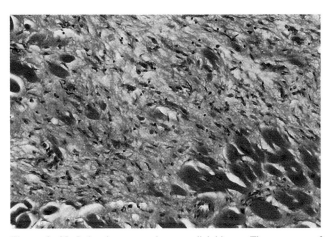

Figure 2–35. Ischemic scar, endomyocardial biopsy. The presence of focal fibrosis with scattered hemosiderin-laden macrophages is indicative of previous ischemic lesion.

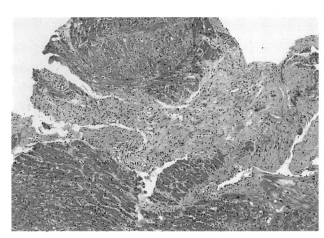

Figure 2–36. Whipple's disease. A patient with malabsorption and restrictive cardiomyopathy underwent endomyocardial and small bowel biopsy. The endomyocardial biopsy sample demonstrates focal interstitial aggregates of foamy histiocytes.

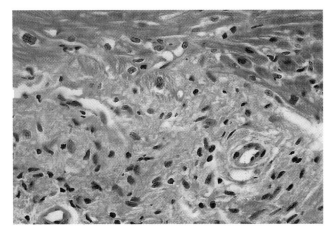

Figure 2–37. Whipple's disease. A higher magnification of the sample in Figure 2–36 demonstrates histiocytic cells with a finely granular, homogeneous cytoplasm. A periodic acid–Schiff stain (not illustrated) demonstrated numerous coarse intracellular bodies.

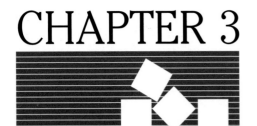

CHAPTER 3

James B. Atkinson, M.D.

Endomyocardial Biopsy of Cardiac Allografts and Transplant Atherosclerosis

ACUTE CARDIAC REJECTION

- The endomyocardial biopsy is the standard by which acute cardiac rejection is evaluated. The clinical signs and symptoms of rejection (arrhythmias, decreased electrocardiographic voltage, left ventricular compliance, echocardiographic dysfunction) do not reliably correlate with the presence or severity of rejection, particularly in cyclosporine-treated patients.
- At least four pieces of myocardium from a standard bioptome (9 French) are required to exclude rejection, and at least 50% of the samples should consist of myocardium and not previous biopsy site or scar tissue. Previous work has demonstrated that, with four pieces of myocardium, there is a 2% false-negative error rate and with three pieces, there is a 5% false-negative error rate. For smaller, disposable bioptomes (7 French), as many as six to eight pieces may be required.
- To evaluate endomyocardial biopsies for acute rejection, multiple sections must represent all levels of the tissue in the paraffin block to be examined. Three to five "step" levels should therefore be cut and stained with hematoxylin and eosin (H and E).
- Complications of endomyocardial biopsy may occur in association with catheter insertion (carotid puncture, vasovagal reactions, bleeding) or while the biopsy samples are being obtained (arrhythmia, conduction abnormalities, perforation). These do not have significant long-term sequelae and, in contrast to patients with cardiomyopathy, clinically significant perforation and death as a complication of endomyocardial biopsy in cardiac transplant patients virtually never occurs.

Histopathology

- The histopathologic features of acute cardiac rejection consist of inflammation with or without myocyte damage. The severity of rejection is classified according to the extent, pattern, and type of inflammation, and the presence or absence of myocyte necrosis. Large, "activated" lymphocytes (predominantly T cells) compose the inflammatory cell infiltrate.
- To establish criteria for treatment of acute rejection, several grading schemes were developed from the original system introduced by Billingham. To standardize the grading of acute rejection, a working formulation was devised by pathologists at a study group sponsored by the International Society for Heart and Lung Transplantation in 1990. This system is based on the original classification, in which mild, moderate, and severe grades are distinguished (Table 3–1).

Additional Histologic Features

- Additional diagnostic categories may be required for biopsy samples that are obtained after episodes of acute rejection:
  - "Ongoing" rejection implies that there is no improvement from the previous biopsy; "resolved" rejection indicates complete resolution and can be graded as 0.
  - "Resolving" acute rejection implies that the degree of inflammation is less than that seen in the previous biopsy, and the biopsy can be assigned a lesser grade.
  - As rejection episodes "resolve," the lymphocytes evolve from large, immunoblastic-like cells to small lymphocytes. In some instances, methyl green pyronin stains may be useful to help determine the relative number of "activated" cells versus small lymphocytes, although this differentiation can usually be made with H and E stain.
- Myocyte damage can be difficult to recognize. The Masson trichrome stain may enhance the recognition of early myocyte damage.
- Immunosuppressive therapy other than standard cy-

Table 3–1
INTERNATIONAL SOCIETY FOR HEART
AND LUNG TRANSPLANTATION GRADING
FOR ACUTE CARDIAC REJECTION*

Grade	Description
0	*No rejection* Normal myocardium with no evidence of inflammation or myocyte damage
1 1A	*Mild rejection* Focal (interstitial or perivascular) lymphocytic infiltration involving one or more pieces and no myocyte damage
1B	Diffuse, sparse lymphocytic infiltrate involving one or more pieces with no myocyte damage.
2	*Focal moderate rejection* One focus with an aggressive, sharply circumscribed infiltrate, usually associated with myocyte damage or architectural distortion of the myocardium. The infiltrate is composed of lymphocytes and immunoblasts, with occasional eosinophils.
3A	*Multifocal moderate rejection* Multifocal lymphocytic inflammatory infiltrates with myocyte damage; eosinophils may be present, and there are areas of normal myocardium between foci of inflammation. These changes can be seen in one or more pieces of myocardium. The distinction of grade 3A from grade 1A (where one or more pieces are involved by inflammation) is made by finding multifocal infiltrates within single pieces in grade 3A rejection, as well as the presence of myocyte damage.
3B	*Diffuse moderate/borderline severe rejection* Diffuse inflammation, with myocyte damage; aggressive lymphocytic infiltrates, which may contain eosinophils and rare neutrophils. There are fewer areas of normal myocardium separating areas of inflammation than in grade 3A.
4	*Severe rejection* Diffuse, aggressive inflammation consisting of lymphocytes, eosinophils and neutrophils; myocyte necrosis is always present; edema, hemorrhage, and vasculitis are also seen.

*From Billingham ME, Cary NRB, Hammond ME, et al. A working formulation for the standardization of nomenclature in the diagnosis of heart and lung rejection: Heart and Lung Rejection Study Group. J Heart Transplant 9:587–593, 1990.

closporine and corticosteroids may influence interpretation of the biopsy:

- Use of the monoclonal antibody OKT3 may be associated with reduced cellularity of the infiltrates, edema, increased vascular rejection, and increased incidence of the Quilty effect.
- Photopheresis is an alternative therapy used in some patients in whom standard therapy is contraindicated or who may be refractory to treatment. The procedure involves administration of autologous lymphocytes treated with 8-methoxypsoralen activated by extracorporally administered ultraviolet-A irradiation. The biopsy sample from these patients may have inflammatory infiltrates that are more extensive and that persist longer despite clinical resolution of acute rejection.

■ Obtaining multiple endomyocardial biopsy samples from infants and young children with cardiac allografts may be difficult due to problems in gaining vascular access. In such patients, there is a tendency for thrombosis and fibrotic occlusion of peripheral and central veins. Efforts are being made to use noninvasive modalities to monitor for acute rejection in this population, but these patients may still require a biopsy diagnosis for confirmation.

■ The initial (and occasionally only) manifestation of acute rejection in biopsies from some infants and children may be interstitial edema, with only a sparse inflammatory infiltrate.

Vascular (Humoral) Rejection

■ Even though most rejection episodes in cardiac allografts are "cellular," Hammond and colleagues have demonstrated a "vascular" form of rejection in some patients. It is postulated that endothelial cells stimulated by activated T cells mediate this form of rejection. Because humoral immune responses and B-cell activation are thought to play an important role, this form of rejection may be referred to as "humoral" rejection.

■ Vascular rejection can be assessed only by immunofluorescence studies on fresh-frozen, unfixed samples using a panel of antibodies against immunoglobulin, components of complement, and fibrinogen.

■ The diagnosis of vascular rejection is suggested when endothelial cells appear activated (large and prominent), and perivascular inflammation or edema is present. Confirmation of the diagnosis is made when immune complexes are demonstrated by immunofluorescence.

■ The prevalence of vascular rejection and its role in subsequent development of graft coronary artery disease remain to be established. It has been suggested that increased HLA-DR staining of blood vessels in endomyocardial biopsies is associated with development of graft coronary artery disease.

■ Vascular rejection should be considered if the allograft is not functioning optimally, particularly in the immediate postoperative period (first 6 weeks after transplantation), if the classic signs of "cellular" rejection are absent in the endomyocardial biopsy, and if other causes of graft dysfunction (postoperative ischemia, infection) have been excluded.

Hyperacute Rejection

■ Hyperacute rejection is seen in less than 1% of cardiac transplant patients; cardiac dilatation and right ventricular failure occur immediately after circulation is established.

■ Hyperacute rejection occurs when there is ABO blood type mismatch, preformed antibodies to the human leukocyte antigen (HLA) system of the allograft, and xenotransplantation.

■ Predisposing factors include prior blood transfusion, multiple pregnancies, multiple cardiac surgeries, and previous transplantation.

■ Preformed antibodies may deposit in allograft endothelial cells and activate the complement, clotting, and fibrinolytic cascades.

■ Grossly, the heart is a deep plum color from diffuse hemorrhage; histologically, there are microvascular thrombi and myocyte necroses.

■ Patients rarely survive for more than a few hours without emergent retransplantation; for this reason, the diagnosis is not made by endomyocardial biopsy.

References

Billingham ME. Cardiac transplantation. In Waller BF (ed). *Contemporary Issues in Cardiovascular Pathology*. Philadelphia, FA Davis, 1988, pp 185–199.

Billingham ME, Cary NRB, Hammond ME, et al. A working formulation for the standardization of nomenclature in the diagnosis of heart and lung rejection: Heart Rejection Study Group. J Heart Transplant 9:587–593, 1990.

Hammond EH, Hansen JK, Spencer LS, et al. Immunofluorescence of endomyocardial biopsy specimens: methods and interpretation. J Heart Lung Transplant 12:S113–S124, 1993.

Hammond EH, Hansen JK, Spencer LS, et al. Vascular rejection in cardiac transplantation: histologic, immunopathologic, and ultrastructural features. Cardiovasc Pathol 2:21–34, 1993.

Rose AG, Cooper DKC, Herman PA, Reichenspurner H, Reichart B. Histopathology of hyperacute rejection of the heart. Experimental and clinical observations in allografts and xenografts. J Heart Lung Transplant 10:223–234, 1991.

Trento AS, Hardesty RL, Griffith BP, Zerbe T, Kormas RL, Bahson HT. Role of the antibody to vascular endothelial cells in hyperacute rejection in patients undergoing cardiac transplantation. J Thorac Cardiovasc Surg 95:37–41, 1988.

NONREJECTION PATHOLOGY

Opportunistic Infections

Clinical Findings

■ Infections constitute the major cause of death in cardiac transplant patients, particularly in the acute postoperative period when episodes of rejection and immunosuppression are the greatest. Although bacterial infections are most common, immunosuppressed patients are at risk for viral, fungal, and protozoal infections as well. The lung is the most common site for infection, followed by the genitourinary and central nervous systems.

■ Infections may occur in the cardiac allograft and can be recognized in endomyocardial biopsy samples. Infection should be suspected when the inflammatory infiltrate in a cardiac biopsy sample is mixed and not characteristic of acute rejection, in which case viral, fungal, and protozoal organisms should be specifically sought.

Specific Organisms and Histopathology

Toxoplasmosis

■ Toxoplasmosis can be acquired from the donor organ or can occur as reactivation of a latent infection.

■ Toxoplasmosis in immunocompromised patients can produce myocarditis as well as necrotizing encephalitis and pneumonia.

■ The endomyocardial biopsy shows a mixed inflammatory infiltrate and tachyzoites or bradyzoites encysted in myocytes.

■ Polymerase chain reaction (PCR) has been used to detect infection with *Toxoplasma* in cardiac biopsy samples. PCR cannot distinguish quiescent infection from active toxoplasmosis, however.

Cytomegalovirus

■ Nearly half of cytomegalovirus (CMV) infections occur by transmission from CMV-seropositive donors to seronegative recipients.

■ Whereas toxoplasmosis has been diagnosed by endomyocardial biopsy, it is rare that CMV inclusions are found in the myocardium. The diagnosis of CMV infection, therefore, is based on typical histologic findings in other organs. Serology may have a high frequency of false-positive and false-negative results.

■ The cytomegalic features of CMV are characteristic and consist of large, basophilic or amphophilic intranuclear inclusions. Intracytoplasmic inclusions may not be seen in every cell but, when present, are composed of small granular basophilic bodies that are positive on periodic acid–Schiff (PAS) staining. Both the nucleus and cytoplasm of infected cells are increased in size. In small biopsy samples, cytopathic changes suggestive of CMV can be confirmed by immunoperoxidase techniques.

■ The use of immunocytochemistry and in situ hybridization techniques to detect CMV in endomyocardial biopsy samples from cardiac allografts has produced mixed results. One group could not detect CMV in cells that did not already have the characteristic cytopathic features (nuclear inclusions, increased size). Arbustini and colleagues, however, found a greater number of infected cells by immunohistochemistry than was seen by conventional staining, and in situ hybridization detected infected cells that did not show evidence of cytopathic effect. PCR was more sensitive, but its interpretation is difficult because PCR-positive biopsies do not necessarily indicate tissue infection and can be the result of amplified sequences derived from circulating leukocytes.

■ Special studies on cardiac biopsy samples (in situ hybridization, PCR) may be warranted if there are suspicious inclusions, or if the inflammatory infiltrate is not typical of that expected for acute rejection.

Neoplasms and Posttransplant Lymphoproliferative Disorders

■ Organ transplant recipients are at increased risk for malignancies; the incidence of neoplastic disease in adult and pediatric heart transplant recipients is between 4% and 13%. Although tumors of low malignant potential (squamous cell and basal cell carcinomas) are most common, these patients have a particularly high risk for hematopoietic-lymphoid neoplasms. Onset may be from months after transplantation to a decade later.

■ Posttransplant lymphoproliferative disorders (PTLDs) compose an aggressive subset of neoplasms that may arise as abnormal polyclonal lymphoid proliferations associated with Epstein-Barr virus infections.

■ PTLDs are composed of B lymphocytes in all stages of differentiation, including plasma cells; progression can occur from a polyclonal population of cells to a monoclonal proliferation in association with clonal immunoglobulin gene rearrangements.

■ PTLDs involve predominantly lymph nodes and extranodal sites, including the central nervous system, gastrointestinal tract, lungs, and soft tissues. Involvement of the cardiac allograft has only rarely been reported.

Artifacts and Caveats

Ischemic Changes

■ It is not uncommon to observe focal ischemic damage in cardiac biopsy samples obtained up to 3 weeks after transplantation. These changes may be particularly prominent in the first biopsy after transplantation and they do not seem to correlate with subsequent clinical outcome.

■ Ischemic changes are recognized by focal myocyte damage or necrosis. There may be a sparse, predominantly neutrophilic, inflammatory infiltrate.

■ Ischemic changes should not be misinterpreted as acute rejection. The distinction can be made by determining the posttransplant interval and by recognizing that, in ischemia, myocyte damage precedes an acute inflammatory response. Therefore, the extent of myocyte damage in ischemia exceeds the degree of inflammation that is otherwise expected with acute rejection.

Previous Biopsy Sites

■ One of the most common pitfalls in diagnosing acute cardiac rejection is misinterpretation of a previous biopsy site.

■ Evidence of a previous biopsy may be seen in 16% of biopsy samples obtained in the immediate postoperative period and may even be more frequent as the number of biopsies increases over time in an individual patient.

■ Changes representing a previous biopsy site range from the presence of fibrin, necrosis, and granulation tissue at or near the endocardial surface (if recent) to fibrosis and disarray of surrounding myocytes if the biopsy site is healed.

■ The location and configuration of previous biopsy sites should provide a clue as to their origin. The presence of fibrin, which is never seen in acute rejection, is a useful marker of a biopsy site.

Quilty Effect

■ In 10% to 14% of patients receiving cyclosporine, the biopsy sample may have a dense endocardial collection of lymphocytes (Quilty effect, named after the first patient noted to have these changes).

■ The infiltrate consists of T lymphocytes surrounding clusters of B cells (unlike the infiltrate of acute rejection), with occasional plasma cells and macrophages. Two subtypes have been defined: Quilty A, in which the infiltrate is confined to the endocardium, and Quilty B, in which the infiltrate encroaches into the myocardium.

■ When the inflammatory infiltrate extends into the subendocardium, the distinction from acute rejection may be difficult. Large Quilty lesions may also make differentiation from a lymphoproliferative disorder problematic. Immunoperoxidase studies can sometimes help make these distinctions.

■ Even though the Quilty effect may, in some way, relate to rejection, it does not portend any known adverse clinical outcome and usually resolves upon subsequent biopsies without specific treatment.

Graft Coronary Artery Disease

Clinical Findings

■ The major limitation to long-term success of cardiac transplantation is the accelerated atherosclerosis that occurs in the coronary arteries of the allograft (Table 3–2). Because the transplanted heart lacks afferent innervation, cardiac transplant recipients may not experience angina, and the first manifestation of coronary artery disease may be silent myocardial infarction, congestive heart failure, or sudden death.

■ The incidence of graft coronary artery disease detected by angiography is approximately 40% at 5 years, although significant narrowing may be detected as early as 1 year after transplantation.

■ The angiographic pattern of graft coronary artery disease usually consists of diffuse concentric narrowing with obliteration of distal vessels. There may be discrete or tubular narrowing with occlusion of major branches, and collateral vessels are poorly developed.

■ The cause of graft coronary artery disease is not known, although immunologic injury to the endothelium may be a common factor. Consistent correlations have not been observed for number of acute rejection episodes, age of the donor heart, or prior history of coronary artery disease. Posttransplant hypertension and hyperlipidemia, both of which are common in patients receiving cyclosporine or corticosteroid immunosuppression therapy, as well as CMV infections may contribute to development of graft coronary artery disease.

Histopathology

■ The histopathologic features of graft coronary artery disease correlate with the angiographic findings. Graft coronary artery disease is characterized by proliferative lesions with both circumferential and longitudinal increases in the intima.

■ Intimal lesions are composed of smooth muscle and myointimal cells and macrophages in an abundant extracellular matrix of fibrous tissue and proteoglycan

Table 3–2
COMPARISON OF HISTOPATHOLOGIC FEATURES FOR GRAFT CORONARY ARTERY DISEASE VERSUS CONVENTIONAL ATHEROSCLEROSIS

Graft Coronary Artery Disease	Conventional Atherosclerosis
Concentric intimal lesion common	Eccentric intimal lesion common
Elastica mostly intact	Elastica damaged
Diffuse	Focal
Branches involved	Spares branches
Intramyocardial arteries involved	Spares intramyocardial vessels
Calcification not extensive	Calcification frequent
Necrotic atheroma rare	Atheroma frequent
Lipid less prominent	Lipid more prominent
Develops rapidly	Develops slowly

ground substance. The internal elastic lamina is intact, in contrast to conventional atherosclerosis, and only small amounts of lipid may be present in early lesions. The intimal lesions are usually concentric but can be eccentric as well.

■ As duration of the cardiac allograft increases, the amount of lipid in the intimal lesions increases, predominantly in foam cells. In long-term survivors, lesions may appear more similar to those seen in conventional atherosclerosis, with extracellular lipid, necrosis, calcification, and an overlying fibrous cap. Rarely, hemorrhage within a lipid-rich plaque or plaque rupture can be seen, such as occurs in unstable lesions of conventional atherosclerosis.

■ The concentric intimal proliferation occurs along the entire extent of the coronary artery, extending into small intramyocardial arteries that may be seen in endomyocardial biopsy samples.

Vasculitis

■ In some cases, active or healed vasculitis can be seen in cardiac allografts. This can involve both the major epicardial and intramyocardial coronary arteries. The finding of concentric intimal thickening in arteries, combined with scant inflammatory infiltrates, suggests that vasculitis may be a precursor to accelerated graft coronary artery disease.

■ The inflammatory infiltrate may be mixed, with lymphocytes, plasma cells, and polymorphonuclear leukocytes, or it may be predominantly lymphocytic. Fibrinoid necrosis involving the arterial wall can

occasionally be seen as can acute or remote (recanalized) thrombosis.

■ In some hearts, a combination of active and healed vasculitis may be present. Healed vasculitis is recognized by sudden segmental fibrous replacement of the media, sometimes involving the intima as well.

■ Vasculitis seems to be more common in children with cardiac allografts than in adults.

References

Arbustini E, Grasso M, Diegoli M, et al. Histopathologic and molecular profile of human cytomegalovirus infections in patients with heart transplants. Am J Clin Pathol 98:205–213, 1992.

Armitage JM, Kormos RL, Stuart RS, et al. Posttransplant lymphoproliferative disease in thoracic organ transplant patients: ten years of cyclosporine-based immunosuppression. J Heart Lung Transplant 10:877–887, 1991.

Atkinson JB, Virmani R. Pathology of heart and combined heart-lung transplantation. In Virmani R, Atkinson JB, Fenoglio JJ (eds). *Cardiovascular Pathology.* Philadelphia, WB Saunders 1991, pp 310–333.

Billingham ME. Cardiac transplant atherosclerosis. Transplant Proc 19(suppl 5):19–25, 1987.

Eisen HJ, Hicks D, Kant JA, et al. Diagnosis of posttransplantation lymphoproliferative disorder by endomyocardial biopsy in a cardiac allograft recipient. J Heart Lung Transplant 13:241–245, 1994.

Holliman R, Johnson J, Savva D, et al. Diagnosis of *Toxoplasma* infection in cardiac transplant recipients using the polymerase chain reaction. J Clin Pathol 45:931–932, 1992.

Johnson DE, Alderman EL, Schroeder JS, et al. Transplant coronary artery disease: histopathologic correlations with angiographic morphology. J Am Coll Cardiol 17:449–457, 1991.

Rose AG, Viviers L, Odell JA. Pathology of chronic cardiac rejection: an analysis of the epicardial and intramyocardial coronary arteries and myocardial alterations in 43 human allografts. Cardiovasc Pathol 2:7–19, 1993.

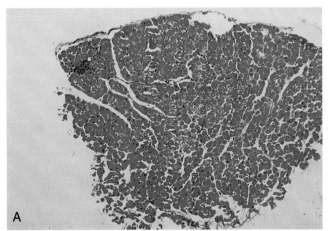 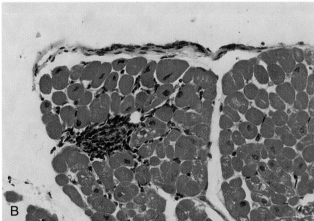

Figure 3–1. *A,* Acute rejection, grade 1A. This piece of myocardium contains a focal infiltrate of lymphocytes and no myocyte damage. Apart from this focus, the biopsy sample is normal. *B,* Acute rejection, grade 1A. A higher magnification of *A* demonstrates the focus of the lymphocytes.

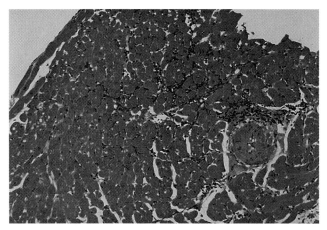

Figure 3–2. Acute rejection, grade 1B. A sparse, interstitial lymphocytic infiltrate without myocyte damage is present in this biopsy sample.

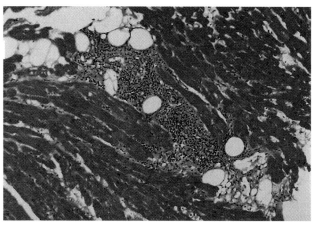

Figure 3–3. Acute rejection, grade 2. Cardiac biopsy showing a well-circumscribed focus of inflammatory cells, which are separating myocytes, indicative of focal moderate (grade 2) rejection.

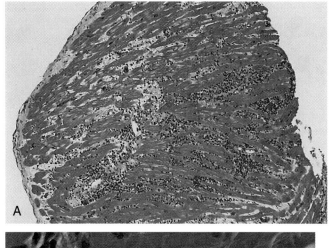

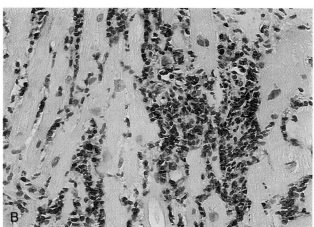

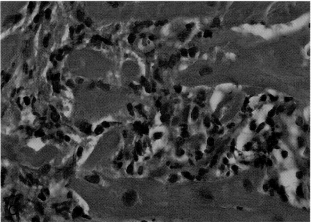

Figure 3–4. *A*, Acute rejection, grade 3A. This biopsy sample has multifocal aggressive infiltrates. *B*, An immunostain for CD3 surface antigen demonstrates that most lymphocytes are T cells. *C*, A higher magnification of *A* demonstrates focal myocyte damage.

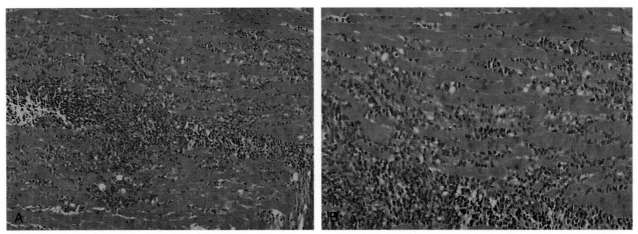

Figure 3–5. *A,* Acute rejection, grade 3B. Endomyocardial biopsy specimen demonstrates diffuse inflammation. *B,* A higher magnification of *A* demonstrates myocyte damage.

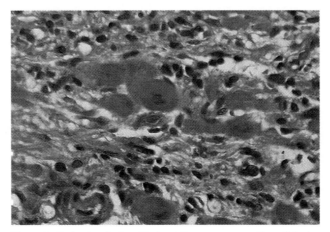

Figure 3–6. Acute rejection. Eosinophils compose a portion of the inflammatory infiltrate.

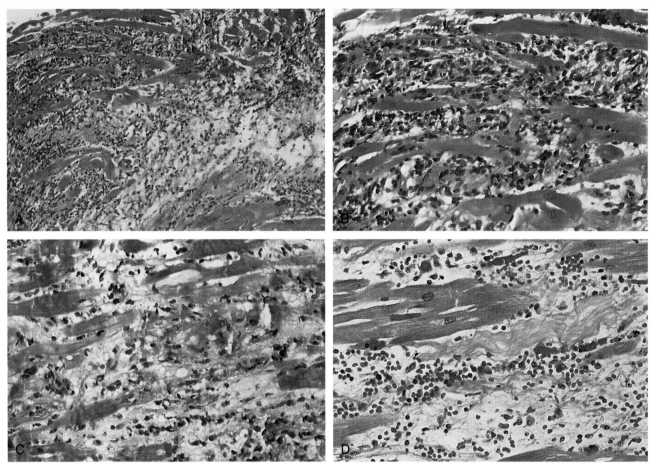

Figure 3–7. *A*, Acute rejection, grade 4. This cardiac biopsy sample exhibits a marked diffuse inflammatory infiltrate. *B*, Acute rejection, grade 4. The infiltrate illustrated in *A* is composed of lymphocytes and neutrophils. *C*, Acute rejection, grade 4. Myocyte necrosis is apparent. *D*, Acute rejection, grade 4. Hemorrhage and edema are features of severe rejection.

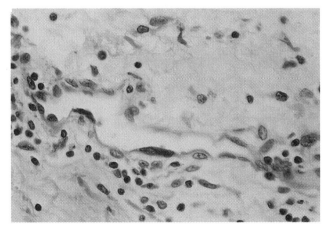

Figure 3–8. Vascular (humoral) rejection. This myocardial vein has prominent, enlarged endothelial cells and perivascular edema and lymphocyte infiltrates.

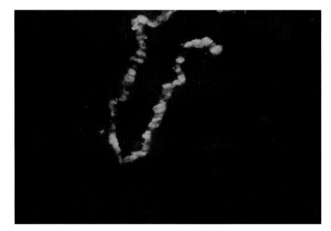

Figure 3–9. Vascular (humoral) rejection. Immunofluorescence reveals uniform vascular staining for antihuman IgG as well as complement (not shown) that are indicative of vascular rejection.

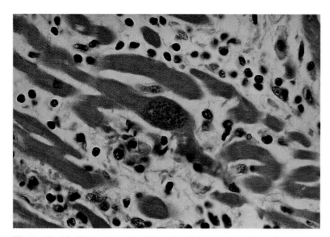

Figure 3–10. Toxoplasmosis. Note the intramyocyte *Toxoplasma* cyst with barely discernible tachyzoites.

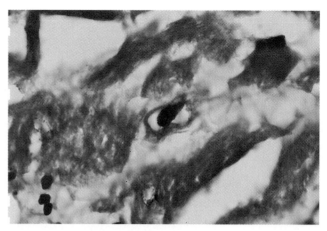

Figure 3–11. Cytomegalovirus infection. Note the characteristic owl's eye nuclear inclusion. (Reproduced from Anderson DW, Virmani R, Reilly JM, et al. Prevalent myocarditis at necropsy in the acquired immune deficiency syndrome. J Am Coll Cardiol 11:792–799, 1988. Reprinted with permission from the American College of Cardiology.)

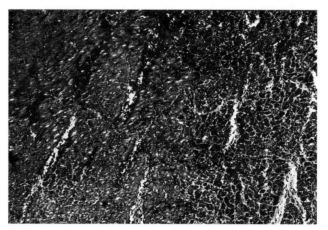

Figure 3–12. Hyperacute rejection. In this autopsy specimen, there is diffuse hemorrhage and necrosis. Hearts with hyperacute rejection do not survive beyond a few hours and therefore are not subjected to endomyocardial biopsy.

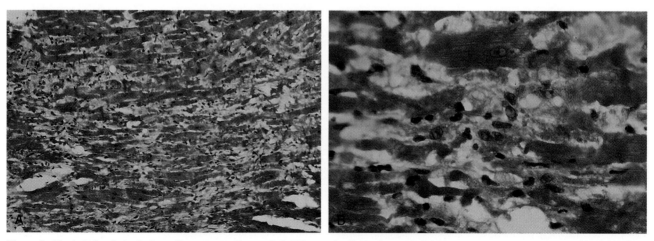

Figure 3–13. *A,* Ischemia in the immediate posttransplant period. This was the first endomyocardial biopsy sample obtained 1 week after transplantation; it shows a focus of myocytes that exhibit ischemic necrosis. *B,* A higher magnification of *A* demonstrates sparse inflammation.

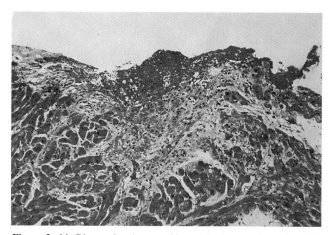

Figure 3–14. Biopsy site. A recent biopsy site is seen along the endocardial surface, with focal loss of cardiac myocytes, scant inflammation, and fibrin overlying the endocardium.

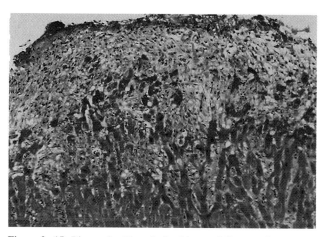

Figure 3–15. Biopsy site. There is focal loss and disarray of myocytes, granulation tissue, and a sparse inflammatory infiltrate.

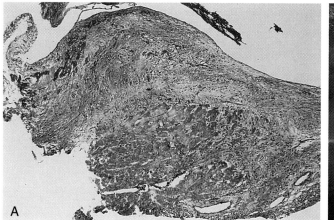

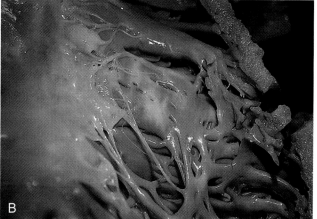

Figure 3–16. *A*, Biopsy site. A well-formed scar, indicative of a remote biopsy site, is located along the endocardial surface of this endomyocardial biopsy sample stained with Masson trichrome stain. *B*, The gross specimen of the lesion depicted in *A* shows multiple endocardial scars on the right ventricular surface of the interventricular septum correlating with the histologic findings of previous biopsy sites. The patient died 3 years after transplantation, and necropsy was performed.

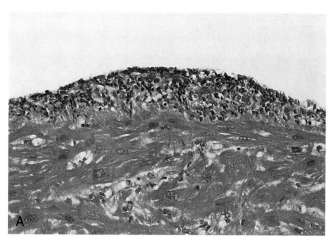

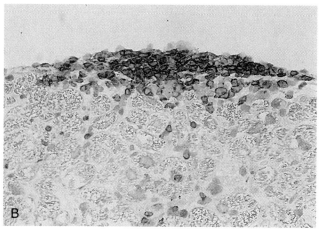

Figure 3–17. *A,* Quilty effect. A sparse endocardial inflammatory infiltrate, characteristic of Quilty effect, is present in this endomyocardial biopsy sample. *B,* An immunostain for CD3 demonstrates that the majority of cells are T cells.

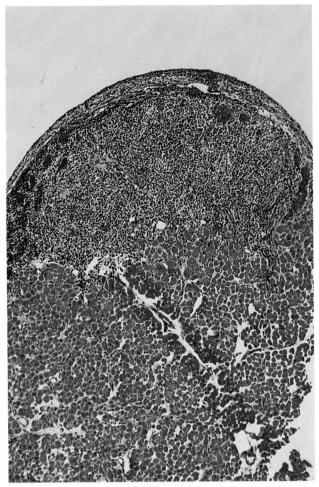

Figure 3–18. The Quilty lesion may demonstrate a more extensive infiltrate. The presence of small capillaries, seen in the endocardial infiltrate in this biopsy sample as well as in that illustrated in Figure 3–17A, is a useful marker to help distinguish the Quilty lesion from acute rejection.

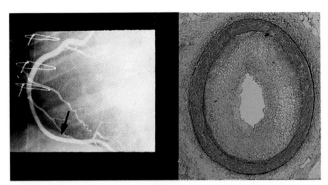

Figure 3–19. Graft coronary artery disease. The left panel shows a coronary angiogram from a 31-year-old woman who underwent cardiac transplantation for dilated cardiomyopathy 18 months earlier. This angiogram was interpreted as normal. One month later, the patient died of graft coronary artery disease. A histologic section obtained at the angiographic site *(arrow)* showed marked narrowing by a concentric proliferative lesion occupying more than 75% of the luminal cross-sectional area (right panel).

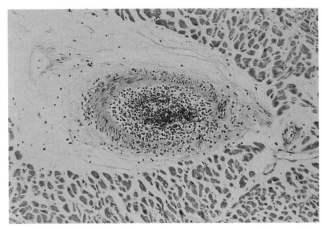

Figure 3–20. Graft coronary artery disease, acute vasculitis. There is an active lymphocytic vasculitis in a 12-month cardiac allograft, with inflammation involving both the intima and media.

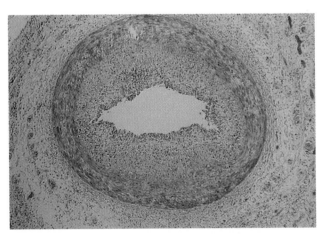

Figure 3–21. Graft coronary artery disease, healing vasculitis. A proliferative fibrointimal lesion contains an inflammatory infiltrate.

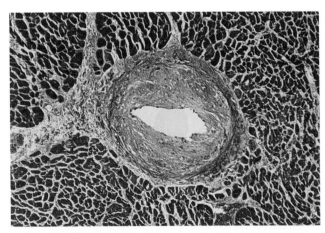

Figure 3–22. Graft coronary artery disease, healed vasculitis. A Masson trichrome–stained section shows an intramyocardial coronary artery with marked fibrosis involving the media and a fibrous, relatively acellular intimal proliferative lesion, indicative of remote vasculitis.

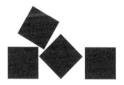

PATHOLOGY OF

NATIVE AND

PROSTHETIC

CARDIAC VALVES

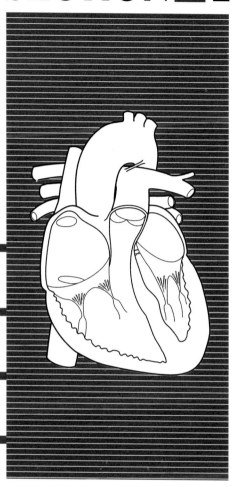

CHAPTER 4

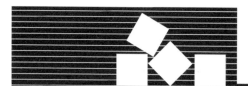

Approach to Cardiac Valves

GROSS EXAMINATION

- Gross examination is the most important aspect of the pathologic examination of valves (Table 4–1).
- An attempt should be made to recreate the intact valve structure in its probable functional condition, estimating the annular circumference, to aid in morphologic observations.
- Whether the entire valve or a portion of valve is submitted should be noted. Valve repair is commonly performed on the mitral valve. Submitted tissue may consist of portions of the valve (anterior and/or posterior leaflet, chordae tendineae, papillary muscles).
- Some valve specimens are submitted in pieces, especially heavily calcified aortic valves. This may impair the ability to make a definitive morphologic diagnosis if, for example, valve cusps and commissures have been surgically fragmented.

Clinical History

The clinical history that should accompany the evaluation of atrioventricular, semilunar, and prosthetic valves is shown in Tables 4–2 through 4–4, respectively.

MICROSCOPIC EXAMINATION

- Histologic evaluation of any aortic tissue submitted with the valve, especially aortic valve, should be performed to look for dissection, cystic medial change, and inflammatory lesions.
- In many cases, microscopic examination of the valve itself is unnecessary and only results in loss of an intact specimen.
- Exceptions in which histologic sections are indicated include the following:

  - Evaluations of vegetations (e.g., endocarditis)
  - Carcinoid heart disease
  - Amyloidosis
  - Connective tissue diseases
  - Ochronosis

GROSS PHOTOGRAPHY

- Gross valve photography is an important tool to document the valve disease for the patient record.

Table 4–2
RECOMMENDED CLINICAL HISTORY
FOR THE EVALUATION OF
ATRIOVENTRICULAR VALVES*

Age
Sex
History of rheumatic fever (yes, no, unknown)
History of endocarditis (yes, no, unknown)
History of mitral prolapse (yes, no, unknown)
Ischemic heart disease (yes, no, unknown)
Other pertinent information
Valve (mitral, tricuspid, other)
Chordal rupture
Stenosis (absent, mild, moderate, severe)
Insufficiency (absent, mild, moderate, severe)

*Modified from Dare AJ, Harrity PJ, Tazelaar HD, Edwards WD, Mullany CJ. Evaluation of surgically excised mitral valves: revised recommendations based on changing operative procedures in the 1990s. Hum Pathol 24:1292, 1993.

Table 4–1
GROSS FEATURES TO RECORD IN THE
SURGICAL PATHOLOGIC EXAMINATION
OF CARDIAC VALVES

Number of excised pieces
Approximate annular circumference (if possible, by apposing leaflets)
Number of commissures; presence of raphes (aortic valve)
Presence of commissural fusion or calcification
The presence of leaflet or cuspal fibrosis (free edge or diffuse), calcification (mild, moderate, severe), destruction or perforation
Congenital malformation
Chordae tendineae (atrioventricular valves): normal, thickened or fused, thinned or elongated, ruptured
Vegetations: presence, size, location, underlying valve destruction, shape (filiform, nodular, irregular)

■ Gross photography is especially indicated in cases that will be sectioned for microscopy.

MICROBIOLOGIC STUDIES

■ Cultures of vegetations should be sent to the laboratory for organism identification and antibiotic sensitivity testing; this should preferably be done in the operating suite.

Table 4–3
RECOMMENDED CLINICAL HISTORY FOR THE EVALUATION OF SEMILUNAR VALVES*

Age
Sex
History of rheumatic fever (yes, no, unknown)
History of endocarditis (yes, no, unknown)
Aortic root dilatation (yes, no, aortitis)
Other pertinent information
Valve (aortic, pulmonary, truncal)
Number of cusps
Stenosis (absent, mild, moderate, severe)
Insufficiency (absent, mild, moderate, severe)

*Modified from Dare AJ, Harrity PJ, Tazelaar HD, Edwards WD, Mullany CJ. Evaluation of surgically excised mitral valves: revised recommendations based on changing operative procedures in the 1990s. Hum Pathol 24:1292, 1993.

Table 4–4
RECOMMENDED CLINICAL HISTORY FOR THE EVALUATION OF PROSTHETIC VALVES*

Age
Sex
Type of prosthesis
Position (e.g., mitral)
Aortic root dilatation (yes, no, aortitis)
Reason for excision
Other pertinent information
Stenosis (absent, mild, moderate, severe)
Insufficiency (absent, mild, moderate, severe)

*Modified from Dare AJ, Harrity PJ, Tazelaar HD, Edwards WD, Mullany CJ. Evaluation of surgically excised mitral valves: revised recommendations based on changing operative procedures in the 1990s. Hum Pathol 24:1292, 1993.

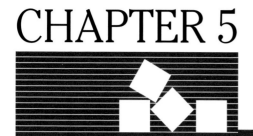

CHAPTER 5

Mitral Valve

SURGICAL PATHOLOGIC APPROACH TO MITRAL VALVE DISEASE

Clinical History

- The preoperative diagnosis is helpful in narrowing the diagnostic categories (Table 5–1).
- In general, mitral stenosis is caused by postinflammatory (postrheumatic) mitral disease.
- Mitral insufficiency may be the result of a wider variety of diseases, including mitral valve prolapse (MVP), postinflammatory disease, ischemic heart disease, and endocarditis.

Approach to the Surgical Specimen

- The type of specimen is helpful in narrowing the diagnostic categories.
- A total valve replacement, resulting in the pathologist's receiving an entire valve, is generally performed on patients with postinflammatory disease, and only infrequently in MVP.
- Only a portion of posterior leaflet is received if there has been valve *repair (valvuloplasty);* this procedure is generally performed for MVP, and less commonly for endocarditis.
- If the specimen consists of the anterior leaflet with or without a portion of the posterior leaflet, the valve replacement may have been for any type of valve disease, including MVP, postinflammatory disease, and ischemic heart disease (Tables 5–2 and 5–3).

- Chordal fragments may constitute the entire specimen; a pathologic diagnosis is impossible, but the likely diagnosis is ischemic papillary muscle disease or MVP.

MITRAL VALVE PROLAPSE

MVP is the congenital myxomatous degeneration of the mitral valve. It is also called floppy mitral valve, a term generally used by pathologists to describe the gross changes of a functionally prolapsing mitral valve.

Incidence and Patient Characteristics

- MVP is the most common congenital valve defect, affecting 0.5% to 3% of the population.
- Asymptomatic MVP is more common in women.
- MVP resulting in progressive mitral regurgitation is more common in men (male:female ratio 3:2).
- The mean age at surgical presentation is 60 years.

Table 5–2
SURGICAL PATHOLOGIC DIAGNOSES, MITRAL VALVE

Classification	Diagnosis	Total (%)	Mean age (years)
Mitral regurgitation	Mitral valve prolapse	15–30*	65
	Postinflammatory disease	10	55
	Ischemic disease	4–8	70
	Endocarditis	2–5	50
	Carcinoid disease	<1	
	Hypertrophic cardiomyopathy	<1	
	Radiation	<1	
	Congenital disease	<1	
	Idiopathic chordal rupture	<1	
Mitral stenosis with or without regurgitation	Postinflammatory disease	25–40*	55
	Ergotamine valve disease	<1	
Mucopolysaccharidosis		<1	
Congenital disease <1			

*The relative proportion of valve replacements for mitral valve prolapse has risen in recent years, with a concomitant drop in the proportion of valves removed for postinflammatory (rheumatic) heart disease.

Table 5–1
RELATIONSHIP OF RESECTED SPECIMEN, PROCEDURE, AND DIAGNOSIS, SURGICALLY EXCISED MITRAL VALVES

Resected Specimen	Procedure	Most Likely Diagnoses
Entire valve	Valve replacement	Postinflammatory
Anterior leaflet plus or minus portion of posterior leaflet	Valve replacement	Postinflammatory, mitral valve prolapse, ischemia
Posterior leaflet	Valve repair	Mitral valve prolapse

Table 5-3
SURGICAL PATHOLOGIC DIAGNOSES,
MITRAL REGURGITATION, BY AGE*

	Incidence (%)	
Diagnosis	*< 60 years*	*> 60 years*
Postinflammatory disease	40	20
Mitral valve prolapse	33	45
Ischemic disease	5	18
Endocarditis	7	5
Other	15	12

*Adapted from Olson LJ, Subramanian R, Ackermann DM, Orszulak TA, Edwards WD. Surgical pathology of the mitral valve: a study of 712 cases spanning 21 years. Mayo Clin Proc 62:22, 1987.

- MVP usually occurs as an isolated cardiac lesion.
- Patients with Marfan syndrome, hypertrophic cardiomyopathy, ostium secundum, atrial septal defect (involving the anterior leaflet), Ehlers-Danlos syndrome, and Ebstein's tricuspid anomaly have an increased incidence of MVP.

Clinical Findings

- Most prolapsing mitral valves function normally.
- Progressive mitral regurgitation occurs in 10% to 15% of patients with MVP.
- MVP is associated with an increased incidence of ventricular and supraventricular arrhythmias.
- In rare cases, MVP results in sudden cardiac death (mechanism unknown).
- There is an increased risk of infectious endocarditis in patients with MVP.
- MVP is occasionally associated with prolapse of the tricuspid or aortic valve, which may also be replaced or repaired at the time of mitral valve surgery.

Surgical Treatment

- MVP is the most common cause of pure mitral regurgitation requiring valve surgery.
- Valve surgery is recommended for patients with severe mitral regurgitation with left ventricular dilatation or dysfunction.
- If technically feasible, valve repair with segmental valve resection (mitral valvuloplasty) and/or placement of a prosthetic ring (annuloplasty) is recommended over total valve replacement.
- The posterior leaflet and chordal attachments to the papillary muscle are often left in place, which improves cardiac systolic performance and reduces left ventricular dilatation.

Gross Pathologic Findings

- Depending on the surgical resection, the surgical specimen may consist of the entire valve, the entire or a large portion of anterior or posterior leaflet and attached chordae, or a wedge resection of valve tissue.
- MVP accounts for most surgically *repaired* mitral

valves; the surgical specimen often consists of a portion of posterior leaflet only.
- There is myxomatous thickening of the valve leaflets with interchordal hooding.
- The middle scallop of the posterior leaflet is often maximally involved.
- Leaflet length is increased and leaflets bulge (prolapse) toward the left atrium.
- Elongation of the chordae associated with abnormal insertion into the leaflet is common.
- Chordae ruptured from their papillary muscle insertion are common (20%-74% of surgically excised mitral valves).
- Multiple ruptured chordae result in a flail leaflet.
- Leaflet calcification may be present near its insertion into its annulus.
- Annular dilatation (circumference > 10 cm) is often present, which worsens mitral regurgitation.
- When only the anterior leaflet is excised, the annular circumference may be estimated as three times the length of the annular cut edge of this leaflet.

Microscopic Pathologic Findings

- Histologic examination is *not* necessary unless endocarditis is suspected.
- Excessive accumulation of proteoglycans in the spongiosa layer results in expansion and elongation of valve leaflets.
- The fibrosa is interrupted by an expansion of the spongiosa by proteoglycan deposition.
- Elastic fiber duplication may occur.

Differential Diagnosis

- In rheumatic mitral valve disease, there is commissural fusion and leaflet retraction with chordal thickening and fusion, which are not features of MVP.
- A precise diagnosis is not always possible, especially if only a portion of valve is resected.

CHRONIC RHEUMATIC MITRAL VALVE DISEASE

Scarring of the mitral valve leaflet and its chordal apparatus is caused by previous acute rheumatic valvulitis.

Relationship to Acute Rheumatic Fever

- A documented history of previous rheumatic fever is present in up to 50% of patients with mitral stenosis; postinflammatory valvular scarring is presumed to be postrheumatic in most cases, unless there is a history of some other nonrheumatic inflammatory disease.
- After acute rheumatic valvulitis, chronic rheumatic valve disease manifests after a latent period (20-25 years), with symptoms typically appearing in the third to fourth decades; in underdeveloped countries, severe postrheumatic valve deformity may occur in adolescents.

- The risk of developing chronic rheumatic valvulitis after an episode of acute rheumatic fever varies and is highest in patients with rheumatic carditis that results in congestive heart failure.

Patient Characteristics and Clinical Findings

- Postrheumatic valvular scarring is more prevalent in women (male:female ratio approximately 0.4:1).
- Valve surgery most often occurs in the fifth decade.
- Rheumatic mitral stenosis is the most important clinical manifestation of chronic rheumatic heart disease; mixed stenosis and regurgitation is common, and pure regurgitation is rare.
- The normal mitral valve area is 4 to 6 cm². Mild stenosis is present with an area of 2 to 4 cm²; moderate stenosis, with 1 to 2 cm²; and severe stenosis, with less than 1 cm².
- Signs and symptoms include dyspnea, congestive heart failure, arrhythmias (especially atrial fibrillation), and pulmonary hypertension; symptoms correlate with a mitral valve area of less than 1.0 cm².
- There is an increased risk of endocarditis.
- Concurrent involvement of the aortic valve is common; involvement of tricuspid and/or pulmonary valves is rare.

Surgical Treatment

- Valve surgery is indicated in symptomatic patients with severe stenosis and/or regurgitation.
- Retention of the posterior leaflet and its chordal attachments to the papillary muscles is associated with improved cardiac function and reduced risk of postoperative left ventricular rupture.

Gross Pathologic Findings

- The surgical specimen consists of either the entire mitral valve or just the anterior leaflet.
- Characteristic findings are commissural fusion; retracted, fibrotic leaflets; and thickened, fibrotic, matted, and shortened chordae tendineae.
- Leaflet calcification may be severe, mild, or absent and is most prominent in the commissures. Marked calcification is more common in men. Calcific nodules may ulcerate through the valve surface.
- From annulus to fused chordae, the stenotic mitral valve is funnel-shaped, and the orifice is shaped like a buttonhole (fish mouth).

Microscopic Pathologic Findings

- Histologic examination is not necessary unless endocarditis is suspected.
- Fibroelastic leaflet thickening is present, with loss of the normal valve architecture.
- Vascularization of the leaflet and associated focal chronic inflammation, predominantly lymphocytes, are seen.
- Dystrophic calcification of leaflet may be present, especially in fused commissures.

MITRAL REGURGITATION SECONDARY TO ISCHEMIC HEART DISEASE

Clinical Findings

- Ischemic mitral regurgitation is more common in men because the incidence of atherosclerotic coronary disease is higher in men.
- Regurgitation may be acute owing to ischemic necrosis and rupture of a papillary muscle in the setting of an acute myocardial infarction, usually resulting in acute pulmonary edema and cardiogenic shock.
- More commonly, regurgitation is chronic, owing to the healed infarction of one or both papillary muscles with left ventricular dilatation and mitral annular dilatation, which further impairs mitral closure.
- The posteromedial papillary muscle has a single blood supply from the posterior descending coronary artery and more frequently becomes infarcted compared with the anterolateral papillary muscle, which has a dual blood supply from diagonal branches (from the left anterior descending coronary artery) and marginal branches (from the left circumflex artery).
- Coronary artery bypass is usually also performed at the time of valve replacement.

Pathologic Findings

- The surgical specimen may consist of the entire valve or just the anterior leaflet.
- The mitral leaflets and chordae are typically unremarkable.
- The pathologic features are present in the papillary muscles, which may or may not be present in the specimen.
- In chronic ischemic mitral regurgitation, the papillary muscle is thin and atrophic; on histologic examination, there is replacement of the papillary muscle by scar tissue.
- In papillary muscle rupture, coagulation necrosis of the papillary muscle is present and associated with a layer of fibrin and platelets along the ruptured muscular surface.

LESIONS OF THE MITRAL VALVE RARELY REQUIRING SURGICAL TREATMENT

Acute Rheumatic Fever

- Rheumatic carditis is caused by group A streptococci.
- In the industrialized world, there has been a marked reduction in the incidence of rheumatic fever, but new outbreaks have occurred in military and civilian populations and have been associated with a virulent, encapsulated, M-protein–rich strain of group A streptococci.
- The diagnosis is confirmed by serologic evidence of a preceding streptococcal infection with either (1) two major Jones criteria (carditis, polyarthritis, chorea, ery-

thema marginatum, subcutaneous nodules) or (2) one major and two minor Jones criteria (fever, arthralgias, previous rheumatic fever or rheumatic heart disease, elevated erythrocyte sedimentation rate, positive C-reactive protein, prolonged P-R interval on electrocardiogram).

- Valve surgery is not performed in the treatment of acute rheumatic fever unless the disease is fulminant, resulting in severe valvular regurgitation and heart failure.
- Pathologically, there are small, verrucous vegetations along the lines of valve closure.
- The mitral and aortic valves are most commonly involved; vegetations are rarely found in the tricuspid or pulmonic valves.
- Histologically, Aschoff's nodules, consisting of foci of fibrinoid necrosis, lymphocytes, macrophages, and occasional plasma cells, may be seen in valve leaflets (or cusps) and within the myocardium of papillary muscles (see Chap. 2).
- The macrophages in Aschoff's nodules consist of Anitschkow's cells (also known as Aschoff's cells, caterpillar cells, and owl eye cells) and multinucleated Anitschkow's cells (Aschoff's giant cells).
- Anitschkow's cells have round to ovoid nuclei, chromatin condensation at the nuclear periphery and in the center, chromatin strands connecting the periphery and center, and clearing elsewhere in the nucleus.

Mitral Annular Calcification

- Mitral annular calcification is a degenerative condition, primarily seen in patients older than 70 years.
- There is a female:male predominance of 4:1.
- Mitral annular calcification occurs at an accelerated rate in patients with MVP.
- There is an increased prevalence of mitral annular calcification in patients with renal failure.
- Mitral annular calcification is often associated with some degree of mitral regurgitation but is rarely severe enough to require surgery.
- Most surgically resected valves with annular calcification have been removed because of MVP or ischemic heart disease.
- Extreme annular calcification may extend into the anterior leaflet and restrict valve opening, resulting in mitral stenosis.
- Pathologically, annular calcification most frequently occurs at the angle between the base of the posterior mitral valve and its attachment to the left ventricular endocardium.
- The dense calcified area may have a central necrotic core that is grossly like putty.
- Histologic examination is not necessary unless endocarditis is suspected.

Rheumatoid Arthritis

- The heart is commonly involved in rheumatoid arthritis, but rarely to the extent so as to produce clinical cardiac dysfunction.
- Cardiac involvement is associated with severe, diffuse joint disease and subcutaneous nodules.
- Rheumatoid involvement of the mitral valve is most common, followed in frequency by involvement of the aortic valve. Tricuspid or pulmonic valve involvement is rare.
- Rheumatoid nodules, most commonly found in the base of the valve leaflet, are usually an incidental finding.
- Valvular regurgitation is produced when large nodules in the leaflets interfere with closure.
- Valvular sclerosis and scarring are present, with focal inflammatory infiltrates containing histiocytes, lymphocytes, plasma cells, and occasional eosinophils.

Systemic Lupus Erythematosus

- Small (3–4 mm) verrucous vegetations (Libman-Sacks vegetations) are found on the atrial and basal ventricular surfaces of the mitral valve extending onto chordae and papillary muscles.
- Libman-Sacks vegetations occur singly or in clusters and are not easily removed from the endocardial surface; they may occasionally result in mitral insufficiency.
- Microscopically, vegetations consist of fibrin, cellular debris, degenerating valve tissue, and inflammatory cells; hematoxylin bodies may be seen.
- Healing lesions result in fibrous thickening of leaflets, and, rarely, mitral stenosis.

Miscellaneous

Case reports document the repair or replacement of mitral valves for the following conditions:

- Amyloidosis
- Whipple's disease
- Postmethysergide therapy
- Mucopolysaccharidosis
- Fabry's disease
- Pseudoxanthoma elasticum
- Congenital mitral stenosis
- Hypertrophic cardiomyopathy
- Hypereosinophilic syndrome
- Trauma
- Postradiation therapy
- Kawasaki disease

References

Dare AJ, Harrity PJ, Tazelaar HD, Edwards WD, Mullany CJ. Evaluation of surgically excised mitral valves: revised recommendations based on changing operative procedures in the 1990s. Hum Pathol 24:1286–1293, 1993.

Hanson TP, Edwards BS, Edwards JE. Pathology of surgically excised mitral valves. One hundred consecutive cases. Arch Pathol Lab Med 109:823–828, 1985.

Olson LJ, Subramanian R, Ackermann DM, Orszulak TA, Edwards WD. Surgical pathology of the mitral valve: a study of 712 cases spanning 21 years. Mayo Clin Proc 62:22–34, 1987.

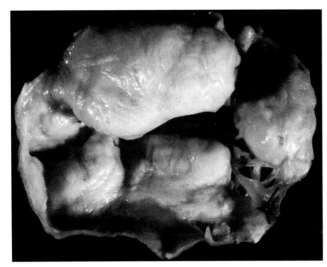

Figure 5–1. Mitral valve prolapse (floppy mitral valve). In this intact surgical specimen, note the billowing and redundancy of all three scallops of the posterior leaflet *(above)* and of the anterior leaflet *(below)*. The commissures are thin and delicate. The trend is to repair rather than replace floppy mitral valves, or to replace the valve and leave the posterior leaflet and its chordal attachments intact.

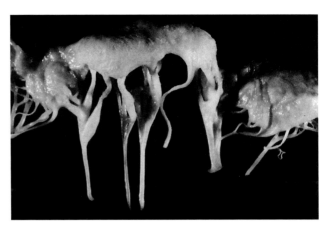

Figure 5–2. Mitral valve prolapse, middle scallop of posterior leaflet and attached chordae. Note the thinning and elongation of the chordae tendineae.

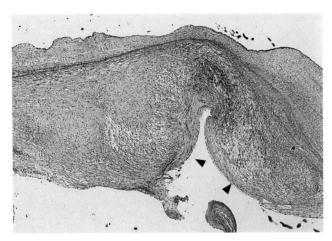

Figure 5–3. Mitral valve prolapse. A histologic section demonstrates expansion of the spongiosa by pools of proteoglycans with disruption of the fibrosa *(arrowheads)*. Microscopic examination generally contributes little to the diagnosis.

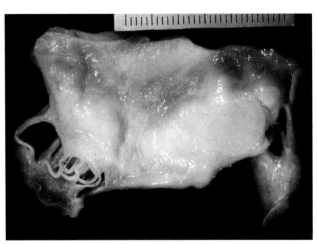

Figure 5–4. Mitral valve prolapse, anterior leaflet. The posterior leaflet of the mitral valve is usually preserved when the valve is replaced. The surgical pathologist receives the anterior leaflet; in this example, portions of the papillary muscle are attached. Note the billowing and redundancy of the valve leaflet. Because changes are usually more pronounced in the posterior leaflet with mitral valve prolapse, the diagnosis of mitral valve prolapse is not always obvious if only the anterior leaflet is excised.

Figure 5–5. Mitral valve prolapse, posterior leaflet. If the valve is *repaired*, the anterior leaflet is left intact, and only a portion of the posterior leaflet is removed. This atrial view demonstrates a thinned, elongated chord and billowing of the leaflet.

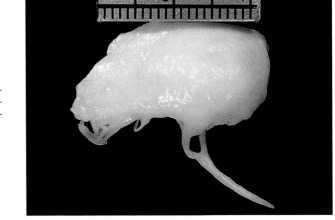

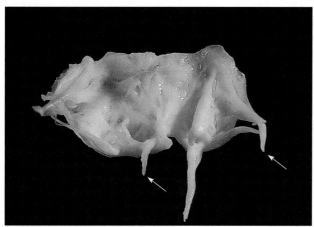

Figure 5–6. Mitral valve prolapse, posterior leaflet. The undersurface, or ventricular surface, of the valve demonstrates irregular chordal insertions and chordal rupture *(arrows)*.

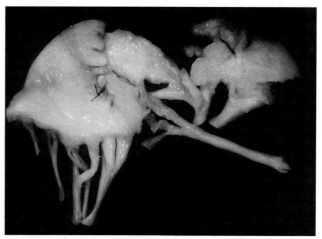

Figure 5–7. Mitral valve prolapse, status after repair. Repair of a mitral valve entails partial removal of the valve (valvuloplasty), suturing of the defect, and placement of an annuloplasty ring (Carpentier ring; see Chap. 9). The patient was a 45-year-old woman with previous annuloplasty and valve repair with recurrent mitral insufficiency.

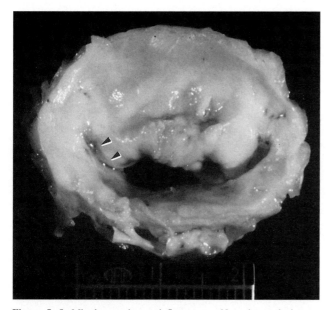

Figure 5–8. Mitral stenosis, postinflammatory. Note the marked commissural fusion *(arrowheads)*. The patient was a 30-year-old woman with a remote history of rheumatic heart disease.

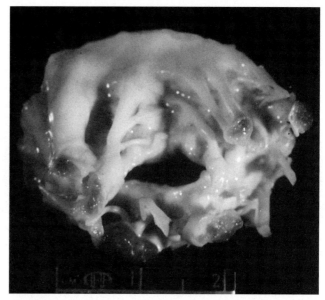

Figure 5–9. Mitral stenosis, postinflammatory. The ventricular view of the valve shown in Figure 5–8 shows thickening of the chordae, with a "sugar coated" appearance. The appearance of a stenotic mitral valve has been linked to that of a fish mouth.

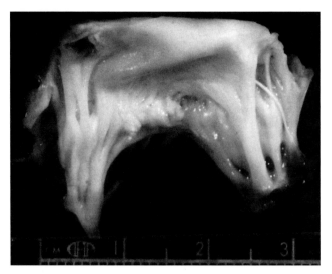

Figure 5–10. Mitral stenosis, postinflammatory. A 72-year-old woman underwent mitral valve replacement for symptomatic mitral stenosis. Note the typical chordal thickening and fusion.

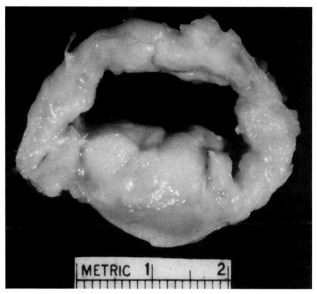

Figure 5–11. Combined mitral stenosis and insufficiency, postinflammatory. The valve leaflet is fibrotic and the valve orifice is relatively large, resulting in lack of closure (incompetence) as well as mild stenosis. Note the marked commissural fusion. The patient was a 43-year-old woman without a history of rheumatic heart disease and with symptomatic mitral insufficiency and stenosis.

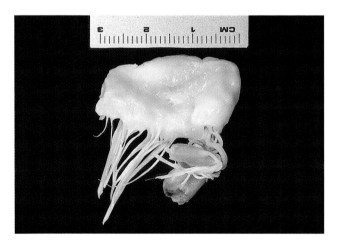

Figure 5–12. Ischemic mitral valve disease. The patient was a 65-year-old man with an acute myocardial infarct and acute mitral regurgitation secondary to the rupture of the posteromedial papillary muscle. The anterior leaflet with ruptured papillary muscle heads was excised.

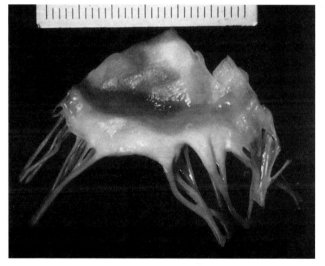

Figure 5–13. Chronic ischemic mitral regurgitation resulting from old papillary muscle infarction and mitral annular dilatation. In most instances, only the anterior leaflet is removed. The valve leaflet appears essentially normal except for age-related mild leaflet fibrosis.

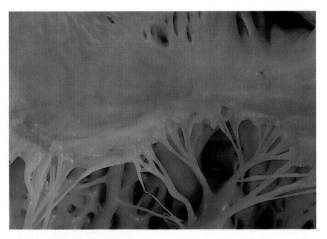

Figure 5–14. Acute rheumatic fever. The mitral and other cardiac valves often show small, firm, multiple vegetations along the lines of closure. The valve is rarely resected during the acute attack. The patient was a 14-year-old boy who died suddenly.

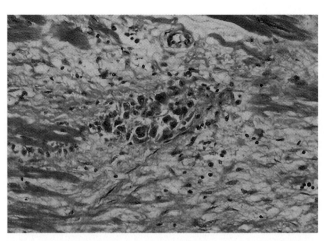

Figure 5–15. Acute rheumatic fever. Aschoff's nodules, interstitial aggregates of Anitschkow's cells with fibrinoid necrosis, are present during the acute attack and may persist for variable periods of time into the chronic phase of disease.

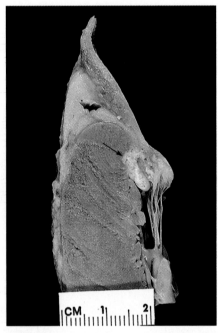

Figure 5–16. Mitral annular calcification. Calcification of the mitral annulus may occur in the elderly, especially in women, and at an accelerated rate on valves that prolapse. The valve is rarely removed for simple annular calcification. This autopsy specimen of the valve annulus demonstrates a mass of pasty calcification just under the valve surface near the valve ring *(arrow)*.

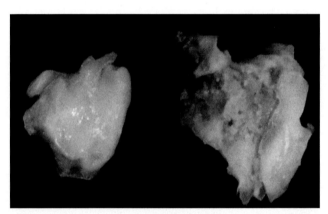

Figure 5–17. Mitral annular calcification. In this valve that was surgically resected for mitral valve prolapse, there were nodules of calcification at the annulus, resulting in a fragmented specimen.

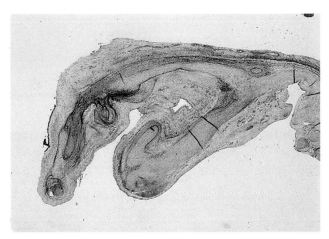

Figure 5–18. Systemic lupus erythematosus, healed Libman-Sacks vegetation. Movat pentachrome stain. Healed vegetations consist of fibrous tissue overlying the valve surface. Note the surface thickening.

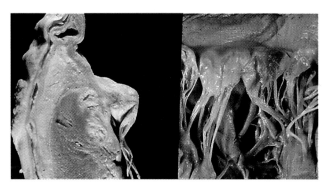

Figure 5–19. Rheumatoid valve disease. Rheumatoid nodules may occur at a site similar to annular calcification. Note the whitish lesions at the base of the leaflet that may lead to valvular incompetence *(left)* and a close-up view of the thickened mitral valve *(right)*.

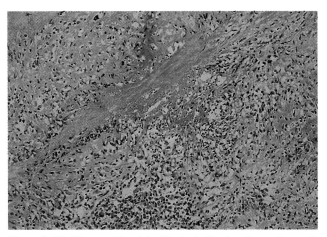

Figure 5–20. Rheumatoid nodule. Histologically, there is zonal necrosis surrounded by palisading histiocytes and chronic inflammatory cells.

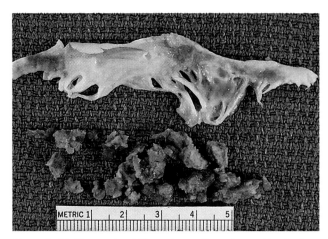

Figure 5–21. Hypereosinophilic syndrome. Generally considered a form of restrictive cardiomyopathy (see Chap. 2), hypereosinophilic syndrome may result in thrombus formation on the ventricular surface, producing adhesion of the mitral valve to the endocardial surface and regurgitation. In this surgically replaced valve, the mitral valve shows areas of attached thrombus. Multiple fragments of endocardial thrombus were removed *(bottom)*.

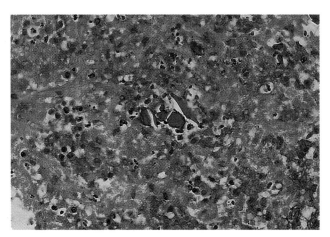

Figure 5–22. Histologic sections of thrombotic material and endocardium demonstrate masses of degranulated eosinophils with crystals composed of eosinophil breakdown products.

CHAPTER 6

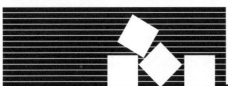

Aortic Valve

APPROACH TO AORTIC VALVE DISEASE

Calcific Valves

- The presence of calcification is indicative of aortic stenosis or combined stenosis and insufficiency. There are three major diagnostic considerations: degenerative disease, congenital bicuspid disease, and postinflammatory (postrheumatic) valve disease.
- Heavily calcified valves may be removed in numerous small pieces; in this case, the diagnosis of fragments of calcified valve cusps, consistent with degenerative aortic stenosis, is made.
- For relatively intact valves with only two cusps present, evidence of a median raphe should be sought in congenitally bicuspid aortic valves. (These patients are generally younger than those with senile calcification.)
- Commissural fusion indicative of postinflammatory aortic stenosis should be sought. In these valves, calcification begins at the commissures and extends onto the cuspal surface. Less often it forms bulky nodules at the base of the cusps as seen in degenerative valve disease. There may be concomitant mitral valve replacement for postrheumatic valve disease.
- Septal myomectomy is performed for hemodynamically significant hypertrophy of the ventricular septum in less than 10% of patients with aortic stenosis and aortic valve replacement. In most cases, the septal hypertrophy is a secondary change. Occasionally, there may be coexistent hypertrophic cardiomyopathy (see Chap. 11).

Noncalcified Valves

- Noncalcified valves are generally insufficient or both stenotic and insufficient.
- Commissural fusion (postinflammatory disease) and median raphe (congenital bicuspid valve) should be sought.
- An increasing number of purely insufficient valves are removed for aortic root disease. In these cases, valves are relatively normal, except there is increased annular circumference (>8 cm) and mild thickening of the leaflet edges (Table 6–1).

- In cases of aortic root dilatation, aortic wall tissue is also often submitted. Histologic evidence of medial degeneration or inflammation should be sought.

AORTIC STENOSIS, CLINICAL FINDINGS

Aortic stenosis is impedance to systolic forward blood flow owing to congenital or acquired lesions of the aortic valve. Normal aortic valve area is greater than 2.0 cm²; mild stenosis, 1.5 to 2.0 cm²; moderate stenosis, 0.8 to 1.5 cm²; severe stenosis, less than 0.8 cm².

General

- Syncope, chest pain (angina), and/or heart failure correlate with severe aortic stenosis, increased mortality, and need for valve replacement.

Congenital Unicuspid and Other Dysplastic Aortic Stenoses

- Congenital unicuspid and other dysplastic aortic stenoses occur in infancy, childhood, or adolescence, and they account for 6% of aortic stenoses in adults.
- Patients are at increased risk for endocarditis.
- Patients with unicommissural valves are at increased risk for aortic dissection.

Congenital Bicuspid Aortic Stenosis

- Congenital bicuspid aortic stenosis occurs in the fifth to seventh decades and is the most frequent cause of aortic stenosis in this age group.
- Congenital bicuspid aortic stenosis accounts for 50% of surgical valve replacements in patients younger than 70 years old.
- Congenital (nondysplastic) bicuspid aortic valves are present in 1% to 2% of the general population.
- The male:female ratio is 1.4 to 4:1.
- Patients are at increased risk for endocarditis and aortic dissection.

Table 6–1
SURGICAL PATHOLOGIC DIAGNOSES,
AORTIC VALVE[1]

Classification	Diagnosis	Total (%)	Mean Age (Years)
Pure aortic stenosis		**66**	**70**
	Degenerative calcification	34[2]	75
	Bicuspid with calcification	23	65
	Postinflammatory disease	6[2]	70
	Miscellaneous	2	
Aortic insufficiency		**24**	**55**
	Aortic root dilatation[3]	12	57
	Postinflammatory disease	3	48
	Bicuspid aortic valve	3	53
	Endocarditis	1	
	Miscellaneous	5	
Aortic stenosis and insufficiency		**10**	**70**
	Degenerative	5[2]	75
	Postinflammatory disease	2[2]	55
	Bicuspid	2	70
	Miscellaneous	1	

[1] Adapted from Dare AJ, Veinot JP, Edwards WD, Tazelaar HD, Schaff HV. New observations on the etiology of aortic valve disease: a surgical pathologic study of 236 cases from 1990. Hum Pathol 24:1330, 1993.

[2] The relative proportion of degenerative aortic valve disease has increased in recent years, and the relative proportion of postinflammatory aortic valve disease has decreased.

[3] Of various causes, including idiopathic (annuloaortic ectasia) and Marfan syndrome (see Chap. 15).

Tricuspid (Acquired) Degenerative Aortic Stenosis

- Occurrence of tricuspid degenerative aortic stenosis in the sixth to eighth decades accounts for more than 50% of surgical valve replacements in patients 70 years old and older.
- Degenerative tricuspid aortic stenosis is more common in men (male:female ratio is 1.6:1).
- Tricuspid degenerative aortic stenosis is the most frequent indication for isolated aortic valve replacement.
- In earlier series, it almost always resulted in aortic stenosis, and only 3% of cases resulted in stenosis and regurgitation; it is now recognized as a relatively common cause of stenosis and regurgitation.

Postinflammatory Aortic Stenosis

- Postinflammatory aortic stenosis is presumed to be postrheumatic, but less than 50% of patients have a history of rheumatic fever.
- It may occur in tricuspid or bicuspid valves.
- It occurs with equal frequency in men and women, although in some series there is a 2:1 male predominance.
- Postinflammatory aortic stenosis accounts for 40% of surgically removed aortic valves in earlier series.
- The proportion of aortic valves removed for postrheumatic disease is declining, because there is a higher rate of operations on elderly patients with degenerative aortic disease and a decrease in the incidence of rheumatic disease.

- Thirty-five percent of valves are purely stenotic; 25% are regurgitant; 40% are stenotic and regurgitant.

Miscellaneous Causes of Aortic Stenosis

- *Ochronosis* is a rare cause of aortic stenosis, resulting in aortic valve replacement (see Chap. 24).
- Other rare causes of aortic stenosis resulting in aortic valve replacement include irradiation, familial hypercholesterolemia, Fabry's disease, and systemic lupus erythematosus.

AORTIC STENOSIS, PATHOLOGIC FINDINGS

Unicuspid and Other Dysplastic Valves

- The most common dysplastic valve is the unicommissural valve with a slit-like opening ("exclamation point") and two aborted commissures.
- The valve leaflet is dysplastic (thickened, myxomatous, fibrotic, with rolled edges).
- Leaflet calcification may or may not be severe. The degree of calcification may increase with previous commissurotomy.
- Histologic evaluation is not necessary unless endocarditis is suspected.
- Less common morphologic conditions of congenital dysplastic aortic stenosis include a dome-shaped valve (acommissural) with three aborted commissures (raphes) or a dysplastic valve with two or three cusps. These patients generally are symptomatic at a young age.

Congenital Bicuspid Aortic Stenosis

Gross Pathologic Findings

- Congenital bicuspid aortic stenosis is characterized by the presence of two separate cusps in intact valve resections.
- A diagnostic feature is the identification of a median raphe (aborted third commissure) in the conjoint cusp, which is present in approximately 60% of cases.
- Most commonly, the two leaflets are of unequal size; in situ, the larger (conjoint) cusp is anterior (64%) and the smaller cusp is posterior. The conjoint cusp is typically less than twice the size of the remaining nonconjoint cusp.
- The two cusps are occasionally of equal size. In these cases, the conjoint cusp cannot be determined and there is no raphe.
- Characteristics of the raphe are as follows:

  - Lack of extension to the free edge of the valve
  - Lack of separation into two cusp margins
  - Relatively straight free edge of the conjoint cusp
  - Frequent dystrophic calcification, beginning in the raphe and extending into the cusp tissue; possible ulceration of the cusp surface by calcific nodules
  - Rarely, raphe consisting of a fibrous strand that extends from the sinus wall to the free cusp edge

Histopathology

- Histologic evaluation is usually not necessary unless endocarditis is suspected.
- The histologic features of the raphe may be helpful in the differential diagnosis with acquired bicuspid valve.

Differential Diagnosis

- Acquired bicuspid valve (postinflammatory commissural fusion) is in the differential diagnosis of congenital bicuspid aortic stenosis. A raphe in a congenitally bicuspid valve is rich in elastic tissue; fused commissures secondary to postinflammatory scarring consist of nonelastic fibrous tissue.
- In valves that are heavily calcified, marked raphal calcification may destroy the elastic tissue, rendering histologic examination useless.
- Occasionally, the raphe in congenitally bicuspid aortic valves may reach the free margin of the cusp or cause partial separation of the raphe into cusp margins; these variants may cause problems in determining whether a congenitally bicuspid valve or an acquired bicuspid valve is present.
- If the valve is fragmented during excision, calcific valves without an identifiable median raphe may be difficult to distinguish from three-leaflet aortic valves.

Postinflammatory (Postrheumatic) Aortic Stenosis

Gross Pathologic Findings

- Commissural fusion is the most important diagnostic feature of postinflammatory aortic stenosis.
- Fusion of two or three commissures may be present; alternatively, there may be fusion of only one of three commissures.
- Commissures may be completely fused from the aortic wall to the free edge, or they may be only partially fused near the aortic wall insertion and remain separate at the free edge.
- The cusps are fibrotically thickened, and variable degrees of cusp calcification may occur, beginning in the fused commissures and extending into the cusp body.

Histopathology

- Histologic examination is rarely necessary or useful in the differential diagnosis, unless it is used to exclude endocarditis.
- The fused commissure consists of fibrous connective tissue with destruction of the underlying valve architecture.
- Cusps are sclerotic and contain foci of calcification, vascularization (small, thick-walled vessels), myxomatous change, and chronic inflammation.

Tricuspid Degenerative Aortic Stenosis

- Heavy calcification may cause fragmentation of the valve during surgical removal.
- Nodular calcification occurs most prominently in the base of the cusps, extending up toward the midportion of the cusp but typically ending proximal to the free edge.
- Commissural fusion is rare.
- Median raphe is absent.
- Histologic examination is not necessary unless endocarditis is suspected.

AORTIC INSUFFICIENCY: CAUSES AND CLINICAL FINDINGS

Aortic insufficiency is the failure of the aortic valve to prevent blood flow from the aorta to the left ventricle during diastole; it may be caused by intrinsic valvular lesions, aortic root disease, or both. Rarely, both valve and aortic root appear normal (see Table 6–1).

Intrinsic Valvular Lesions

- In postrheumatic scarring, a definitive history of rheumatic fever is uncommon (< 10% of cases) and declining in incidence.
- Congenital bicuspid aortic valves account for 7% to 20% of cases of pure aortic insufficiency.
- Congenital unicuspid aortic valve is rare. These valves usually result in stenosis, but may, especially in association with aortic root dilatation, result in pure insufficiency.
- Infectious endocarditis occurs in 10% of cases.
- Decalcification procedures for calcific aortic stenosis may result in aortic insufficiency but are currently only rarely performed.
- Myxomatous aortic valves may be seen in the Marfan syndrome and, rarely, in patients with mitral valve prolapse; histologically, the spongiosa of the valve leaflet is expanded by proteoglycans, resulting in discontinuity of the zona fibrosa.
- Connective tissue diseases are often associated with aortic root disease.
- Prolapse of the right aortic cusp into the left ventricular outflow tract may occur in a membranous ventricular septal defect.
- Rare causes of aortic insufficiency are quadricuspid valves; large, noninfected fenestrations; Fabry's disease; and Hurler's syndrome.

Disease of the Ascending Aorta

- Disease of the ascending aorta is the most common cause of pure aortic insufficiency resulting in valve replacement (see Chap. 15).
- The cause is often not apparent on examination of the valve; histologic examination of the aortic wall may reveal nonspecific medial degenerative changes, evidence of dissection, or aortitis.
- Causes are as follows:

  - Idiopathic dilatation of the aortic root (annuloaortic ectasia): 70% to 90% of cases
  - Marfan syndrome (younger age at presentation compared with annuloaortic ectasia)

- Hypertension
- Aortic dissection
- Traumatic aortic laceration
- Ehlers-Danlos syndrome
- Osteogenesis imperfecta
- Pseudoxanthoma elasticum
- Aortitis (inflammatory and syphilitic)
- Aortic root dilatation in patients with chronic congenital heart disease, especially tetralogy of Fallot

Normal Aortic Valve and Normal Ascending Aorta

- Rarely, idiopathic aortic incompetence occurs in the absence of obvious valvular or aortic disease.
- In patients with membranous or subpulmonic ventricular septal defects, aortic incompetence may lead to surgical resection of the aortic valve.
- In patients with hypertrophic cardiomyopathy and prior myomectomy, aortic insufficiency may result.

Clinical Findings

- Aortic root dilatation and bicuspid valves are more common in men; postinflammatory disease is more common in women.
- In older individuals (60–80 years old), dilatation of the aorta is most often idiopathic (annuloaortic ectasia; see Chap. 15) or related to systemic hypertension.
- In younger persons (20–40 years old), Marfan syndrome and congenital heart disease are most frequent.
- Acute severe regurgitation (most commonly caused by infectious endocarditis, aortic dissection, or trauma) often requires urgent surgery.
- Chronic severe regurgitation may be well tolerated for decades, with surgical intervention indicated for patients with symptoms of heart failure or objective evidence of left ventricular dysfunction.

AORTIC INSUFFICIENCY, PATHOLOGIC FINDINGS

Postinflammatory (Postrheumatic) Scarring

- Diffuse fibrosis of valve cusps results in contracture and shortening with mild commissural fusion.
- Calcification is typically mild or absent.
- If commissural fusion is present, the valve lesion is likely to be mixed stenotic and regurgitant.
- Histologic examination is usually not necessary unless endocarditis is suspected.

Aortic Root Dilatation

- Valve cusps may be thin and stretched or only mildly fibrotic and thickened.
- The cusp free edges may be rolled secondary to chronic severe regurgitation.
- Occasionally, foci of chronic inflammation may be encountered in the valve cusps as part of the accompanying aortitis (e.g., collagen vascular disease).

- In acute aortic insufficiency secondary to aortic dissection, the dissecting hematoma extending to commissural attachments or into the valve cusps results in cuspal malalignment.
- In traumatic laceration of the proximal aorta, there may be avulsion of the commissural attachment to the sinus of Valsalva wall.
- Histologic evaluation of any aortic tissue submitted with the aortic valve should be performed to seek dissection, cystic medial change, and inflammatory lesions.
- Refer to Annuloaortic Ectasia in Chapter 15.

Bicuspid Aortic Valve

- The valve consists of two aortic cusps, unequal in size.
- A median raphe is frequently present in the conjoint (larger) cusp.
- An uncommon variant is a raphal cord that extends from the sinus wall to the free edge that produces cusp retraction.
- The valve cusps show varying degrees of fibrous thickening and rolled edges, and valvular prolapse is common in pure aortic regurgitation secondary to a congenitally bicuspid valve (16%–24% of all cases of aortic incompetence).
- There is an increased incidence of structural abnormalities of the aortic root (cystic medial change), so that valvular regurgitation may be primarily caused by aortic root dilatation rather than lesions in the valve cusps themselves.
- Histologic study is usually not necessary unless endocarditis is suspected.

COMBINED AORTIC STENOSIS AND INSUFFICIENCY

Clinical and Etiologic Considerations

- Combined significant aortic stenosis and aortic regurgitation previously accounted for 25% to 30% of aortic valve surgery cases; with an increase in the incidence of valve replacement for senile degenerative stenosis, this proportion has decreased in the United States.
- The age range at time of surgery is 40 to 80 years, with a male:female ratio of 1.5:1.
- Symptoms and signs are similar to those of aortic stenosis or regurgitation.
- Postinflammatory disease was previously the most common cause (approximately 70% of cases); currently, there has been an increase in degenerative aortic valve disease resulting in combined stenosis and insufficiency.
- Congenitally bicuspid valves account for up to 25% of cases.
- The remaining cases are caused by miscellaneous conditions (congenital unicuspid valve, infectious endocarditis, congenitally abnormal tricuspid aortic valve, quadricuspid aortic valve).
- Prior surgical decalcification of calcified valves and prior mediastinal radiation therapy may result in combined aortic stenosis and insufficiency.

Postinflammatory (Postrheumatic) Combined Aortic Stenosis and Regurgitation

▪ Valvular stenosis is produced by leaflet calcification, fibrosis, and commissural fusion that restrict cusp excursion.

▪ The degree of calcification is generally less extensive than in postinflammatory valve disease that results in pure stenosis.

▪ Regurgitation is produced by leaflet fibrosis and retraction that prevents closing edges from aligning in diastole.

▪ One, two, or all three commissures may be fused.

▪ Histologic examination is not necessary unless endocarditis is suspected.

Congenital Bicuspid Aortic Valve Producing Combined Aortic Stenosis and Regurgitation

▪ A median raphe is present in most cases.

▪ Stenosis and regurgitation are produced by cusp fibrosis and calcification, especially along the raphe.

▪ The degree of calcification is generally more extensive than in postinflammatory valve disease.

▪ Partial commissural fusion may be present.

▪ Histologic examination is not necessary unless endocarditis is suspected.

CONNECTIVE TISSUE AND MISCELLANEOUS DISEASES THAT RARELY REQUIRE SURGICAL TREATMENT

Seronegative Spondyloarthropathies

▪ Seronegative spondyloarthropathies include ankylosing spondylitis, Reiter's syndrome, and psoriatic arthritis.

▪ They are associated with HLA-B27 histocompatibility antigen.

▪ They occasionally involve the aortic root and aortic valve cusps to produce significant aortic regurgitation.

▪ The valve cusps are scarred and fibrotically thickened, particularly in their basal portion, which results in cusp retraction.

▪ Foci of chronic inflammation may be seen in histologic sections.

▪ Refer to Chapter 16.

Systemic Lupus Erythematosus

▪ Functional valve abnormalities are uncommon in systemic lupus erythematosus and consist of mild insufficiency during the acute phase and stenosis from scarring and valve deformity during the chronic phase.

▪ Libman-Sacks vegetations may be found near the commissures of the aortic valve on the ventricular surface, but mitral valve involvement is more common (see Chap. 5).

▪ Microscopically, vegetations consist of fibrin, cellular debris, degenerating valve tissue, and inflammatory cells. Hematoxylin bodies may be seen.

Rheumatoid Arthritis

▪ Aortic regurgitation is rarely produced by rheumatoid nodules.

▪ Rheumatoid nodules, most commonly found in the base of the valve leaflet, are usually an incidental finding.

▪ Valvular regurgitation is produced when large nodules in the leaflets interfere with closure.

▪ Valvular sclerosis and scarring are present with focal inflammatory infiltrates containing histiocytes, lymphocytes, plasma cells, and occasional eosinophils.

Miscellaneous Conditions

▪ Case reports of valve repair or replacements have been published for Behçet's syndrome, hypereosinophilic syndrome, mucopolysaccharidosis (Hunter-Hurler phenotype), amyloidosis, radiation therapy, and postmethysergide therapy.

References

Carlson RG, Mayfield WR, Normann S, Alexander JA. Radiation-associated valvular disease. Chest 99:538–545, 1991.

Dare AJ, Veinot JP, Edwards WD, Tazelaar HD, Schaff HV. New observations on the etiology of aortic valve disease: a surgical pathologic study of 236 cases from 1990. Hum Pathol 24:1330–1338, 1993.

Hanson TP, Edwards BS, Edwards JE. Pathology of surgically excised mitral valves. One hundred consecutive cases. Arch Pathol Lab Med 109:823–828, 1985.

Kim YI, Daenen W. Aortic valve replacement in cardiac ochronosis. Eur J Cardiothorac Surg 6:625–626, 1992.

Olson LJ, Subramanian R, Edwards WD. Surgical pathology of pure aortic insufficiency: a study of 225 cases. Mayo Clin Proc 59:8935–8941, 1984.

Passik CS, Ackermann DM, Pluth JR, Edwards WD. Temporal changes in the causes of aortic stenosis: a surgical pathologic study of 646 cases. Mayo Clin Proc 62:119–123, 1987.

Peterson MD, Roach RM, Edwards JE. Types of aortic stenosis in surgically removed valves. Arch Pathol Lab Med 109:829–832, 1985.

Subramanian R, Olson LJ, Edwards WD. Surgical pathology of combined aortic stenosis and insufficiency: a study of 213 cases. Mayo Clin Proc 60:247–254, 1985.

Subramanian R, Olson LJ, Edwards WD. Surgical pathology of pure aortic stenosis: a study of 374 cases. Mayo Clin Proc 59:683–690, 1984.

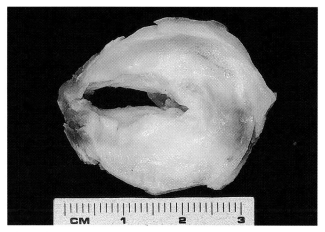

Figure 6–1. Aortic stenosis, unicuspid aortic valve. These patients are generally the youngest to undergo valve replacement for aortic stenosis. Note the eccentric valve orifice that has been described as an exclamation point or teardrop; there is a single commissure at the left of the photograph.

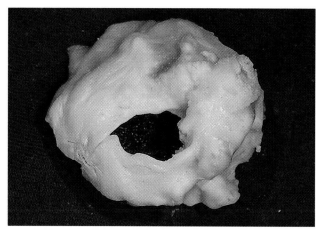

Figure 6–2. Aortic stenosis, unicuspid aortic valve. The patient was a 20-year-old man with critical aortic stenosis. In this example, there is no well-formed commissure. The differential diagnosis includes congenital bicuspid aortic valve with extensive commissural fusion (superimposed postinflammatory changes). Because of the patient's young age, the diagnosis of acommissural unicuspid aortic valve is most likely in this case. Note the nodular calcification.

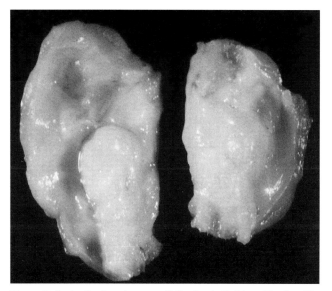

Figure 6–3. Aortic stenosis, congenitally dysplastic bicuspid valve. The patient was a 5-year-old boy with previous commissurotomy. There are two valve leaflets that are obviously dysplastic and malformed; note the irregular, thickened cusps.

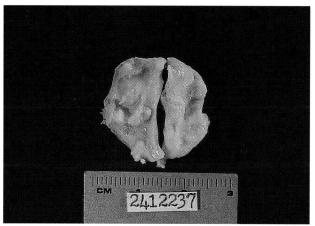

Figure 6–4. Aortic stenosis, congenital bicuspid valve. Most bicuspid valves are not dysplastic and become stenotic only in adulthood when secondary calcification occurs. The patient was a 70-year-old woman. Despite the absence of an obvious median raphe, the diagnosis of congenital bicuspid valve may be made if the specimen is intact and two valve leaflets are identified.

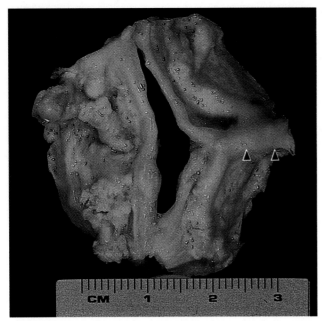

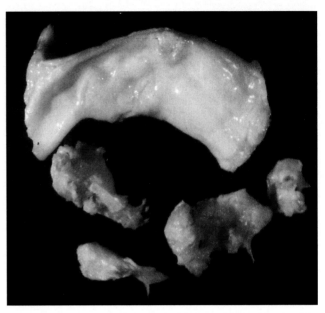

Figure 6–5. Aortic stenosis, congenital bicuspid valve, aortic view. Note the median raphe *(arrowheads)*. Although the distinction between raphe and fused commissure may be difficult, especially in surgically resected valves, the size of the conjoint cusp is less than twice the size of the nonconjoint cusp, and the free edge of the conjoint cusp is relatively straight.

Figure 6–6. Aortic stenosis, presumed congenital bicuspid valve. The patient was a 54-year-old man. If the valve is removed in pieces, only a nonspecific diagnosis of calcific aortic stenosis can be rendered. Because of the patient's age and the suggestion of two leaflets, one conjoint and the other fragmented, the likely diagnosis is congenital bicuspid valve.

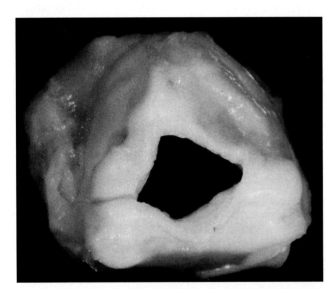

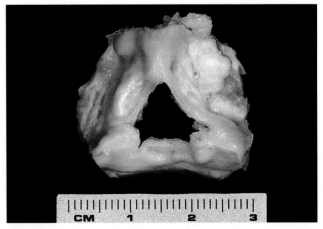

Figure 6–7. Aortic stenosis, postinflammatory (postrheumatic), aortic view. The patient was a 29-year-old woman with critical aortic stenosis. Note the extensive fusion of all commissures, and the fibrosis. Calcification is variable in postinflammatory valves; in this case, it is not grossly evident.

Figure 6–8. Aortic stenosis, postinflammatory (postrheumatic), aortic view. Note the marked commissural fusion and nodular calcification. The patient also underwent mitral valve resection (not shown).

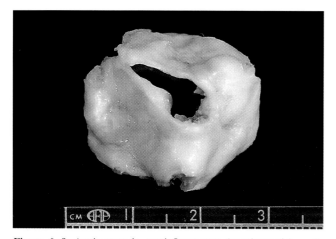

Figure 6–9. Aortic stenosis, postinflammatory (postrheumatic), aortic view. In some cases, there is unequal involvement of commissures; in this example, two commissures show marked fusion, and one is relatively spared. The patient was a 60-year-old woman with mitral and aortic stenosis.

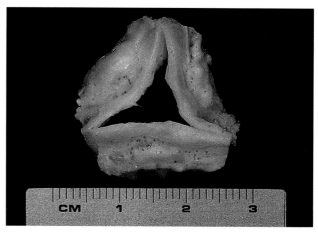

Figure 6–10. Degenerative aortic stenosis, aortic view. Note the nodular calcification at the base of the cusps.

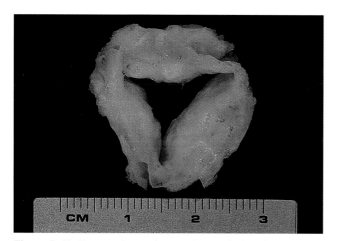

Figure 6–11. Degenerative aortic stenosis, ventricular view. Note the leaflet thickening, which may result in a lack of valve closure; occasionally, there is a degree of incompetence in addition to aortic stenosis in calcified degenerative aortic valves.

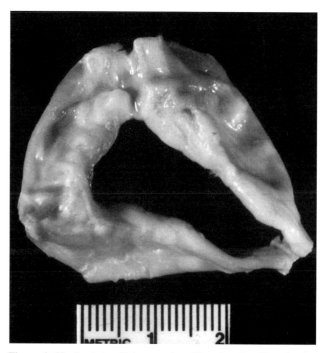

Figure 6–12. Aortic insufficiency, unicuspid aortic valve. Note the single commissure and two aborted commissures and the typical teardrop-shaped orifice. In rare cases, insufficiency develops instead of the typical stenosis of the unicuspid aortic valve. In this 48-year-old man, there was concomitant aortic root dilatation secondary to cystic medial degeneration (not shown) contributing to aortic insufficiency. Weakening of the aortic wall is associated with congenital bicuspid and unicuspid valves.

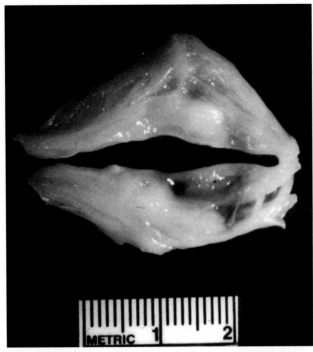

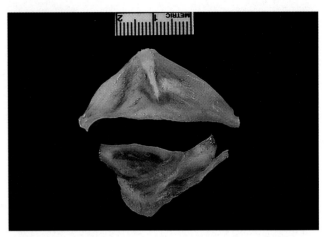

Figure 6–13. Aortic insufficiency, bicuspid aortic valve. Approximately 20% of bicuspid aortic valves are removed because of regurgitation. In this regurgitant valve removed from a 20-year-old man, there is increased annular circumference and nonspecific fibrosis and myxomatous valvular degeneration. The mechanism of aortic regurgitation is often a result of aortic root dilatation secondary to structural weakness of the aortic wall.

Figure 6–14. Aortic insufficiency, bicuspid aortic valve. Note the increased annular circumference, median raphe, and lack of extensive calcification or fibrosis. The patient was a 39-year-old man with aortic insufficiency and aortic root dilatation. The median raphe is broadest near the annulus and is calcified (lower leaflet). It does not extend to the free margin of the conjoint cusp, which is relatively straight.

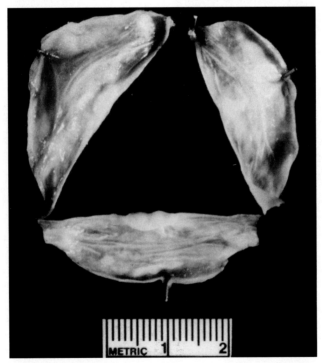

Figure 6–15. Aortic insufficiency secondary to aortic root dilatation. Note the three valve cusps that are relatively normal, except for their increased annular circumference. The patient was a 51-year-old man with idiopathic aortic root dilatation.

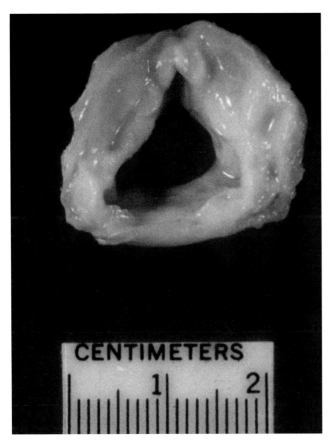

Figure 6–16. Combined aortic insufficiency and stenosis, postinflammatory. It may be difficult to distinguish purely stenotic valves from those that are both stenotic and insufficient, on the basis of gross examination. In this aortic valve that was removed for combined stenosis and incompetence, the leaflets are fibrotic and relatively immobile, resulting in lack of valve closure (incompetence) as well as a decreased valve orifice area (stenosis). Note the commissural fusion that is typical of postinflammatory (postrheumatic) aortic valve disease.

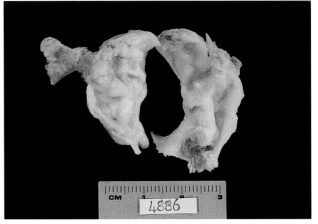

Figure 6–17. Congenital bicuspid aortic valve, combined stenosis and insufficiency. Note the heavy calcification of two distinct leaflets. An obvious median raphe was not identified in this case.

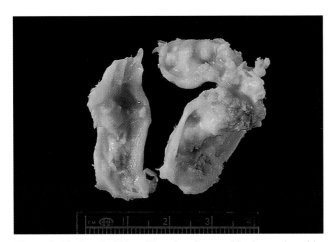

Figure 6–18. Acquired bicuspid aortic valve, combined stenosis and insufficiency, aortic view. Note the heavy calcification and fusion of one commissure. In contrast to a raphe, the free margin at the site of the fused margin is indented, not straight, suggesting previous separation into two valve cusps (see Fig. 6–5 for comparison). The cause of single commissural fusion is presumably postinflammatory.

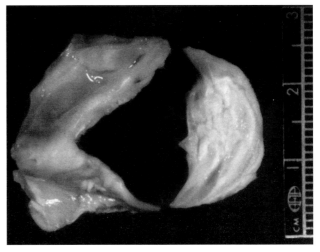

Figure 6–19. Acquired bicuspid aortic valve, combined stenosis and insufficiency. Because of the indentation of the leaflet margin at the site of cuspal fusion, the cause is likely postinflammatory, not congenital (raphe). The mitral valve removed at the same time demonstrated typical postinflammatory changes (not shown), supporting the diagnosis of an acquired (postrheumatic) lesion for the aortic valve.

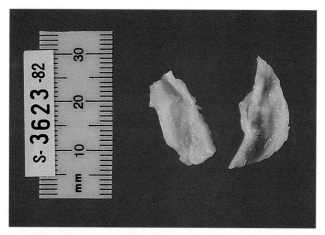

Figure 6–20. Aortic insufficiency, Reiter's syndrome. The gross features are nonspecific and consist of mild fibrosis. Only two leaflets were submitted for pathologic evaluation.

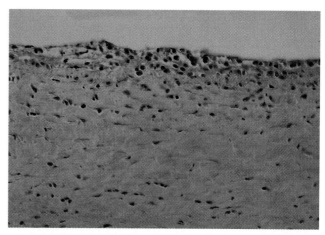

Figure 6–21. Aortic insufficiency, Reiter's syndrome. Because of a history of Reiter's syndrome, histologic examination was performed. There is a mononuclear inflammatory infiltrate on the valve surface, and acute and chronic inflammation extended into the valve.

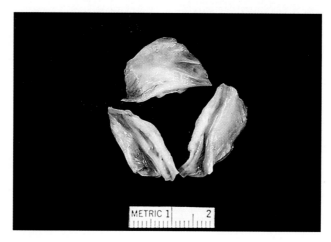

Figure 6–22. Aortic insufficiency, syphilis. The three complications of syphilitic aortitis are aneurysm, coronary ostial stenosis, and aortic insufficiency. The valve demonstrates fibrosis and rolled free margins secondary to aortic regurgitation. These changes are nonspecific; the diagnosis of syphilis depends on clinical data.

CHAPTER 7

Tricuspid Valve, Pulmonary Valve, and Miscellaneous Native Valves

TRICUSPID VALVE

Approach to Tricuspid Valve Resection

Anatomically Normal Valves

- The underlying condition necessitating tricuspid valve resection in anatomically normal valves is pulmonary hypertension.
- Pulmonary hypertension results in right-sided heart failure and tricuspid regurgitation.
- The annular circumference is usually increased (>12 cm).

Anatomically Abnormal Valves

- Tricuspid insufficiency is more common than stenosis (Table 7–1).
- Conditions include rheumatic (postinflammatory) disease, congenitally floppy (myxomatous) valves, and Ebstein's anomaly.
- Commissural fusion and normal or smaller annular circumference are features of rheumatic disease.
- Increased annular circumference (>12 cm) is associated with Ebstein's anomaly and tricuspid valve prolapse.
- Resected myxomatous tricuspid valves are often accompanied by resected myxomatous mitral valves.

Postinflammatory (Postrheumatic) Tricuspid Valve Disease

Clinical Findings

- Clinically significant postrheumatic scarring of the tricuspid valve is rare; however, postrheumatic disease is the most common indication for surgical removal of the tricuspid valve.

- Postrheumatic disease results in tricuspid regurgitation (56%), combined stenosis and tricuspid regurgitation (41%), and, rarely, isolated tricuspid stenosis (3%).
- Postrheumatic scarring of the tricuspid valve never occurs as an isolated valve lesion, and tricuspid involvement occurs much less frequently than mitral or aortic disease.
- Symptomatic patients have right-sided heart failure (ascites, hepatomegaly, anasarca, fatigue).
- Significant tricuspid stenosis is more common in women.
- Surgical treatment (valvotomy or valve replacement for stenosis, annuloplasty for regurgitation) is performed at the time of mitral valve replacement.

Pathologic Findings

- Valvular stenosis is caused by commissural fusion, which is most often seen in the anteroseptal commissure.
- Valve leaflet fibrosis is almost always diffuse in stenotic valves, but may be limited to lines of valve closure in incompetent valves.
- Chordal changes consisting of fusion, thickening, and shortening are not typically severe, and leaflet calcification is rare.
- Histologic evaluation is not necessary unless endocarditis is suspected.

Ebstein's Anomaly

Ebstein's anomaly is a congenital cardiac lesion in which the tricuspid valve is displaced downward, resulting in atrialization of the inflow portion of the right ventricle.

Table 7–1
SURGICAL PATHOLOGIC DIAGNOSES,
TRICUSPID VALVE*

Classification	Diagnosis	Total (%)
Tricuspid insufficiency		**74**
	Postinflammatory disease	30
	Pulmonary hypertension	15
	Congenital (non-Ebstein's) anomaly	12**
	Ebstein's anomaly	10
	Endocarditis	3
	Tricuspid valve prolapse	2
	Carcinoid syndrome	<1
Tricuspid stenosis and insufficiency		**23**
	Postinflammatory disease	22
	Congenital disease	<1
	Carcinoid syndrome	<1
Tricuspid stenosis		**2**
	Postinflammatory disease	2
	Congenital disease	<1
	Carcinoid syndrome	<1

*Adapted from Hauck AJ, Freeman DP, Ackermann DM, Danielson GK, Edwards WD. Surgical pathology of the tricuspid valve: a study of 363 cases spanning 25 years. Mayo Clin Proc 63:851–863, 1988.
**This value is higher than that from other series, likely due to referral patterns at the Mayo Clinic.

Pathologic Findings

■ There is downward displacement of the septal and posterior leaflets.
■ The broad and sail-like anterior leaflet produces tricuspid regurgitation or stenosis and, occasionally, pulmonary outflow tract obstruction.
■ Most surgically resected cases are secondary to pure tricuspid incompetence.
■ The broad anterior tricuspid leaflet contains abnormal fibrous strands and may be focally muscularized and fenestrated.

Miscellaneous Congenital Tricuspid Valve Disease

Types and Incidence

■ Myxomatous degeneration (floppy tricuspid valve) accounts for 2% to 5% of cases of tricuspid insufficiency that result in valve replacement.
■ Floppy tricuspid valve is often accompanied by mitral valve prolapse (see Chap. 5); isolated tricuspid valve prolapse is rare.
■ A number of other congenital heart diseases unrelated to Ebstein's anomaly may result in tricuspid incompetence and valve replacement.
■ Underlying diseases include complete transposition of the great arteries, tetralogy of Fallot, pulmonary stenosis and atresia, dysplastic tricuspid valve, and other congenital heart diseases.

Pathologic Findings

■ There is a wide variety of pathologic changes reflecting the spectrum of congenital heart disease that occurs as underlying conditions.
■ In most instances, the valves are regurgitant.
■ The myxomatous tricuspid valve is similar in appearance to the more common mitral valve prolapse syndrome (see Chap. 5); there is dilatation of the valve annulus and increase in leaflet area.
■ Annular dilatation with minimal valvular changes is common in many of the complex congenital heart disease syndromes.
■ Hypoplasia and dysplasia of tricuspid valves may occur in many different types of complex congenital heart disease.

Pulmonary Venous Hypertension Resulting in Tricuspid Insufficiency

Clinical Findings

■ Pulmonary venous hypertension commonly results in tricuspid incompetence; however, surgical replacement is rarely required.
■ In most patients, the pulmonary hypertension is secondary to mitral valve disease.
■ Types of mitral valve disease include stenosis, regurgitation, and combined stenosis and regurgitation.

Pathologic Findings

■ The tricuspid regurgitation is generally a result of annular dilatation.
■ There are minimal gross changes in the valve, consisting primarily of focal leaflet thickening.

Carcinoid Tricuspid Valve Disease

Clinical Findings

■ Carcinoid heart disease occurs in 20% to 50% of patients with carcinoid syndrome, secondary to a metastatic carcinoid tumor.
■ Carcinoid heart disease is an important cause of morbidity and mortality in these patients, and valve replacement is occasionally necessary.
■ Significant accumulation of carcinoid plaques deposited on the valve surface results in tricuspid regurgitation with or without stenosis and rarely in pure stenosis.
■ Tricuspid valve plaques occur with the same frequency as pulmonary valve plaques; rarely, the mitral valve is involved as well.

Pathologic Findings

■ The pathogenesis of carcinoid plaques is unknown but may be related to endothelial injury from vasoactive agents produced by the carcinoid tumor.
■ White carcinoid plaques first accumulate on the ventricular endocardial surface.
■ In severe cases, the atrial and ventricular surfaces of the tricuspid valve are involved, resulting in leaflet and chordal thickening.

- Histologically, carcinoid plaques consist of smooth muscle cells within a proteoglycan matrix; these are deposited on the underlying normal valve tissue.

PULMONARY VALVE

Congenital Pulmonary Stenosis

Table 7–2 shows the most frequent indications for surgical resection of pulmonary valves.

Clinical Findings

- Congenital pulmonary stenosis accounts for more than 90% of excised pulmonary valves.
- Isolated pulmonary stenosis accounts for approximately 10% of congenital heart disease; survival into adulthood is common.
- Congenital pulmonary stenosis may occur as an isolated valve lesion or as part of other forms of complex congenital heart disease.
- Percutaneous balloon valvuloplasty has been used to successfully treat pulmonary stenosis, especially the isolated form, obviating the need for valve repair or replacement.
- Most resected pulmonary valves arise in hearts with other anomalies, particularly tetralogy of Fallot.
- Less common types of congenital heart disease associated with surgically resected stenotic pulmonary valves include double outlet right ventricle, tricuspid atresia, atrioventricular canal, double inlet left ventricle, pulmonary atresia, and transposition of the great arteries.

Pathologic Findings

- The pulmonary valve may be tricuspid, bicuspid, unicuspid, or acommissural.
- A bicuspid or tricuspid valve is usually present in tetralogy of Fallot.
- A dome-shaped valve with fused commissures is most often found in isolated pulmonary stenosis; it frequently has a keyhole shape and a unicommissural valve and is often dysplastic; this morphologic condition is amenable to balloon dilatation and therefore rarely requires replacement.
- Dysplastic leaflets and annular hypoplasia are common features.
- Valvular calcification is often seen in older individuals.

Miscellaneous Conditions

- Carcinoid heart disease may result in pulmonary stenosis or in combined pulmonary stenosis and insufficiency. The clinical and pathologic findings of carcinoid pulmonary disease are similar to those of tricuspid valve disease, with carcinoid lesions seen on the arterial surface.
- Rheumatic heart disease rarely affects the pulmonary valve and is a rare cause of pulmonary valve resection.

TRUNCAL AND COMMON ATRIOVENTRICULAR VALVES

Truncal Valve

The truncal valve is a semilunar valve that connects the heart with the truncus arteriosus (single great artery supplying the coronary arteries, aorta, and pulmonary arteries).

Clinical Findings and Incidence

- Truncus arteriosus is a rare form of congenital heart disease, accounting for 1% to 4% of cardiac deformities in congenital heart disease.
- Valve replacement may be performed in cases of severe incompetence of the truncal valve.
- Most patients are between 5 and 21 years of age at the time of operation.

Pathologic Findings, Surgically Excised Valves

- The truncal valve is most often tricuspid but may be bicuspid, quadricuspid, or unicommissural.
- A raphe is often present.
- Cuspal thickening, mild calcification, and mild commissural fusion may be seen.
- Cuspal perforations indicative of previous endocarditis are rare.
- Histologically, there may be expansion of the spongiosa, with nodular thickening and disruption of the fibrosa, resulting in a dysplastic valve.

Common Atrioventricular Valve

The common atrioventricular valve connects both atria or a single atrium to both ventricles; it is present in complete atrioventricular canal defect.

Clinical Findings

- In most cases of atrioventricular canal defect, the valve may be repaired at surgery with little resultant regurgitation.

Table 7–2
SURGICAL PATHOLOGIC DIAGNOSES, PULMONARY VALVE*

Classification	Diagnosis	Total (%)
Pulmonary stenosis		**91**
	Tetralogy of Fallot	52
	Other congenital diseases	20
	Isolated pulmonary stenosis	16
	Carcinoid disease	3
Pulmonary insufficiency		**4**
	Tetralogy of Fallot	3
	Endocarditis	<1
Pulmonary stenosis and insufficiency		**3**
	Congenital heart disease	1
	Carcinoid disease	2

*Adapted from Altrichter PM, Olson LJ, Edwards WD, Danielson GK. Surgical pathology of the pulmonary valve: a study of 116 cases spanning 15 years. Mayo Clin Proc 64:1352–1360, 1989.

- In selected patients, especially those with double orifice mitral component, replacement of the entire valve may be necessary.
- Most patients are younger than 25 years old at the time of surgery (mean age 8 years); occasionally, valve replacement is performed in infants.
- Valves are purely regurgitant preoperatively.

Pathologic Findings

- The number of leaflets in excised specimens ranges from 5 to 8.
- Mild commissural fusion, thickening, and hooding deformities may be present.
- Calcification and destructive lesions are rare.
- Histologically, there may be thickening of the spongiosa and focal fibrosis.

References

Alrichter PM, Olson LJ, Edwards WD, Puga FJ, Danielson GK. Surgical pathology of the pulmonary valve: a study of 116 cases spanning 15 years. Mayo Clin Proc 64:1352–1360, 1989.

Fuglestad SJ, Danielson GK, Puga FJ, Edwards WD. Surgical pathology of the common atrioventricular valve: a study of 11 cases. Am J Cardiovasc Pathol 2:49–55, 1988.

Fuglestad SJ, Puga FJ, Danielson GK, Edwards WD. Surgical pathology of the truncal valve: a study of 12 cases. Am J Cardiovasc Pathol 2:39–47, 1988.

Hauck AJ, Freeman DP, Ackermann DM, Danielson GK, Edwards WD. Surgical pathology of the tricuspid valve: a study of 363 cases spanning 25 years. Mayo Clin Proc 63:851–863, 1988.

Kriwisky M, Froom P, Ribak J, Cyjon A, Lewis B, Gross M. Isolated tricuspid valve prolapse. Cardiology 75:145–148, 1988.

Waller BF. Etiology of pure tricuspid regurgitation. Cardiovasc Clin 17:53–95, 1987.

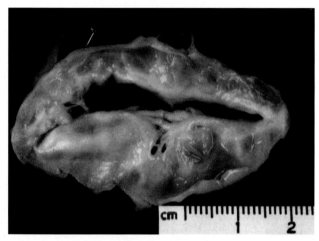

Figure 7–1. Tricuspid stenosis, postinflammatory. There is commissural fusion with leaflet fibrosis. The patient, a 45-year-old woman, had concurrent tricuspid insufficiency and mitral stenosis.

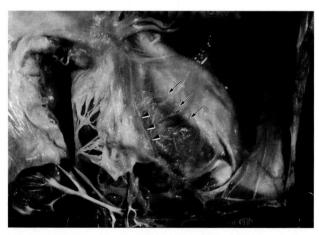

Figure 7–2. Congenital tricuspid valve, Ebstein's anomaly. This autopsy specimen demonstrates downward displacement of the septal tricuspid valve leaflets *(arrowheads)* and paper-thin change of the ventricle (so-called atrialization) between the true tricuspid annulus *(arrows)* and the effective tricuspid annulus. Surgical repair includes plication of the atrialized ventricle, valve repair, or valve replacement. The gross and histologic changes of excised valves are nonspecific, and diagnosis depends on clinical information.

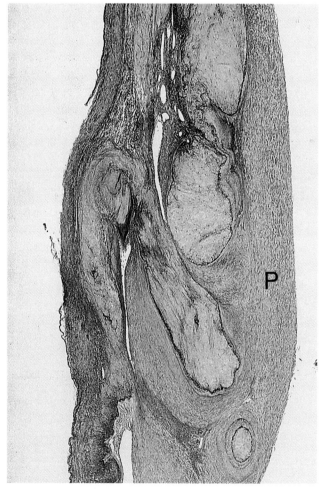

Figure 7–3. Tricuspid valve, carcinoid syndrome. Note the carcinoid plaque (P), consisting of a diffuse proliferation of smooth muscle cells in a proteoglycan matrix, overlying the normal valve surfaces and encircling the chordae tendineae.

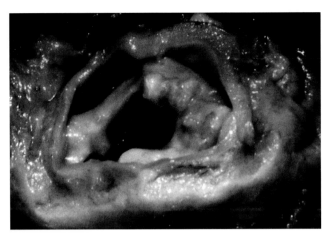

Figure 7–4. Pulmonary stenosis, status after commissurotomy. Most types of isolated pulmonary stenosis are acommissural dome-shaped valves that are not replaced but are treated with balloon dilatation (previously, with open commissurotomy). The patient was a 58-year-old man who died from traumatic consequences of an accident; commissurotomy for isolated pulmonary stenosis had been performed decades previously.

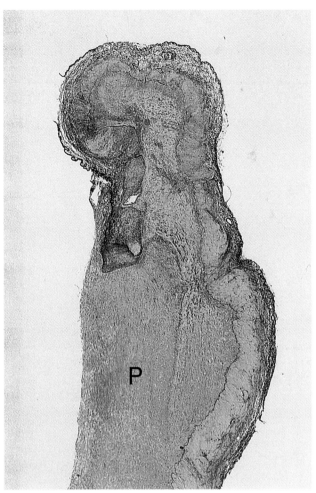

Figure 7–6. Carcinoid heart disease, pulmonary valve. The valve was removed at the same time as the tricuspid valve illustrated in Figure 7–3. Note the similar features of carcinoid plaque (P): smooth muscle cells in a proteoglycan matrix deposited on the arterial surface of the valve, resulting in functional stenosis.

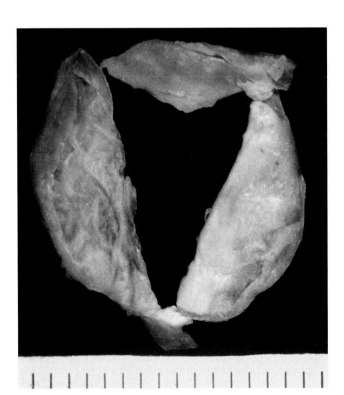

Figure 7–5. Most pulmonary valve resections are performed for patients with congenital heart disease, especially tetralogy of Fallot. The valves are rarely dome shaped, but are bileaflet or trileaflet valves. This valve was removed from a 46-year-old woman with tetralogy of Fallot; ventricular septal defect repair had been accomplished years previously. Note the normal appearance of the trileaflet valve with a small annular circumference.

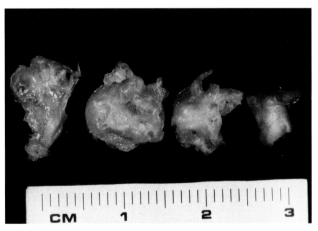

Figure 7–7. Common atrioventricular valve. The patient was a 5-month-old infant with common atrioventricular valve and valvular regurgitation. The tricuspid valve was reconstructed and the mitral valve replaced. In some cases of complete atrioventricular canal, repair of both valves is not possible. Note the redundant, dysplastic valve leaflets.

CHAPTER 8

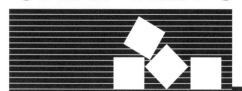

Endocarditis/Valvular Vegetations

INFECTIOUS ENDOCARDITIS

Table 8–1 shows the various anatomic substrates that underlie valvular endocarditis in children and adults.

Clinical Findings

- Most cases of adult infectious endocarditis occur in the setting of an anatomically abnormal valve as follows:

  - 29% mitral valve prolapse
  - 21% degenerative lesions (i.e., calcification)
  - 13% bicuspid aortic valve and other rare congenital conditions
  - 6% postrheumatic valves (earlier series much higher)

- The remaining 31% of infectious endocarditis cases occur on normal valves; many of these cases arise in patients with predisposing noncardiac conditions.
- Predisposing noncardiac conditions include drug abuse (especially intravenous), alcoholism, cirrhosis, immunosuppression, and colon cancer.
- Cardiac signs and symptoms include new valvular regurgitation murmurs, congestive heart failure secondary to severe regurgitation, infectious pericarditis, and heart block. Valvular stenosis secondary to a bulky vegetation is rare.
- Noncardiac signs and symptoms include fever, anemia, musculoskeletal pain, glomerulonephritis, emboli (e.g., myocardial infarction, stroke, renal infarction, limb artery occlusion), and septic shock.
- Indications for valve surgery include significant heart failure, valve annular abscess, heart block, major organ embolization, and persistent bacteremia.

Pathogenesis and Sites of Involvement

- Certain microorganisms are associated with specific clinical settings, such as the following:

  - *Staphylococcus aureus:* drug abuse, and now becoming more prevalent in other settings as well
  - *Streptococcus viridans:* subacute cases and rheumatic valves

- Enterococci: highly virulent, occur on normal valves
- *Streptococcus bovis:* colon carcinoma
- *Streptococcus pneumoniae:* alcoholism and pneumococcal sepsis
- Gram-negative organisms: drug abuse and diabetes mellitus
- Fungi: immunocompromised patients and drug abuse

- The pathogenesis of infectious endocarditis may initially involve formation of a sterile thrombus on an abnormal valve endocardial surface, followed by colonization, reproduction of microorganisms, and invasion of valve tissue.
- The mitral and aortic valves are most often involved.
- Valves with an underlying defect that predisposes the patient to endocarditis are more likely regurgitant than stenotic, probably secondary to increased bidirectional flow, precipitating endocardial damage.
- The tricuspid valve is involved in up to 50% of cases of endocarditis in intravenous drug abusers; tricuspid endocarditis in other patients is rare.

Gross Pathologic Findings

- Friable vegetations usually start at the line of closure and are most often found on the atrial surface of the atrioventricular valves and on the ventricular surface of the semilunar valves.
- Vegetations may be associated with valve leaflet ulceration or perforation or rupture of chordae tendineae or papillary muscles.
- Spread of infection from the closing edge of one valve leaflet to its apposing side results in "kissing lesions."
- Weakening of the leaflet by infection can result in leaflet aneurysm formation, which bulges toward the left atrium (with mitral valve endocarditis) or left ventricle (with aortic endocarditis). Regurgitation may acutely worsen when there is perforation of the aneurysm.
- Appearance of active vegetations varies from soft gray-pink to firm yellow-brown. In "healed" lesions, there may be focal leaflet fibrotic thickening, calcification, and/or perforation.

Table 8-1

INCIDENCE OF PREDISPOSING VALVULAR LESIONS AND MICROBIAL ISOLATES IN PATIENTS WITH ENDOCARDITIS ON NATIVE VALVES*

	Children (%)	Adults < 60 yrs (%)	Adults > 65 yrs (%)	Pregnant Women (%)	IV Drug Addicts (%)
Predisposing Lesion					
Postrheumatic	1.5-10	25-30	8	74**	
Congenital	75-100	10-20	2	74**	10
Mitral valve prolapse		20-50	10		
Degenerative			30		
IV drug abuse				8	100
Other		10-15	10		10
None		25-50	40	18	
Organisms					
Streptococci	40-50	50-70	30	60	6-12
Enterococci	4	10	15	6	8
Staphylococcus aureus	25	20	30	16	60
Staphylococcus epidermidis	5	5	15	2	1
Gram-negative bacilli	5	<1	5		10
Fungi	1	<1			5
Diphtheroids		<1			2
Polymicrobials				4	5
Other		<1		6	
Culture-negative organisms	0-15	5-10	5	4	4-10

*Adapted from Korzeniowski OM, Kaye D. Infective endocarditis. In Braunwald E (ed). *Heart Disease*, 4th ed. Philadelphia. WB Saunders, 1992, p 1079.

**74% includes both postrheumatic and congenital heart disease.

■ A portion of excised vegetation should be sent to the laboratory for organism identification and antibiotic sensitivity testing.

Histologic Findings

■ Brown and Hopps and Gomori's methenamine silver (or periodic acid–Schiff) staining of histologic sections should be performed to identify microorganisms.
■ Brown and Brenn stain may be superior for gram-positive organisms, which, upon death, may stain reddish with the Brown and Hopps stain.
■ Acute vegetations consist of platelets, fibrin, neutrophils, and microorganisms.
■ Organizing vegetations contain chronic inflammatory cells (lymphocytes, macrophages, giant cells) and fewer neutrophils.
■ Healed vegetations consist of focal valve fibrosis, smooth-edged perforations, and/or aneurysms.

NONINFECTIOUS ENDOCARDITIS (MARANTIC ENDOCARDITIS, NONBACTERIAL THROMBOTIC ENDOCARDITIS)

Clinical Findings

■ Noninfectious endocarditis most often occurs in the setting of an underlying malignancy, chronic inflammatory disease, or coagulopathy.

■ Tricuspid or pulmonic vegetations may occur secondary to central venous catheter–induced trauma.
■ The cause of noninfectious endocarditis is unknown but may involve platelet and fibrin deposition on valves that have endothelial injury in the setting of a hypercoagulable state (e.g., lupus anticoagulant, antiphospholipid antibodies, underlying adenocarcinoma, disseminated intravascular coagulation).
■ Embolization is not uncommon and is the usual indication for surgery.

Pathologic Findings

■ The aortic and mitral valves are the most common valves affected.
■ Vegetations may be large or small and are gray-pink, friable, soft or firm masses along the valvular line of closure, without associated valvular ulceration or perforation.
■ Vegetations consist predominantly of fibrin and platelets, with a few trapped erythrocytes and rare acute and chronic inflammatory cells.
■ The underlying valve is usually normal.

VEGETATIONS OF COLLAGEN VASCULAR DISEASE

Systemic Lupus Erythematosus

■ Libman-Sacks vegetations may occur on the mitral, tricuspid, and, less commonly, aortic valves.

■ These are rarely present in excised valve specimens (see Chap. 5).

Acute Rheumatic Fever

■ During the acute illness, small, uniform, firm vegetations occur on cardiac valves.
■ The vegetations occur on the lines of closure of the valve leaflet and may occur on any valve, although the mitral and aortic are most often involved.
■ These valves are rarely excised surgically (see Chap. 5).

PAPILLARY FIBROELASTOMA

Clinical Findings

■ Incidental nodules on valve surfaces are found at echocardiography or at autopsy (see Chap. 11).
■ Left-sided tumors may cause embolic symptoms (stroke, cardiac ischemia).

Pathologic Findings

■ The mitral valve is most commonly involved, although any valve or area of the endocardium may be affected.
■ The papillary nature of the excrescence may not be readily appreciated grossly unless the valve is submerged in water.
■ Histologically, the papillae are avascular (unlike myxoma excrescences); relatively acellular, containing occasional fibroblasts and smooth muscle cells; and lined by endothelial cells.
■ Most tumors show proteoglycan deposition and elastic fibers, although the latter feature may be variable.

Differential Diagnosis

■ Marantic vegetations—the gross appearance may mimic nonbacterial endocarditis, especially if there is superimposed fibrin platelet thrombus; for this reason, an elastic stain may be helpful in ascertaining papillary fibroelastoma as the cause of a vegetation.
■ Myxoma—these tumors rarely arise on the valve surface; they contain capillaries and myxoma cells, unlike papillary fibroelastoma.

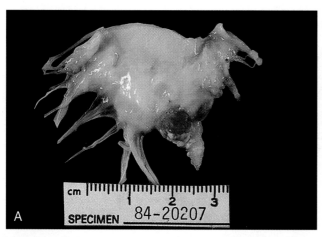
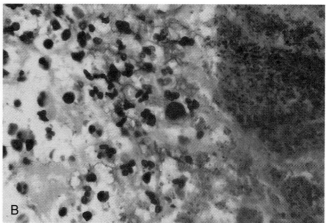

Figure 8–1. *A,* Acute bacterial endocarditis, mitral valve. The anterior leaflet of the mitral valve demonstrates a bulky vegetation and chordal rupture. The underlying valve demonstrates changes of mitral valve prolapse. *B,* Infectious endocarditis, mitral valve, Brown and Hopps stain. A histologic section of the vegetation demonstrates acute inflammation and bacterial colonies.

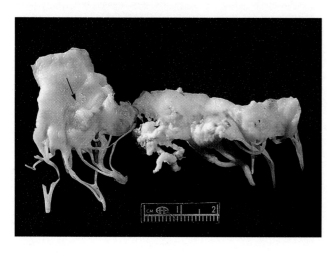

Figure 8–2. Mitral valve prolapse, infectious endocarditis. The patient was a 54-year-old man with mitral regurgitation, low-grade fevers, and a vegetation demonstrated by echocardiography. Chordae were thinned and haphazard, and there was leaflet billowing consistent with mitral valve prolapse. There was a bulky vegetation on the posterior leaflet *(right)* with focal valve destruction and chordal rupture. The anterior leaflet shows a "kissing lesion" *(arrow).* Histologically, there were acute inflammation and underlying granulation tissue (not shown).

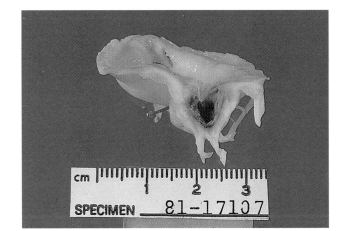

Figure 8–3. Postinflammatory mitral stenosis with healing endocarditis. A section through the valve demonstrates a hemorrhagic fibrinous exudate on the atrial surface of the fibrotic valve.

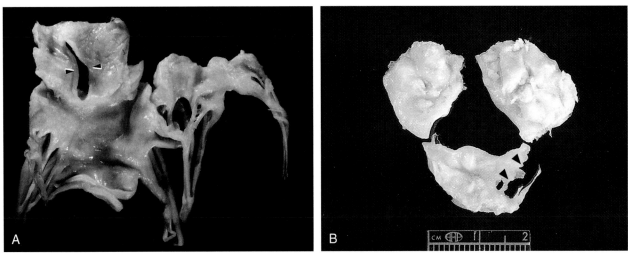

Figure 8–4. *A,* Healed endocarditis, mitral valve. The patient was a middle-aged man with coronary artery atherosclerosis, mitral regurgitation, endocarditis treated with antibiotics, and aortic stenosis. The patient underwent combined aortic and mitral valve replacement as well as coronary artery bypass grafting. The mitral valve demonstrated a perforation *(arrowheads)* of an aneurysmally dilated portion of the anterior leaflet. *B,* Healed endocarditis, aortic valve. This valve was removed at the same time as the valve illustrated in *A.* Note the perforation of the aortic cusp *(arrowheads).* There are calcific deposits present on all cusps.

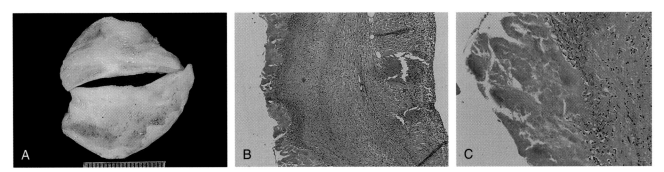

Figure 8–5. *A,* Infectious endocarditis, bicuspid aortic valve. A 38-year-old man was diagnosed with bacterial endocarditis, bicuspid aortic valve, worsening aortic insufficiency, and left ventricular dilatation. An aortic valve replacement demonstrated a bicuspid aortic valve. The surface was irregular and shaggy, but there were no discrete destructive lesions. *B,* Infectious endocarditis, bicuspid aortic valve. A histologic section of the valve illustrated in *A* demonstrates a diffuse acute and chronic inflammatory infiltrate with fibrin accumulation on the valve surface. *C,* Infectious endocarditis, bicuspid aortic valve. A higher magnification of *B* demonstrates acute inflammation, fibrin deposits, and bacterial colonies.

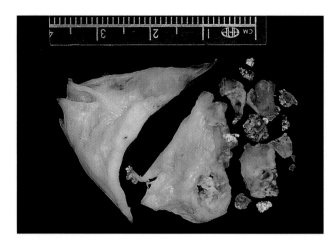

Figure 8-6. Infectious endocarditis, bicuspid aortic valve. A 30-year-old man suffered from infectious endocarditis with blood cultures positive for *Streptococcus viridans*. Note the destructive lesion of one of the valve leaflets and the multiple friable vegetations.

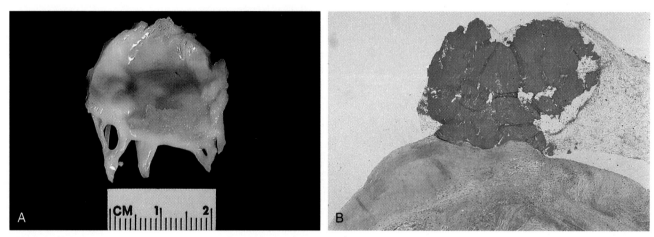

Figure 8-7. *A*, Marantic endocarditis, anterior leaflet of mitral valve. Note the vegetations along the lines of valve closure, without associated valve perforation. *B*, Marantic endocarditis. There is a fibrin-platelet, acellular vegetation on the atrial surface of the valve, without destruction of the underlying valve.

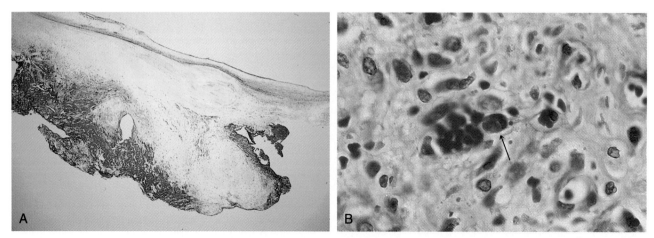

Figure 8-8. *A*, Systemic lupus erythematosus, Libman-Sacks vegetation. These lesions may rarely achieve large dimensions, resulting in valvular incompetence and the need for surgical removal. Note the fibrotic mitral valve; on the undersurface of the valve leaflet there is organizing fibrinous vegetation. *B*, Systemic lupus erythematosus, Libman-Sacks vegetation. A lupus erythematosus cell may occasionally be identified *(arrow)*.

CHAPTER 9

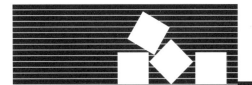

Prosthetic Valves, Aortocoronary Bypass Grafts, and Vascular Prostheses

PROSTHETIC HEART VALVES

Definitions

- Xenograft = heterograft; indicates grafting of treated tissue from a nonhuman species.
- Homograft = allograft; indicates grafting of tissue from human donors; allograft specifically indicates genetic variability between the donor and recipient.
- Autograft = grafting of tissue from an individual to a different site in the same individual (donor = recipient).

Types of Valves

Tissue Valves

- Porcine valves

  • Carpentier-Edwards*
  • Hancock*

- Pericardium (bovine) valves**
- Human homograft valves*

Mechanical Valves

- Caged-ball valves

  • Starr-Edwards valve*

- Caged-disk valves
- Tilting disk valves

  • Bjork-Shiley valve
  • Omniscience valve*
  • Medtronic-Hall valve*

---

* Approved for use in the United States
** Under clinical trial

- Bileaflet valves

  • St. Jude valve*

Complications

- Early complications of prosthetic valve surgery include transient disturbances in the conduction system, occlusion of a normal or anomalous coronary artery, and long sutures, knots, and fragments of chordae obstructing valve movement.
- Early infections are usually secondary to perioperative contaminants.
- Infections after 60 days result from bacteremic seeding.
- Endocarditis with or without ring abscesses occurs at a rate of 5% at 5 years and is more frequent in prosthetic valves placed in patients with previous infective endocarditis.
- Thrombosis occurs at a rate of 1% to 4% per year (at a greater rate in patients with atrial fibrillation or heart block).
- Organizing thrombus, or pannus, is desirable over the sewing ring, but thrombus extending to valve surfaces may compromise blood flow or result in thromboembolism.
- Paravalvular leaks can result from noninfectious tissue retraction, incomplete surgical seating, or endocarditis. The resected valve may appear to be normal.
- Flow gradients across the prosthesis may result in hemolysis and renal hemosiderosis, the severity of which varies by type of valve.
- Prosthetic disproportion by the placement of inappropriately large valves may result in septal irritation, interference to left ventricular emptying, and decreased occluder motion.
- Porcine and mechanical valve prostheses are compared in Table 9–1.

Table 9–1
COMPARISON OF PORCINE AND
MECHANICAL VALVE PROSTHESES

Porcine Valves	Mechanical Valves
Undergo eventual degeneration	Relatively durable
Cuspal calcification, especially in children	Do not calcify
No systemic anticoagulation necessary	Require systemic anticoagulation
Ring abscesses may occur	Ring abscesses may occur
Valve cusp may become infected	Surfaces resistant to infection

Tissue Valves

- Cuspal degeneration and calcification
- Cuspal infections

Mechanical Valves

- Long sutures or knots occluding movement of disk
- Strut or disk fracture
- Ball variance (older models of caged-ball valves)
- Frayed cloth coverings occluding valve or coronary ostia (older models of mechanical valves)

Porcine Bioprosthetic Valves

- Aortic porcine valve
- Glutaraldehyde-treated tissue mounted on a mechanical stent
- Carpentier-Edwards: slightly noncircular Elgiloy stent
- Hancock: circular polypropylene stent

Indications for Placement

- Patients older than 65 years of age for aortic valve replacement
- Patients older than 70 years of age for mitral valve replacement
- Women of childbearing age and other patients in whom anticoagulation is contraindicated
- As replacements for thrombosed mechanical valves

New Generation Bioprosthetic Valves

- Undergoing clinical trials
- Tissue preservation at low or zero pressure
- Preserved in the presence of calcium mitigation agents
- Altered stent profiles that are reduced or even absent
- Hancock II valve: Delrin ring replaces polypropylene
- Other models: Carpentier-Edwards supra-annular porcine, St. Jude-Bioimplant porcine, Medtronic Intact porcine, and Carpentier-Edwards stentless porcine

Pathologic Changes

- Calcification and degeneration resulting in valve failure occur in 50% of valves by 15 years.
- Calcification is accelerated in children.
- Tears are classified by site: cuspal tears (type I), crescentic tears at the bases of the sinus not involving the free margin (type II), irregular tears in the center of the valve cusp (type III), multiple small perforations (type IV). Type III degeneration is often caused by infection.
- Thrombotic occlusion is relatively uncommon in bioprosthetic valves compared with mechanical valves.

Bovine Pericardial Valves

- Bovine pericardial valves consist of treated bovine pericardium applied to a stent.
- Older types were especially prone to degeneration and were withdrawn from use.
- Bovine pericardial valves undergo tissue degeneration and cuspal tears, similar to porcine valves.
- New generation valves include Mitroflow pericardial and Carpentier-Edwards pericardial; these valves are in clinical trials.

Human Cadaver Homograft Valves

Indications for Placement

- Used in the semilunar position
- In children and in patients with congenital malformations
- In adults for reimplantation of an infected prosthetic aortic valve
- Alternative to mechanical valves in aortic valve replacement in adults younger than 50 years of age
- Limited supply

Preservation

- Irradiation and high concentrations of antibiotics in the 1960s led to a high rate of valve degeneration.
- Improved cryopreservation techniques developed in the 1970s have led to a resurgence of their use.
- Cryopreserved valves have a long shelf-life and are preferentially harvested from donors with a warm ischemic time of less than 12 to 24 hours.
- Fresh valves may be harvested from beating heart donors or transplant recipients, are usually stored in nutrient media with low concentrations of antibiotics, and must be used soon after harvesting.

Advantages

- Do not require stenting in the semilunar position
- Are resistant to thrombosis

Pathologic Changes and Complications

- Calcification and tissue degeneration occur at a rate similar to that with xenograft prostheses.
- Obstruction at anastomotic sites may result in outflow tract obstruction, but the valve itself may be normal.

Caged-Ball Mechanical Valves

- Starr-Edwards caged-ball valve is the most common type of caged-ball mechanical valve and is the only one currently approved for use in the United States.
- These valves have separate models for aortic and mitral positions.
- Compared with other valves, caged-ball mechanical valves have been in longest continual clinical use.

- Carbon-coated graphite (pyrolytic carbon) surfaces for struts and occluders do not require cloth coverings.

Complications

- Caged-ball mechanical valves have a relatively high rate of thromboembolic complications and have high pressure gradients in small sizes.
- Abnormal disk movement or ball variance, due to swelling and distortion of the silicone rubber disk, occurred in early types of caged-ball and caged-disk valves.
- Cloth coverings of previously used valves decreased thrombogenicity and noise, but potentiated hemolysis, became worn and frayed, and rarely occluded coronary ostia.

Tilting Disk Valves

- Bjork-Shiley convexo-concave and spheric valves were popular tilting disk valves but are no longer used.
- The Bjork-Shiley Monostrut prosthesis is in clinical trials.
- The Omniscience valve is a monoleaflet prosthesis with a titanium orifice ring and a pyrolytic carbon disk controlled by short struts; the opening angle is 80°.
- The Medtronic-Hall pyrolytic carbon disk opens to 70° (mitral) and 75° (aortic), and the ring and strut combination is machined from a single piece of titanium. The strut passes through a hole in the center of the disk; the disk is rotatable within the sewing ring.

Complications

- Strut fractures occur rarely but were relatively common in Bjork-Shiley 60° and 70° convexo-concave valves, leading to catastrophic disk escape; these valves are no longer implanted.

Bileaflet Valves

- The St. Jude bileaflet valve is in widespread use and is composed of pyrolytic carbon-coated graphite. The leaflets open to 85°.
- No other bileaflet valve is approved for use in the United States.

Complications

- Complications are similar to those of other mechanical valves.

References

Albertucci M, Wong K, Petrou M, et al. The use of unstented homograft valves for aortic valve reoperations. Review of a twenty-three-year experience. J Thorac Cardiovasc Surg 107:152–161, 1994.
Brudon RA, Miller DC, Oyer PE, et al. Durability of porcine valves at fifteen years in a representative North American patient population. J Thorac Cardiovasc Surg 103:238–251, 1992.
Ishihara T, Ferrans VJ, Boyce SW, et al. Structure and classification of cuspal tears and perforations in porcine bioprosthetic cardiac valve implanted in patients. Am J Cardiol 48:665, 1981.
Kirklin JK, Smith D, Novick W, et al. Long-term function of cryopreserved aortic homografts. A ten-year study. J Thorac Cardiovasc Surg 106:154–165, 1993.
Platt MR, Mills LJ, Estrera AS, Hillis LD, Buja LM, Willerson JT. Marked thrombosis and calcification of porcine heterograft valves. Circulation 62:862, 1980.
Schoen FJ. Cardiac valve replacement. In *Interventional and Surgical Cardiovascular Pathology*. Philadelphia, WB Saunders, 1989, pp 124–172.
Silver MD, Butany J. Mechanical heart valves: methods of examination, complications, and modes of failure. Hum Pathol 18:577–585, 1987.
Turina J, Hess OM, Turina M, Krayenbuehl HP. Cardiac bioprostheses in the 1990s. Circulation 88:775–781, 1993.

AORTOCORONARY BYPASS GRAFTS

Early Closure of Saphenous Vein Grafts (Within 30 Days)

- Early closure of saphenous vein grafts results from mechanical problems, inadequate size of coronary vessels, and poor runoff.
- Mechanical problems include eversion or compression of the graft during suturing.
- Severe atherosclerosis in the distal segment of the bypassed coronary artery may result in poor runoff.
- Luminal thrombi are found in one third of grafts that fail within 30 days.
- Dissection is a rare cause of early graft closure.
- Grafts closing within 30 days become cordlike with diffuse obliteration of the lumen.

Late Closure of Saphenous Vein Grafts (30 Days to 1 Year)

- Fibrointimal proliferation occurs in all grafts and is concentric, with gradual narrowing of the lumen.
- The proliferative cell is a smooth muscle cell, which stains positively for muscle-specific actin.
- Smooth muscle proliferation occurs in a matrix rich in proteoglycans and collagen.
- The pathogenesis of fibrointimal proliferation may be related to endothelial damage, damage to the vasavasorum, exposure to arterial pressures, and/or loss of vascular pedicle.

Late Closure of Saphenous Vein Grafts (After 1 Year)

- Fibrointimal proliferation is present in approximately 90% of grafts.
- Atherosclerosis occurs in less than 25% of cases and may be associated with recent thrombus.
- The morphology of graft atherosclerosis is characterized by plaque rich in lipid, having numerous cholesterol clefts with a giant cell reaction and a thin fibrous cap.
- The plaque is generally soft and friable; dense fibrosis and calcification, typical of native coronary arteries, are rarely seen.
- Atherosclerotic aneurysms occur in less than 1% of grafts, generally after 5 years; these are often multiple, and there is medial atrophy with loss of elastic tissue.
- Risk factors dictate the type of morphologic change seen in vein grafts. Hypertension is associated with fibrointimal proliferation, whereas diabetes mellitus and

hypercholesterolemia are associated with atherosclerosis.

Internal Mammary Artery Graft

- Internal mammary artery (IMA) grafts are superior to vein grafts, with better survival rate and better cumulative event-free survival.
- Histologic studies demonstrate a low incidence of atherosclerosis and fibrointimal proliferation occurring over the long term.

SYNTHETIC CONDUITS

Materials

- The most commonly used synthetic materials are Dacron and Gore-Tex (polytetrafluoroethylene, PTFE)
- Gore-Tex grafts are generally used for smaller muscular arteries; Dacron is used for larger muscular and elastic arteries.
- Cardiac reconstructive surgery in the 1970s and early 1980s used porcine heterografts in extracardiac conduits until a high rate of calcification and failure precluded their continued use.
- Subsequently, most extracardiac conduits were nonvalved.
- Currently, cryopreserved homograft valves are used with extracardiac conduits.

Indications for Placement

- Synthetic conduits for coronary bypass surgery, especially Gore-Tex grafts, have been used in a limited fashion as an alternative to saphenous veins; short-term pat-ency is approximately 60% from 3 to 12 months, an unacceptable rate compared with that of IMA and saphenous vein grafts.
- Extracardiac conduits for congenital heart disease are used primarily in the following conditions:

  - Truncus arteriosus
  - Tetralogy of Fallot with severe outflow tract obstruction and pulmonary atresia
  - Transposition of the great arteries with left ventricular outflow tract obstruction
  - Tricuspid atresia
  - Subaortic stenosis

Complications

- Generally, complications include anastomotic obstruction, obstruction of the conduit due to fibrous peels (neointima) or thrombosis, degeneration of the valve in valved conduits, endocarditis, and anastomotic pseudoaneurysms.
- Compression of the conduit between the sternum and the heart occurs if the conduit is not placed lateral to the sternum.
- Obstruction at the proximal anastomosis may be caused by abnormal angulation of the conduit.
- Symptomatic calcific degeneration of porcine valves within extracardiac conduits occurs at a rate of greater

than 30% in 1 year; asymptomatic obstruction occurs in up to 60% of patients.
- Cryopreserved homograft valved conduits fare better and are free of obstruction in approximately 90% of patients at 3.5 years.
- The luminal fibrous peel, or neointima, occurs in all extracardiac conduits.
- The fibrous peel may be loosely attached to the conduit layer.
- Occasionally, the peel may cause obstruction, due to diffusely thick neointima, thrombotic separation of the neointima from the conduit, or formation of a flap valve after dislodgment of the neointima from the conduit.
- Histologically, fibrous peels consist of a luminal region of dense collagen and a conduit portion composed of active granulation tissue with proliferating fibroblasts, neovascularization, and inflammation.

Reference

Edwards WD, Agarwal KC, Feldt RH, et al. Surgical pathology of obstructed, right-sided, porcine-valved extracardiac conduits. Arch Pathol Lab Med 107:400–405, 1983.

AORTOFEMORAL BYPASS GRAFTS

Complications

- Significant late complications occur in approximately 2% of patients who receive aortofemoral bypass grafts.
- Graft infection and graft limb stenoses are the most common complications requiring reoperation.
- The most common organism involved in late graft infections is *Staphylococcus epidermidis;* the mean postoperative interval of diagnosis is 3 to 4 years.
- Clinically, graft infections are suggested by anastomotic aneurysms, perigraft exudate, draining groin mass, perigraft gas, or aortoduodenal fistulas.
- False aneurysms (pseudoaneurysms) are the most common overall complication and are detected in more than 50% of grafts by sonography; they account for 20% to 40% of reoperations.
- Although generally asymptomatic, anastomotic pseudoaneurysms rupture in rare cases, resulting in generally fatal exsanguination into the retroperitoneum, bowel, or urinary tract.
- Approximately 20% of anastomotic aneurysms are dissections.
- Predisposing factors to femoral anastomotic aneurysms include hypertension, superficial femoral artery occlusion, and flow turbulence.
- Other common complications that are often asymptomatic include perigraft hematoma and accumulations of sterile serous fluid (seromas).
- Thrombotic occlusion of the graft or native artery near the anastomosis is uncommon.

Pathologic Diagnosis

- Graft infections tend to be associated with acute inflammation and granulation tissue.

- Occasionally, the histologic diagnosis of infection can be difficult, and organisms are difficult to identify in tissue sections or routine culture.
- The optimal method of diagnosing *S. epidermidis* infection is by aerobic culture of the prosthetic fabric in broth media.

Treatment and Outcome

- Patients with gastrointestinal complications have higher mortality and morbidity than patients with simple graft infection or pseudoaneurysm.

- Complete graft excision with extra-anatomic bypass is recommended for patients with graft infections.

References

Drury JK, Leiberman DP, Gilmour DG, Pollock JG. Operation for late complications of aortic grafts. Surg Gynecol Obstet 163:251–255, 1986.

McCann RL, Schwartz LB, Georgiade GS. Management of abdominal aortic graft complications. Ann Surg 217:729–734, 1993.

Plate G, Hollier LA, O'Brien P, Pairolero PC, Cherry KJ, Kazmier FJ. Recurrent aneurysms and late vascular complications following repair of abdominal aortic aneurysms. Arch Surg 120:590–594, 1985.

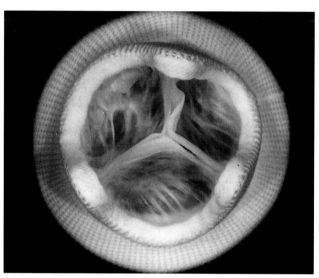

Figure 9–1. Hancock porcine xenograft valve, aortic view. Porcine valves are made from biochemically treated tissue mounted on a mechanical stent; 0.2% to 0.6% glutaraldehyde is used for preservation. The valves are mounted on a stent, which is attached to a sewing ring. In Hancock valves, the stents are circular and made of polypropylene.

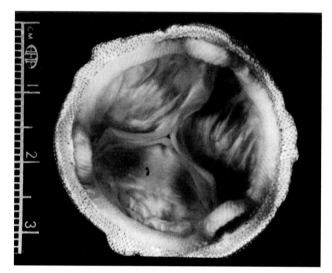

Figure 9–2. Carpentier-Edwards porcine valve, aortic view. The stent is made of Elgiloy and is slightly noncircular to accommodate the muscular shelf attached to the right coronary cusp in the native porcine aortic valve.

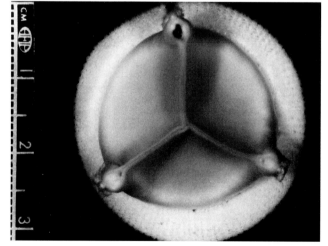

Figure 9–3. Bovine pericardial valve, Ionescu-Shiley. Introduced in the mid-1970s, these valves had a higher rate of tissue failure than porcine valves and are no longer approved for use in the United States.

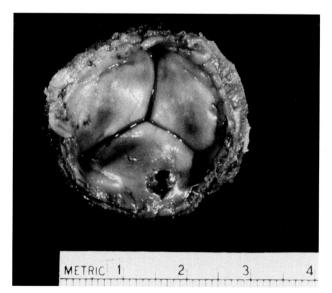

Figure 9–4. Explanted porcine valve. Valve failure resulted from a cuspal tear near the sewing ring. There is a normal degree of pannus overgrowth on the sewing ring. Because of the discrete nature of the tear and the relatively normal appearance of the two other cusps, an infectious cause for this tear must be ruled out by history and, if necessary, by culture and histologic study.

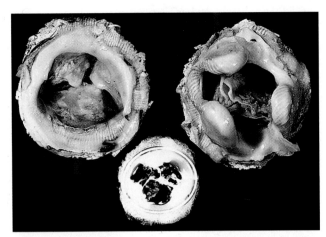

Figure 9–5. Degenerative calcific changes, Hancock porcine valve. This explanted valve is shown from the aortic view *(upper left)* and ventricular view *(upper right)*. Distortion of the leaflets prevents proper closure, resulting in incompetence. A radiograph of the valve *(below)* demonstrates the extent of calcification on the valve cusps.

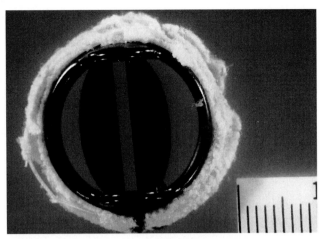

Figure 9–6. Mechanical valve, bileaflet. The most common bileaflet valve, and the only bileaflet valve currently approved in the United States, is the St. Jude valve. It is composed of pyrolytic carbon–coated graphite; the leaflets open to 85°.

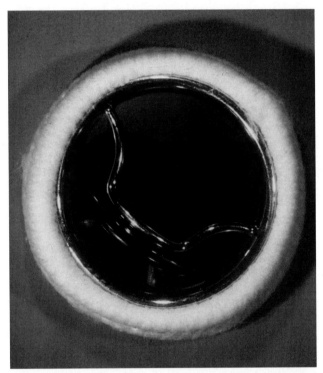

Figure 9–7. Mechanical valve, tilting disk. The Bjork-Shiley valve was extremely popular but is no longer in use in this country. The Bjork-Shiley Monostrut prosthesis (not shown) is in clinical trials. A major and a minor strut are welded to a titanium ring, to which is attached the cloth sewing ring. Fractures in the welds may be imperceptible to the naked eye and result in disk escape, with catastrophic results.

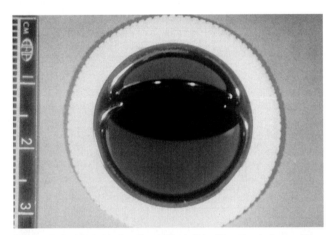

Figure 9–8. Mechanical valve, tilting disk. The Omniscience tilting disk valve is a monoleaflet prosthesis with a titanium orifice ring and a pyrolytic carbon disk controlled by short struts. The opening angle is 80°.

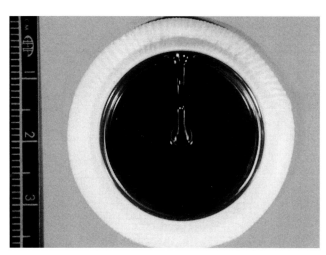

Figure 9–9. Mechanical valve, tilting disk. The Medtronic-Hall pyrolytic carbon disk opens to 70° (mitral) and 75° (aortic), and the ring and strut combination is machined from a single piece of titanium. The strut passes through a hole in the center of the disk. The valve disk is rotatable within the sewing ring.

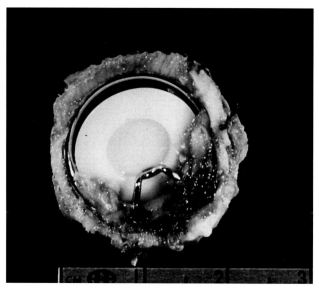

Figure 9–10. Bjork-Shiley mechanical valve, thrombosis. The most common complication of mechanical valves is thrombosis, which may propagate from the sewing ring and obstruct disk movement, resulting in valve failure from incompetence and stenosis.

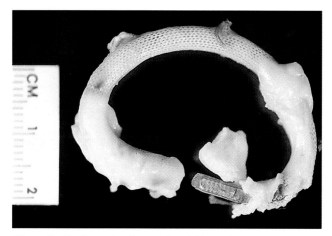

Figure 9–11. Carpentier ring, explant. This surgical specimen was removed from a patient with persistent mitral incompetence after annuloplasty with ring placement. There is focal neointimal growth on the ring surface.

SECTION ■ 3

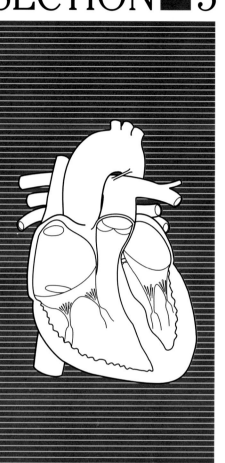

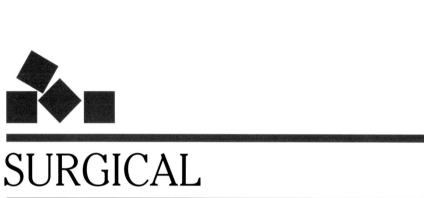

SURGICAL

PATHOLOGY OF

CARDIAC MASSES

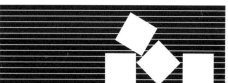

CHAPTER 10

Approach to Cardiac Tumors

INCIDENCE

- Approximately 2000 primary cardiac tumors have been reported. The incidence of cardiac tumors in autopsy series is between 0.001% and 0.03%. Metastatic cardiac tumors are between 40 and 500 times more common than primary tumors in autopsy series; however, in surgical series of cardiac tumors, primary benign and malignant cardiac tumors outnumber metastatic neoplasms.
- Eighty percent of surgically resected cardiac tumors are myxomas. However, because better imaging techniques reveal more incidental lesions and because surgeons are more aggressive than previously in removing malignant and infiltrating tumors, the average surgical pathologist probably encounters cardiac tumors other than the myxoma, some of which may be clinically and histologically confused with myxoma.

METHODS OF SAMPLING

- Most cardiac tumors are excised after initiation of cardiopulmonary bypass, because the cardiac chambers are entered.
- For primarily epicardial tumors and those limited to atrial appendages, extracorporeal circulation is not required.
- Occasionally, in large inoperable tumors, the biopsy specimen is taken for tissue diagnosis using a needle.
- Recently, cardiac tumors, especially those that are right-sided, have been diagnosed by endomyocardial biopsy.
- Endomyocardial biopsy is ideal for the diagnosis of metastatic tumors, which are largely right-sided and in which a tissue diagnosis has already been made.
- The histologic diagnosis of a primary cardiac sarcoma may be difficult on the basis of an endomyocardial biopsy, because there are sampling limitations.

SURGICAL PATHOLOGIC EVALUATION

- There are several general principles in the histopathologic evaluation of cardiac tumors. For all tumors, especially myxomas and other polypoid tumors, it is best to ink surgical margins at the endocardial attachment site, to determine completeness of excision. Although some data refute that there is an increased risk of recurrence with incomplete excision of cardiac myxoma, the surgeon often requests information on adequacy of surgical excision of myxomas as well as of sarcomas.
- Myxomas, especially of the right atrium, may be calcified, necessitating decalcification. In addition, left atrial sarcomas may have areas of osteoid and bone formation, also necessitating decalcification.
- Sterile dissection of cardiac sarcomas and preservation of a portion of tumor in culture medium allow cytogenetic studies that are occasionally helpful in the differential diagnosis of sarcomas. Prognostication based on DNA ploidy has not been studied for primary sarcomas of the heart because they are rare. However, data from noncardiac soft-tissue sarcomas may be extrapolated to cardiac tumors and provide potentially valuable data. Therefore, an unfixed portion of a malignancy for DNA ploidy studies and flow cytometry should be saved for its research or potential clinical relevance.

CLINICOPATHOLOGIC CORRELATES

- Simple clinical data greatly help to narrow the differential diagnosis of a cardiac tumor removed surgically.
- It is especially important to know the patient's age at occurrence, the site, and, if possible, clinical data re-

Table 10–1
SURGICALLY EXCISED CARDIAC TUMORS

Parameter	More Common	Less Common
Age		
Intrauterine	Rhabdomyoma	Teratoma
Infant/newborn	Fibroma, rhabdomyoma, teratoma	Histiocytoid cardiomyopathy
Children	Fibroma, rhabdomyoma	Sarcoma, myxoma, teratoma
Adults	Myxoma, primary sarcoma, metastatic tumor	Papillary fibroelastoma, lipomatous hypertrophy of interatrial septum, fibroma, hemangioma
Site		
Left atrium	Myxoma	Primary sarcoma
Right atrium	Myxoma, angiosarcoma, metastatic tumor	Lipomatous hypertrophy of atrial septum, other sarcoma
Left ventricular/ right ventricular wall	Fibroma, rhabdomyoma, hemangioma	Sarcoma
Multiple sites	Rhabdomyoma, sarcoma, familial myxoma	Histiocytoid cardiomyopathy, lymphoma
Valve	Papillary fibroelastoma	Myxoma, hamartoma, sarcoma, hemangioma, blood cyst
Left ventricular/ right ventricular endocardium	Papillary fibroelastoma, metastatic melanoma	Hemangioma, myxoma
Atrioventricular nodal area	Atrioventricular nodal tumor	Teratoma

garding rare clinical syndromes associated with certain congenital lesions (Table 10–1). Certain myxomas may be familial, occur in younger patients, or be associated with a syndrome of spotty skin pigmentation, endocrine abnormalities, and noncardiac myxomas; these tumors are invariably friable and myxoid in gross appearance. Patients with tuberous sclerosis have a high incidence of cardiac rhabdomyoma. Cardiac fibromas are more likely to develop in patients with Gorlin's syndrome (osteomas, sebaceous cysts).

■ Magnetic resonance imaging and computed tomography scans determine exact location of the tumor in the heart, multiplicity of tumors, and tissue density. These technologies are helpful in predicting the type of tumor that may be encountered and possibly whether the process is benign or malignant.

References

Blondeau P. Primary cardiac tumors—French studies of 533 cases. Thorac Cardiovasc Surg 38:192–195, 1990.

Dein JR, Frist WH, Stinson EB, et al. Primary cardiac neoplasms. Early and late results of surgical treatment in 42 patients. J Thorac Cardiovasc Surg 93:502–511, 1987.

Miralles A, Bracamonte L, Oncul H, et al. Cardiac tumors: clinical experience and surgical results in 74 patients. Ann Thorac Surg 52:886–895, 1991.

Murphy MC, Sweeney MS, Putnam JB, et al. Surgical treatment of cardiac tumors: a 25-year experience. Ann Thorac Surg 49:612–617, 1990.

Reece IJ, Cooley DA, Frazier OH, Hallman GL, Powers PL, Montero CG. Cardiac tumors. J Thorac Cardiovasc Surg 88:439–446, 1984.

Tazelaar HD, Locke TJ, McGregor CG. Pathology of surgically excised primary cardiac tumors. Mayo Clin Proc 67:957–965, 1992.

Verkkala K, Kupari M, Maamies T, et al. Primary cardiac tumours—operative treatment of 20 patients. Thorac Cardiovasc Surg 37:361–364, 1989.

CHAPTER 11

Benign Cardiac Tumors

MYXOMA

A myxoma is a benign endocardial neoplasm composed of "myxoma" cells within a myxoid matrix. The origin of the myxoma cell is controversial; possibilities include primitive endocardial cushion cell and endothelial cell. The thrombotic theory of origin of cardiac myxoma is generally discounted. Greater than 75% of surgically excised benign cardiac masses are myxomas (Table 11–1).

Clinical Findings

- Cardiac myxomas often cause varied, confusing symptoms that may lead to a delay in diagnosis.
- Left atrial myxomas constitute 80% of cardiac myxomas; they cause symptoms of mitral stenosis, ischemia of extremities or brain (embolization), arrhythmias, syncope, sudden death, and constitutional symptoms (fever, weight loss, anorexia).
- Right atrial myxomas account for most of the remaining 20% of cardiac myxomas and may cause recurrent pulmonary emboli, tricuspid valve obstruction, endocarditis, and constitutional symptoms.
- Diagnosis depends on echocardiography, which may be supplemented by magnetic resonance imaging (MRI) and computed tomography (CT) scans.
- Emboli may rarely form fusiform aneurysms, especially in cerebral circulation; these are diagnosed by angiography.
- Typical auscultatory findings (tumor "plop") occur in less than 50% of cases.
- Myxoma syndrome is characterized by familial, multiple, recurrent myxomas in young individuals. Often, there is spotty skin pigmentation and endocrine abnormalities; myxomas may be found anywhere on endocardial surfaces (Table 11–2).
- Recurrence occurs in 2% of sporadic cases and does not appear to be related to the extent of the surgical excision.

Gross Pathologic Findings

- Myxomas may connect to the atrial septum by a broad stalk (atrial patching may be necessary) or by a narrow pedicle.

- Myxomas are usually variegated, with hemorrhagic fibrotic and myxoid areas.
- Myxomas may be smooth (fibrotic) or friable (gelatinous, myxoid); the latter are more likely to embolize.
- Myxomas of the myxoma syndrome are always of the friable, gelatinous type; these are more likely to occur in areas remote from the atrial septum, including valves and ventricular surfaces.

Microscopic Pathologic Findings

- Diagnosis depends on the presence of "myxoma" cells; these are unique to cardiac myxomas.
- Myxoma cells (sometimes referred to as lepidic cells) are stellate or ovoid, with eosinophilic cytoplasm and indistinct cell borders.
- The nuclei of myxoma cells contain open chromatin. Nucleoli are indistinct or prominent.
- Myxoma cells form rings, cords, and nests that seem to emanate from and merge imperceptibly with capillaries, which are often infiltrated by lymphocytes and histiocytes.
- The myxoid background is infiltrated by a sparse or focally dense collection of histiocytes, plasma cells, mast cells, and lymphocytes. Hemosiderin is invariably present within macrophages.
- The surfaces of myxomas are lined by myxoma cells

Table 11–1

SURGICAL RESECTIONS OF BENIGN CARDIAC TUMORS*

Tumor Type	Number (n)	Percent (%)
Myxoma	221	76
Fibroma	22	8
Rhabdomyoma	14	5
Lipoma**	13	5
Hemangioma	12	4
Papillary fibroelastoma	9	3
Histiocytoid cardiomyopathy	1	
Total	**292**	

*Data from Dein et al, Miralles et al, Reece et al, Tazelaar et al.
**Includes lipomatous hypertrophy of atrial septum.

with endothelial differentiation; these cells may rarely contain mitotic figures.

- Smooth, fibrotic myxomas are characterized by fibrosis, relatively little myxoid matrix, and degenerative changes.
- Degenerative changes include calcification, which is present in 15% of left-sided myxomas and in 55% of right-sided myxomas, and ossification, which is present in approximately 8% of myxomas.
- Gamna bodies (calcific elastic fiber degeneration) are present in approximately 17% of cardiac myxomas and are occasionally extensive.
- Extramedullary hematopoiesis is present in approximately 7% of cardiac myxomas.
- Approximately 1% of myxomas have intestine-like glands that express cytokeratin, carcinoembryonic antigen, and intracytoplasmic mucin vacuoles; these are often present at the base of the tumor.
- Embolic foci in rare cases grow locally beyond the arterial wall, but metastases of myxoma to lymph nodes or viscera do not occur.
- Immunohistochemical studies are not particularly helpful in the differential diagnosis; myxoma cells may express a variety of antigens, but are generally cytokeratin negative, variably S-100 positive, and variably positive for smooth muscle and endothelial markers.

Treatment and Clinical Course

- Approximately 2% of cardiac myxomas recur after surgical treatment; in these cases, the diagnosis of myxoma syndrome should be considered.
- There is no evidence that inadequacy of surgical excision is related to recurrence.
- The long-term course of patients with myxomas and cerebral aneurysms is unknown, but patients may remain asymptomatic for long periods.

Differential Diagnosis

- Sarcomas of various types may have a prominent myxoid background, but lack characteristic myxoma cells, contain cellular areas with pleomorphism and atypical mitotic figures, and lack abundant hemosiderin.
- Papillary fibroelastoma tumors are avascular, do not contain myxoma cells, and are usually present on valves.

Table 11–2
FEATURES OF MYXOMA SYNDROME

Skin and mucous membrane lesions
  Ephelides (spotty pigmentation/lentiginosis)
  Blue nevi
  Myxoma
Cardiac myxomas, often multiple or recurrent
Mammary myxofibroadenomas
Endocrine lesions
  Nodular adrenal cortical hyperplasia
  Acromegaly/pituitary adenomas
  Sertoli cell tumors, testis
  Psammomatous melanotic schwannoma

- Hemangiomas, when intracavitary, may have a myxoid background, and the vascular background of capillary hemangioma may mimic myxoma; however, there are branching capillary structures and generally areas of cavernous hemangioma. Myxoma cells and abundant hemosiderin are absent.
- Organized thrombus lacks myxoma cells, Gamna bodies, and extensive calcification. Occasionally, the distinction between fibrotic myxoma and organized thrombus is difficult.
- The 1% of myxomas with glandular structures have been misdiagnosed as metastatic carcinoma. Glandular structures of myxoma do not have mitoses, necrosis, or cellular atypia.

References

Attum AA, Johnson GS, Masri Z, Girardet R, Lansing AM. Malignant clinical behavior of cardiac myxomas and "myxoid imitators." Ann Thorac Surg 44:217–222, 1987.

Burke AP, Virmani R. Cardiac myxomas: a clinicopathologic study. Am J Clin Pathol 100:671–680, 1994.

Carney JA, Gordon H, Carpenter PC, Shenoy BV, Go VL. The complex of myxomas, spotty pigmentation, and endocrine overactivity. Medicine 64:270–283, 1985.

Coard KC, Silver MD. Gamna body of the heart. Pathology 16:459–461, 1984.

Dein JR, Frist WH, Stinson EB, et al. Primary cardiac neoplasms. Early and late results of surgical treatment in 42 patients. J Thorac Cardiovasc Surg 93:502–511, 1987.

Lie JT. The identity and histogenesis of cardiac myxomas. A controversy put to rest (editorial). Arch Pathol Lab Med 113:724–726, 1989.

Markel ML, Waller BF, Armstrong WF. Cardiac myxoma. A review. Medicine 66:114–125, 1987.

Miralles A, Bracamonte L, Oncul H, et al. Cardiac tumors: clinical experience and surgical results in 74 patients. Ann Thorac Surg 52:886–895, 1991.

Reece IJ, Cooley DA, Frazier OH, Hallman GL, Powers PL, Montero CG. Cardiac tumors. J Thorac Cardiovasc Surg 88:439–446, 1984.

Roeltgen DP, Weimer GR, Patterson LF. Delayed neurologic complications of left atrial myxoma. Neurology 31:8–13, 1981.

Tazelaar HD, Locke TJ, McGregor CG. Pathology of surgically excised primary cardiac tumors. Mayo Clin Proc 67:957–965, 1992.

Trotter SE, Shore DF, Olsen EG. Gamna-Gandy nodules in a cardiac myxoma. Histopathology 17:270–272, 1990.

FIBROMA

Cardiac fibroma is a congenital, solitary, mural hamartoma of fibrous tissue.

Clinical Findings

- Fibromas occur from birth to adulthood, usually in infancy or childhood; the mean age at presentation is approximately 13 years.
- Eighty-six percent of tumors occur in children, one third of whom are younger than 1 year of age.
- Symptoms include arrhythmias, sudden death, and congestive heart failure; patients may present with asymptomatic murmurs.
- Diagnosis rests on imaging studies, echocardiography, MRI, and CT scan.

- Calcification may be seen on radiograph, MRI, and CT scan.
- There is occasional association with Gorlin's syndrome (nevoid basal cell carcinoma syndrome); manifestations include enlarged occipital circumference, odontogenic keratocysts of the jaws, epidermal cysts, rib anomalies, and multiple basal cell carcinomas of the skin.
- Surgical resection is curative.

Gross Pathologic Findings

- Bulging, whorled masses of rubbery white tissue resemble a uterine "fibroid."
- About one half of cardiac fibromas are grossly circumscribed.
- Sites of involvement, in order of decreasing frequency, are left ventricular free wall, right ventricle, and atria.
- Fibromas are generally mural lesions.
- Rarely, fibromas may bulge into the ventricular outflow, resulting in subaortic stenosis.

Microscopic Pathologic Findings

- In infants, cardiac fibromas are cellular with relatively little collagen; mitoses are rare or absent.
- In children and adults, there is extensive collagen deposition; some tumors histologically resemble scars.
- Elastic fibers are often prominent.
- Calcification is present in approximately one third of cases.
- Small vessel thickening is frequent in tumors.
- Inflammation is sparse and generally limited to perivascular regions and those at the margin of the tumor, usually mononuclear.
- Infiltration of surrounding muscle is present, even if the tumor is grossly circumscribed.

Treatment and Clinical Course

- Surgical therapy is the preferred treatment of fibromas. This can cause normalization of cardiac rhythm in patients with ventricular tachyarrhythmias.
- In some patients, tumors are not resectable, and partial excision is performed with good long-term prognosis.
- There appears to be little propensity for growth of cardiac fibroma after infancy; several reports have documented spontaneous regression of cardiac fibroma.

Differential Diagnosis

- Rhabdomyoma tumors are usually multiple, are composed of vacuolated striated muscle cells, and do not calcify.
- In adults, the histologic appearance is similar to scarring; however, unlike scars, fibromas are tumors that bulge on section and infiltrate into surrounding tissues.
- In infants, it may be difficult to distinguish cellular fibroma from fibrosarcoma; in our experience, most fibrous infantile cardiac tumors do not spread and are best classified as fibromas. Mitoses are not frequent in fibroma, unlike in sarcoma.

References

Burke AP, Rosado-de-Christenson M, Templeton PA, Virmani R. Cardiac fibroma. Clinicopathologic correlates and surgical treatment. J Thorac Cardiovasc Surg 108:862–870, 1994.

Ceithaml E, Midgley FM, Perry LW, Dullum MK. Intramural ventricular fibroma in infancy: survival after partial excision in 2 patients. Ann Thorac Surg 50:471–472, 1990.

Coffin CM. Congenital cardiac fibroma associated with Gorlin syndrome. Pediatr Pathol 12:255–262, 1992.

Reul GJ, Howell JF, Rubio PA, Peterson PK. Successful partial excision of an intramural fibroma of the left ventricle. Am J Cardiol 36:262–265, 1975.

Williams DB, Danielson GK, McGoon DC, Feldt RH, Edwards WD. Cardiac fibroma. J Thorac Cardiovasc Surg 84:230–236, 1982.

RHABDOMYOMA

Cardiac rhabdomyoma is a hamartoma that occurs exclusively in the heart, often as multiple nodules. It is composed of altered cardiac myocytes with large vacuoles and abundant glycogen.

Incidence and Clinical Findings

- Rhabdomyomas are the most common tumor of the heart in infants and children in autopsy series; they are second most common, after fibroma, in surgical series.
- Rhabdomyomas are rare in patients older than 10 years.
- There is a high association (approximately 50%) with tuberous sclerosis (intracranial hamartomas, facial angiofibromas, subungual fibromas, linear epidermal nevi, renal angiomyolipomas, other hamartomas).
- Virtually 100% of infants with tuberous sclerosis have echocardiographic evidence of cardiac rhabdomyoma; because of spontaneous regression, this number decreases to 60% in children and less than 25% in adults.
- Most rhabdomyomas of the heart are multiple, especially those in patients with tuberous sclerosis.
- Symptoms include congestive heart failure, arrhythmias, fetal hydrops, and sudden death.
- Up to 90% of cardiac tumors diagnosed in utero are rhabdomyomas.

Gross Pathologic Findings

- Pale, circumscribed nodules range from 1 mm to several centimeters in size.
- Rhabdomyomas in patients with tuberous sclerosis are usually multiple, mural lesions that do not obstruct blood flow and are not surgically resected. When innumerable small tumors are present, the term "rhabdomyomatosis" has been used.
- Solitary tumors are more frequent in sporadic cases, which account for most surgical resections. Patients without tuberous sclerosis tend to have bulky tumors that project into the cardiac chambers, obstructing blood flow.

Microscopic Pathologic Findings

- There are well-demarcated nodules of clear cells that have cross-striations.
- The typical cell of rhabdomyoma is the "spider cell,"

possessing vacuolated cytoplasm, with strands of cytoplasm extending from the periphery of the cell to the nucleus.

▪ Ultrastructurally, cells are similar to myoblasts, with intercalated disk-like structures around the cell periphery. Glycogen and contractile elements are plentiful.

Differential Diagnosis

▪ Rhabdomyoma is a distinctive tumor that rarely causes diagnostic problems.
▪ Glycogen storage disease (especially Pompe's disease) results in diffuse vacuolization of myocytes with central vacuoles and peripheral location of myofibrils; discrete tumors and spider cells are absent.
▪ Whipple's disease rarely affects the heart; the involved cells are histiocytes, not myocytes, and show characteristic periodic acid–Schiff (PAS)–positive granules (see Chap. 2).
▪ In histiocytoid cardiomyopathy, cells resemble histiocytes with fine vacuoles; tumors are usually smaller than those of rhabdomyoma (1–3 mm). There are few contractile elements and abundant mitochondria, unlike in rhabdomyoma.
▪ In adults, there is occasionally a poorly circumscribed tumor of mature, hypertrophied, disorganized myocytes with scarring; these are best described as hamartomas of cardiac muscle.

References

Burke AP, Virmani R. Cardiac rhabdomyoma, a clinicopathologic study. Mod Pathol 4:70–74, 1991.
Chan HS, Sonley MJ, Moes CA, Daneman A, Smith CR, Martin DJ. Primary and secondary tumors of childhood involving the heart, pericardium, and great vessels. A report of 75 cases and review of the literature. Cancer 56:825–836, 1985.
Fenoglio JJ Jr, McAllister HA, Ferrans VJ. Cardiac rhabdomyoma: a clinicopathologic and electron microscopic study. Am J Cardiol 38:241–251, 1976.
Groves AM, Fagg NL, Cook AC, Allan LD. Cardiac tumors in intrauterine life. Arch Dis Child 67:1189–1192, 1992.
Shrivastava S, Jacks JJ, White RS, Edwards JE. Diffuse rhabdomyomatosis of the heart. Arch Pathol Lab Med 101:78–90, 1977.
Smythe JF, Dyck JD, Smallhorn JF, Freedom RM. Natural history of cardiac rhabdomyoma in infancy and childhood. Am J Cardiol 66:1247–1249, 1990.

HISTIOCYTOID (ONCOCYTIC) CARDIOMYOPATHY (PURKINJE CELL HAMARTOMA)

Histiocytoid cardiomyopathy is a congenital hamartoma of multiple microscopic clusters of modified myocytes with an appearance similar to that of histiocytes.

Clinical Findings

▪ Histiocytoid cardiomyopathy occurs in infancy and early childhood at a mean age of 12 months.
▪ Symptoms include tachyarrhythmias, sudden death, and congestive heart failure.
▪ There is a female predominance of 4:1.
▪ Patients may respond to surgical removal.

Gross Pathologic Findings

▪ Nodules (1–15 mm, usually <3 mm) are raised and yellowish.
▪ All portions of the heart are involved, including valves and conduction system, subendocardially and subepicardially.

Microscopic Pathologic Findings

▪ Cells look like histiocytes but are positive for muscle markers (actin) and negative for histiocytoid markers (KP-1) by immunohistochemistry.
▪ Collections of large, pale, vacuolated, rounded or oval cells are faintly PAS positive.
▪ Ultrastructurally, there are poorly developed intercellular junctions, a marked increase in mitochondria, and few contractile elements, resembling oncocytes.

Differential Diagnosis

▪ Rhabdomyoma (described previously).
▪ Whipple's disease (see Chap. 2) shows strong PAS positivity and patients are adults.
▪ S-100 positivity, adult patients, and epicardial location differentiate granular cell tumor from histiocytoid cardiomyopathy.

Reference

Malhotra V, Ferrans VJ, Virmani R. Infantile histiocytoid cardiomyopathy: report of three cases and review of literature. Am Heart J 128:1009–1021, 1994.

PAPILLARY FIBROELASTOMA (FIBROELASTIC PAPILLOMA)

Papillary fibroelastoma is a benign tumor (probable hamartoma) composed of avascular papillary excrescences resembling Lambl's excrescences. Unlike Lambl's excrescences, papillary fibroelastomas may occur at any location on the valve and may achieve large size.

Clinical Findings

▪ Most papillary fibroelastomas do not cause symptoms and are incidental findings at autopsy, during surgery for other conditions, or on echocardiography.
▪ Left-sided tumors may be symptomatic and are increasingly detected echocardiographically and removed surgically.
▪ Symptoms include angina and transient ischemic attacks.
▪ Symptoms are caused by embolization (tumor fragments or attached thrombi) or by prolapse into coronary ostia (aortic valve tumors).
▪ Papillary fibroelastomas are usually located on aortic and mitral valves. Less commonly, they are on atria, ventricles, and tricuspid and pulmonic valves.

Gross Pathologic Findings

▪ Classic tumors look like sea anemones and are best appreciated by immersing the specimen in water.

- Surface thrombi may render the gross appearance similar to that of marantic vegetation.

Microscopic Pathologic Findings

- Papillary fronds are lined by endothelial cells.
- Elastic tissue and collagen are present in the core of the fronds, with the surrounding myxomatous matrix being lined by endothelial cells.
- Occasionally, there is little or no stainable elastin.
- Fronds lack capillaries.
- Surface thrombi may form and organize, obscuring the lesion unless stained with elastic stains.

Differential Diagnosis

- Marantic endocarditis—papillary fibroelastoma and nonbacterial thrombotic endocarditis may coexist; in cases of nonbacterial thrombotic endocarditis, underlying papillae should be sought using elastic stains.
- Myxoma—myxoma cells and capillaries are absent in papillary fibroelastoma; most myxomas lack elastic tissue.

References

Almagro UA, Perry LS, Choi H, Pinar K. Papillary fibroelastoma of the heart: report of six cases. Arch Pathol Lab Med 106:318–321, 1982.
Boone S, Higginson LA, Walley VM. Endothelial papillary fibroelastomas arising in and around the aortic sinus, filling the ostium of the right coronary artery. Arch Pathol Lab Med 116:135–137, 1992.
Edwards FH, Hale D, Cohen A, Thompson L, Pezzella AT, Virmani R. Primary cardiac valve tumors. Ann Thorac Surg 52:1127–1131, 1991.
Fishbein MC, Ferrans VJ, Roberts WC. Endocardial papillary elastofibromas. Arch Pathol 99:335–341, 1975.
McFadden PM, Lacy JR. Intracardiac papillary fibroelastoma: an occult cause of embolic neurologic deficit. Ann Thorac Surg 43:667–669, 1987.
Tazelaar HD, Locke TJ, McGregor CGA. Pathology of surgically excised primary cardiac tumors. Mayo Clin Proc 67:957–965, 1992.
Valente M, Basso C, Thiene G, et al. Fibroelastic papilloma: a not-so-benign cardiac tumor. Cardiovasc Pathol 1:161–166, 1992.

HEMANGIOMA

Benign proliferation of blood vessels may be of many histologic types; whether these lesions are neoplasms, hamartomas, or malformations is unclear.

Clinical Findings

- Hemangiomas of the heart may cause arrhythmias, syncope, sudden death, pericardial effusion, or shortness of breath. Occasionally, hemangiomas may be incidental findings on chest radiograph or echocardiography.
- Surgical excision is curative.

Gross Pathologic Findings

- Spongy or hemorrhagic masses are variably circumscribed either within myocardium or as subendocardial material projecting into a cardiac chamber.
- Tumors may occur in either ventricle or in the atrium.

Microscopic Pathologic Findings

- Hemangioma may resemble capillary, cavernous, or arteriovenous hemangiomas; often, there is a combination of histologic patterns.
- Mural hemangiomas are similar to extracardiac intramuscular hemangiomas, with the presence of fat and occasionally fibrous tissue; these are poorly circumscribed infiltrative tumors.
- Cavitary hemangiomas are more likely capillary or cavernous; a myxoid background is typical.
- There may be areas of papillary endothelial hyperplasia mimicking angiosarcoma.

Differential Diagnosis

- In angiosarcoma, clearly malignant areas with mitotic activity, cellular atypia, and necrosis are usually found.
- Capillary hemangiomas that extend into the lumen often have a myxoid background; unlike in myxoma, myxoma cells are absent, and the site of endocardial attachment is usually not near the fossa ovalis.

Reference

Burke AP, Johns J, Virmani R. Hemangiomas of the heart: a clinicopathologic study of 10 cases. Am J Cardiovasc Pathol 3:283–290, 1991.

LIPOMATOUS HYPERTROPHY, ATRIAL SEPTUM

Lipomatous hypertrophy of the atrial septum is a hamartomatous lesion composed of vacuolated "fetal" fat cells, mature fat, and hypertrophied myocytes.

Clinical Findings

- Patients are middle-aged or elderly and often obese.
- There is an association with cardiac hypertrophy.
- Supraventricular arrhythmias, sudden death, and congestive heart failure may occur.
- Imaging demonstrates a right atrial mass of fat density by MRI; transesophageal echocardiography demonstrates attachment to atrial septum better than can be demonstrated by transthoracic echocardiography.

Gross Pathologic Findings

- Lipomatous hypertrophy is generally within the atrial septum and is poorly circumscribed; it may become massive and extend into the mediastinum. The atrial septal component is not always recognizable.
- Lipomatous hypertrophy usually bulges into the right atrium; for this reason, surgically removed examples are typically described as right atrial tumors.
- Lipomatous hypertrophy is a fatty lesion; sometimes streaks of myocardial tissue are evident.

Microscopic Pathologic Findings

- A triad of cells include vacuolated brown fat cells, hypertrophic myocytes, and normal fat cells.

- Thick-walled vessels and fibrous tissue are occasionally present.
- Scattered lymphocytes may be seen.

Differential Diagnosis

- Liposarcomas are rare in the heart; hypertrophied bizarre myocytes and vacuolated fat cells should not be mistaken for malignant cells or lipoblasts.
- Cardiac lipomas are circumscribed fatty neoplasms composed of mature fat without interspersed brown fat or myocytes; these are much more rare than lipomatous hypertrophy and are usually epicardial, not intra-atrial.
- Lipomatous infiltrates may occur in cardiac hemangiomas, but these are generally mural lesions.
- Rare lipomatous hamartomas of the mitral valve occur.

Reference

Shirani J, Roberts WC. Clinical, electrocardiographic and morphologic features of massive fatty deposits ("lipomatous hypertrophy") in the atrial septum. J Am Coll Cardiol 22:226–238, 1993.

MISCELLANEOUS TUMOR-LIKE LESIONS, PSEUDOTUMORS, AND CYSTS

Hypertrophic Cardiomyopathy

- Fifty percent of patients with hypertrophic cardiomyopathy have significant left ventricular outflow tract obstruction with a significant hemodynamic gradient.
- In these patients, surgeons may resect asymmetric septum adjacent to the anterior leaflet of the mitral valve in the aortic outflow (septal myotomy/myectomy).
- Gross features of myectomy specimens demonstrate areas of endocardial fibrosis (left ventricular outflow tract plaque), which correspond to friction lesions from the mitral valve.
- Microscopic features are endocardial fibrosis and myofiber disarray.
- Histologically, hypertrophic cardiomyopathy has four major components: myocyte hypertrophy, interstitial fibrosis, disorganized branching myocytes, and intramural coronary artery thickening.
- Because these features are most prominent in the inner one third of the septum, they are not seen close to the endocardial plaque and may not be prominent in myectomy specimens.
- Septal myectomy is occasionally performed in patients with aortic stenosis and aortic valve replacement to widen the left ventricular outflow tract.
- Up to 10% of patients with aortic valve stenosis and secondary septal hypertrophy require septal myectomy at the time of aortic valve replacement (see Chap. 6).
- Most patients with aortic stenosis and septal hypertrophy do not have evidence of primary hypertrophic cardiomyopathy; histologic sections do not demonstrate myofiber disarray or other features of hypertrophic cardiomyopathy.

Monocyte/Macrophage Incidental Cardiac Excrescence

- Monocyte/macrophage incidental cardiac excrescence (MICE) is a collection of detached mesothelial cells, histiocytes, and other blood cells that are most often artifacts from bypass surgery extracorporeal circulation.
- Generally, MICE is an incidental finding within atria or ventricles, usually during open heart surgery for other conditions; occasionally, MICE is seen attached to myxomas or other tumors.
- Microscopically, there is an absence of stroma or vascular supply in detached clusters of mesothelial cells, monocytes, and mononuclear inflammatory cells.
- Mesothelial cells are strongly cytokeratin positive; monocytes express macrophage markers, such as KP-1.

Calcifying Intracardiac Pseudoneoplasms

- Symptoms of calcifying intracardiac pseudoneoplasms include embolic phenomena and shortness of breath.
- Patients often have underlying diseases, such as antiphospholipid syndrome, that predispose them to thrombosis or calcification.
- Calcifying intracardiac pseudoneoplasms may occur in any of the four cardiac chambers.
- Histologically, there are nodular calcium and surface fibrin thrombi in relatively acellular lesions.

Lipomatous Hamartoma of Valves

- Lipomatous hamartomas of valves are rare lesions; approximately 10 have been reported.
- Poorly demarcated masses of fat and fibrous tissue that affect the mitral or tricuspid valve result in valvular incompetence.

Ectopic Thyroid

- Heterotopic thyroid tissue may be present within the heart and be functional.
- Often, in ectopic thyroid, there is ventricular outflow tract obstruction, typically of the right ventricle.

Intracardiac Cysts

- Intracardiac cysts in the region of the atrioventricular node and tricuspid valve are usually of endodermal origin and are classified as atrioventricular (AV) nodal tumors.
- An AV nodal tumor (previously termed mesothelioma) is an endodermal rest in an AV nodal area that causes sudden death or heart block. It is generally diagnosed at autopsy, although several have been surgically excised. Fifty percent are large enough to cause visible cysts. AV nodal tumors must be considered in the differential diagnosis of cardiac cysts that occur near the tricuspid valve.
- Rarely, bronchogenic cysts and other foregut cysts may be entirely intramyocardial (see Chap. 14).
- Foregut cysts are typically invested by a layer of smooth muscle and may show evidence of bronchogenic differentiation.

- Inflammatory processes (such as hydatids or echinococcal cysts) must be considered in the differential diagnosis of cardiac cysts.
- Blood cysts of the tricuspid and mitral valves are common incidental findings at infant autopsy. Rarely, they may persist and achieve a size of several centimeters, resulting in tricuspid stenosis. They are dark red, thin-walled, unicavitary cysts that, on microscopic examination, are simple endothelium-lined cysts filled with blood.

References

Courtice RW, Stinson WA, Walley VM. Tissue fragments recovered at cardiac surgery masquerading as tumoral proliferations; evidence suggesting iatrogenic or artifactual origin and common occurrence. Am J Surg Pathol 18:167–174, 1994.

Crotty TB, Edwards WD, Oh JK, Rodeheffer RJ. Lipomatous hamartoma of the tricuspid valve: echocardiographic–pathologic correlations. Clin Cardiol 14:262–266, 1991.

RARE BENIGN NEOPLASMS

- Paragangliomas are generally present in the atria or on the epicardial surfaces (see Chap. 14). They are rarely malignant, and 50% are functional, causing hypertension. Histologic and immunohistochemical findings are identical to those of extracardiac paragangliomas. The term "pheochromocytoma" is occasionally used for functional tumors.
- Neurofibroma and schwannoma may be present in patients with neurofibromatosis and may cause ventricular outflow obstruction. They are extremely rare in the heart.
- Granular cell tumors are epicardial nodules, usually near the left main coronary artery, that are seen as incidental autopsy findings. They are probably underdiagnosed but are not clinically significant.

- Cardiac teratoma occurs in utero or in newborns, most often in the pericardial space (see Chap. 14) or in the ventricular septum extending into the right ventricular outflow tract. Rare malignant cases have been reported.
- Lipomas are usually asymptomatic epicardial tumors. Occasionally, they are large and multiple. They may be excised to relieve congestive heart failure.
- Inflammatory pseudotumors are benign neoplasms of myofibroblastic derivation that occur rarely in the heart without site predilection. Synonyms include plasma cell granuloma, inflammatory fibrous histiocytoma, and inflammatory myofibroblastic tumor. They may be associated with hypergammaglobulinemia and fever. Histologically, there is a proliferation of compact spindle cells with intermingled lymphocytes, plasma cells, and eosinophils, resembling fibrous histiocytoma or nodular fasciitis. The immunohistochemical profile is nonspecific, with positivity for muscle-specific actin and vimentin.

References

Abad C, Jimenez P, Santana C, et al. Primary cardiac paraganglioma. Case report and review of surgically treated cases. J Cardiovasc Surg 33:758–772, 1992.

Betancourt B, Defendini EA, Johnson C, et al. Severe right ventricular outflow tract obstruction caused by an intracavitary cardiac neurilemoma: successful surgical removal and postoperative diagnosis. Chest 75:522–524, 1979.

Fenoglio JJ Jr, McAllister HA Jr. Granular cell tumors of the heart. Arch Pathol Lab Med 100:276–278, 1976.

Gopalakrishnan R, Ticzon AR, Cruz PA, et al. Cardiac paraganglioma (chemodectoma). A case report and review of the literature. J Thorac Cardiovasc Surg 76:183–189, 1978.

Hui G, McAllister HA, Angelini P. Left atrial paraganglioma: report of a case and review of the literature. Am Heart J 113:1230–1234, 1987.

Johnson TL, Shapiro B, Beierwalters WH, et al. Cardiac paragangliomas. A clinicopathologic and immunohistochemical study of four cases. Am J Surg Pathol 11:827–834, 1985.

Tractos S, Turi G, Bienpica L. Primary cardiac neurilemoma. Cancer 37:883–886, 1976.

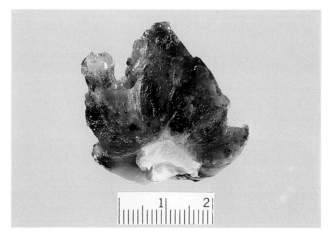

Figure 11–1. Cardiac myxoma. There is a mucoid mass attached to a portion of the atrial septum by a broad-based stalk.

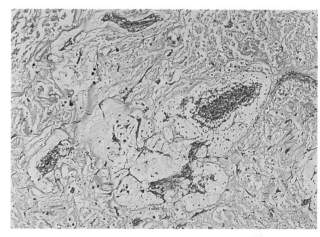

Figure 11–2. Cardiac myxoma. The diagnostic feature of cardiac myxoma is the myxoma cell, which forms elongated cords and rings clustered around capillaries.

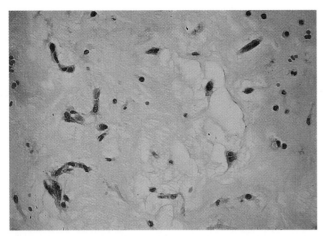

Figure 11–3. Cardiac myxoma. Myxoma cells are stellate, are multinucleate, and have a propensity to form cords and rings. There is abundant cytoplasm with poorly demarcated borders, and bland, oval nuclei.

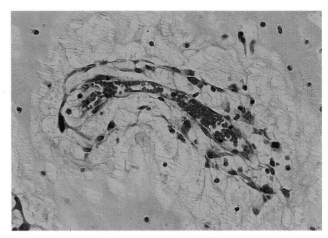

Figure 11–4. Cardiac myxoma. Myxoma cells typically form rings, which surround capillaries; these structures are often infiltrated by mononuclear inflammatory cells.

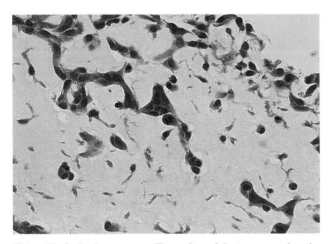

Figure 11–5. Cardiac myxoma. The surface of the tumor may be relatively cellular, and there are branching structures of multinucleated myxoma cells.

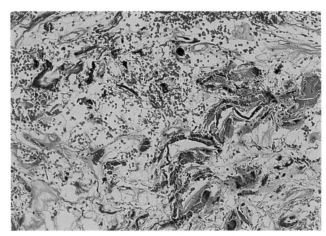

Figure 11–6. Cardiac myxoma. Degenerative changes are common; in this example, there are elongated structures impregnated with iron and elastic fibers (Gamna bodies).

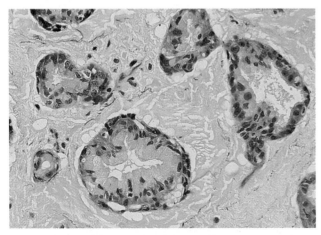

Figure 11–7. Cardiac myxoma, Movat pentachrome. One percent of cardiac myxomas possess glands lined by goblet cells; unlike in metastatic adenocarcinoma, there are no mitotic figures or atypia.

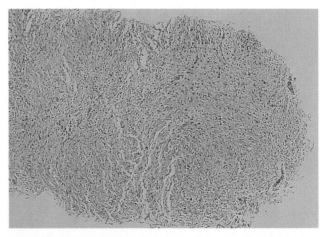

Figure 11–8. Cardiac fibroma. A needle biopsy was performed on a large, infiltrating cardiac mass that could not be resected. The mass is moderately cellular.

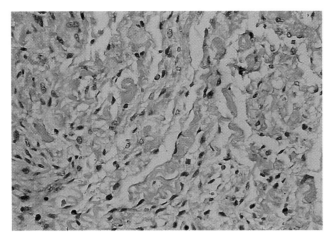

Figure 11–9. Cardiac fibroma. A higher magnification of Figure 11–8 demonstrates fibroblasts in a collagenous background.

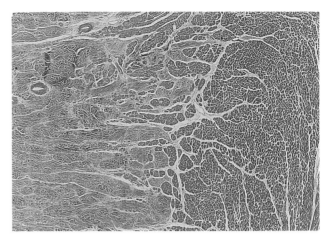

Figure 11–10. Cardiac fibroma. A Masson trichrome stain demonstrates a fibrous mass infiltrating adjacent myocardium. Fibromas in adults and children are much less cellular than those of infants.

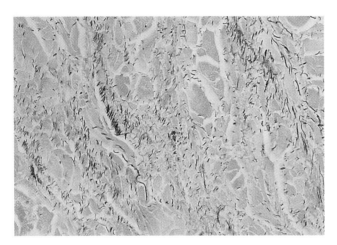

Figure 11–11. Cardiac fibroma. An elastic van Gieson stain demonstrates elastic fibers in the tumor illustrated in Figure 11–10.

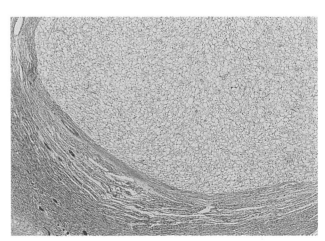

Figure 11–12. Cardiac rhabdomyoma. These are circumscribed, noninfiltrating tumors composed of clear, vacuolated cells.

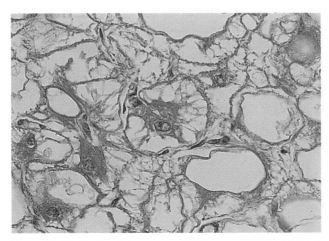

Figure 11–13. Cardiac rhabdomyoma. A higher magnification of Figure 11–12 demonstrates the diagnostic "spider cell" with circumferential cytoplasmic vacuoles surrounding a centrally located nucleus; note the strands of retracted cytoplasm.

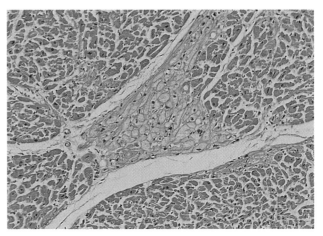

Figure 11–14. Histiocytoid cardiomyopathy. Note the collection of small clear cells. The collections are usually smaller than tumors of rhabdomyoma and are not as well demarcated.

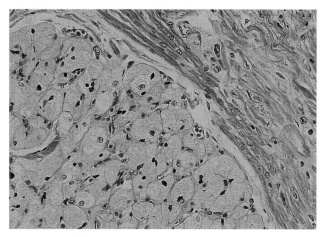

Figure 11–15. Histiocytoid cardiomyopathy. In contrast to cells of rhabdomyoma, the cells resemble histiocytes, have small vacuoles, and lack evident myofilaments.

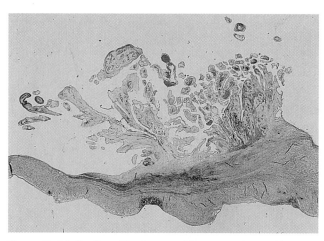

Figure 11–16. Papillary fibroelastoma, Movat pentachrome. Numerous papillary fronds emanate from the valve surface. There are focal areas of elastic fibers, stained black.

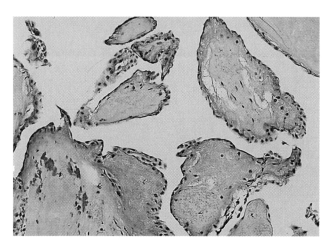

Figure 11–17. Papillary fibroelastoma. The papillary fronds are avascular, are lined by endothelial cells, and contain sparse spindle cells within the core.

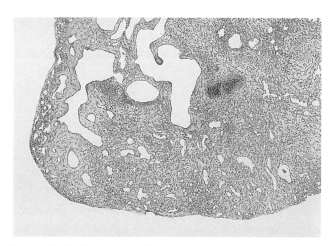

Figure 11–18. Hemangioma. This tumor, which projected into the ventricular cavity, is composed of vascular channels of various sizes.

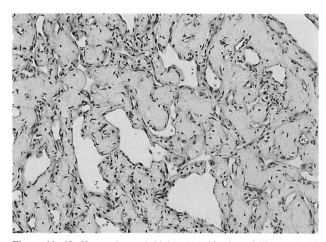

Figure 11–19. Hemangioma. A higher magnification of Figure 11–18 demonstrates a mixture of cavernous and capillary spaces.

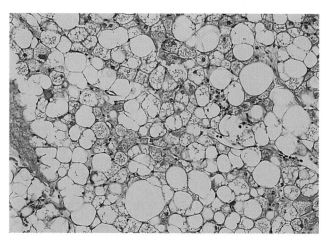

Figure 11–20. Lipomatous hypertrophy, atrial septum. Hypertrophied myocytes are present among mature and multivacuolated (brown) fat cells.

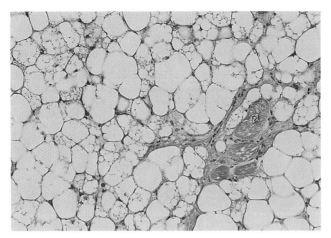

Figure 11–21. Lipomatous hypertrophy, atrial septum. A higher magnification of Figure 11–20 demonstrates hypertrophied myocytes.

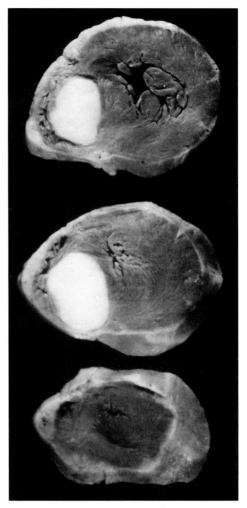

Figure 11–22. Lipoma. Rarely, lipomas may be intramyocardial or intracavitary lesions, as in this example; more commonly, they are located on the epicardial surface. (Courtesy of Dr. Leroy Riddick.)

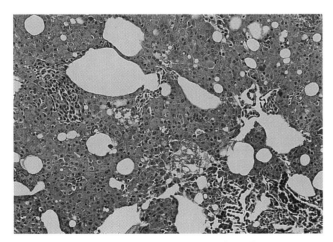

Figure 11–23. Monocyte/macrophage incidental cardiac excrescence. There are detached clusters of cells with interspersed fat globules.

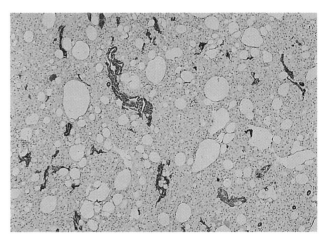

Figure 11–24. Monocyte/macrophage incidental cardiac excrescence. Immunohistochemical stain for cytokeratin demonstrates positivity in mesothelial cells; histiocytes and fat cells do not stain.

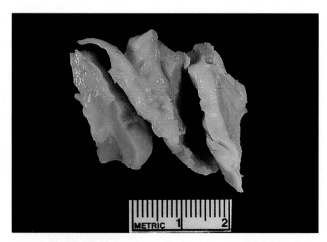

Figure 11–25. Hypertrophic cardiomyopathy, myectomy specimen. Note the pieces of myocardium with marked endocardial thickening.

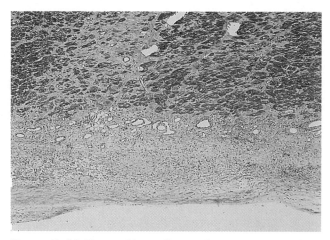

Figure 11–26. Hypertrophic cardiomyopathy, myectomy specimen. There is marked endocardial fibrosis. Photomicrograph of specimen illustrated in Figure 11–25.

CHAPTER 12

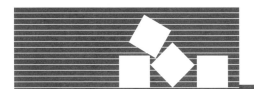

Malignant Cardiac Tumors

OVERVIEW OF CARDIAC SARCOMAS

Primary malignant cardiac neoplasms are of connective tissue origin (Table 12–1).

Patient Characteristics and Clinical Findings

- There is no sex predilection for cardiac sarcomas as a group.
- The mean age at presentation is 41 years, although diagnosis may be made at any age.
- In infants and children, cardiac sarcomas are rare and are usually undifferentiated sarcomas or rhabdomyosarcomas.
- Symptoms and complications include dyspnea, chest pain, pericardial effusion, syncope, hemoptysis, sudden death, metastatic masses, fever, obstruction of hepatic vein, and superior vena caval obstruction.
- Diagnosis is best made by echocardiography in conjunction with magnetic resonance imaging (MRI) or computed tomography (CT) scans.

Pathologic Findings

- The left atrium is the site of 50% of cardiac sarcomas; these often project into the cavity, mimicking myxoma.
- Unlike myxoma, left atrial sarcomas are often multinodular or multiple, infiltrating the atrial wall or valves.
- Occasionally, cardiac sarcomas are pedunculated, intracavitary lesions with little gross myocardial infiltration; therefore, the distinction between a benign and malignant tumor is not always possible on gross or radiographic findings.
- Right atrial tumors are generally angiosarcomas; these are multiple, hemorrhagic masses that usually extend into the pericardium.
- Left atrial tumors generally are malignant fibrous histiocytoma (MFH), leiomyosarcoma, or osteosarcoma.
- Cystic, hemorrhagic, and necrotic areas may impart a variegated gross appearance on biopsy section, or the tumor may be relatively homogeneous, white, and firm.

- Calcification is especially frequent in left atrial sarcomas; often, these areas correspond to malignant osteoid (osteosarcoma).
- Focal areas of myxoid stroma are common in cardiac sarcomas, especially in tumors arising in the left atrium, such as fibrosarcoma, malignant fibrous histiocytoma, and leiomyosarcoma.

Tumor Grading

- There is no universal grading of cardiac sarcoma.
- Tumors with necrosis are considered high grade, regardless of mitotic rate.
- Tumors with more than 1 mitosis/high-power field in the most mitotically active area of tumor are considered high grade.
- Tumors with fewer than 1 mitosis/high-power field are considered low grade.

Survival, Metastatic Sites

- Survival appears to be independent of histologic type.
- Mean survival for most types of cardiac sarcomas is approximately 9 months.
- The presence of tumor necrosis and high mitotic rates are indicative of relatively poor prognosis.
- Metastatic sites include lung, vertebrae, liver, brain, bowel, lymph nodes, long bones, spleen, adrenal glands, and skull.

Differential Diagnosis

- The most common pitfall is the misdiagnosis of myxoid cardiac sarcoma as myxoma; both lesions typically occur in the left atrium and are endophytic masses projecting into the atrial cavity.
- Sarcomas often have multiple attachment sites, not necessarily at the fossa ovalis, often grow within the cardiac wall, histologically lack myxoma cells and abundant hemosiderin, and generally contain easily identifiable mitotic figures.
- Metastatic spindle cell carcinoma, especially of renal cell origin, must always be considered in the differential diagnosis of right atrial tumors; renal cell carcino-

Table 12–1
CARDIAC SARCOMAS

Histologic Type	M:F	Mean Age	Total Cases (%)	Favored Site
Angiosarcoma	2.5:1	40	25–40	Right atrium, pericardium
Malignant fibrous histiocytoma	1:1	44	10–30	Left atrium
Fibrosarcoma or myxosarcoma	1:1.5	40	10–20	Left atrium
Unclassified sarcoma	1:1	35	5–20	Left atrium, ventricle
Leiomyosarcoma	1:1	35	5–10	Left atrium
Rhabdomyosarcoma	1.4:1	25	5–10	None (ventricles or atria)
Osteosarcoma	1:1	35	3–10	Left atrium
Liposarcoma	1:1	60	2–5	Atria
Synovial sarcoma	4:1	40	1–3	Ventricles, pericardium
Neural sarcoma			<1	Epicardial surfaces
Miscellaneous*			<1	Diverse sites

*Malignant mesenchymoma, malignant Triton tumor (neurofibrosarcoma with rhabdomyosarcoma), malignant rhabdoid tumor, and malignant hemangiopericytoma.

mas contain glycogen, epithelial membrane antigen, and, generally, cytokeratin.

■ Although extracardiac sarcomas metastasize to the heart in the end stage of disease in up to 25% of cases, it is rare for an extracardiac sarcoma to present as a cardiac mass. Nevertheless, metastatic sarcoma should always be considered in the differential diagnosis of primary cardiac sarcoma, especially if the tumor is in the right atrium and the histologic pattern is not that of angiosarcoma.

References

Bear PA, Moodie DS. Malignant primary cardiac tumors. The Cleveland Clinic experience, 1956 to 1986. Chest 92:860–862, 1987.

Burke AP, Cowan D, Virmani R. Cardiac sarcomas. Cancer 69:387–395, 1992.

Flipse TR, Tazelaar HD, Holmes DR Jr. Diagnosis of malignant cardiac disease by endomyocardial biopsy. Mayo Clin Proc 65:1415–1422, 1990.

McAllister HA, Fenoglio JJ Jr. *Tumors of the Cardiovascular System.* Washington, DC, Armed Forces Institute of Pathology, 1978, pp 81–102.

Murphy MC, Sweeney MS, Putnam JB Jr, et al. Surgical treatment of cardiac tumors: a 25-year experience. Ann Thorac Surg 49:612–617, 1990.

Putnam JB Jr, Sweeney MS, Colon R, Lanza LA, Frazier OH, Cooley DA. Primary cardiac sarcomas. Ann Thorac Surg 5:906–910, 1991.

Reece IJ, Cooley DA, Frazier OH, Hallman GL, Powers PL, Montero GC. Cardiac tumors: clinical spectrum and prognosis of lesions other than classical benign myxoma in 20 patients. J Thorac Cardiovasc Surg 88:439–446, 1984.

Tazelaar HD, Locke TJ, McGregor CG. Pathology of surgically excised primary cardiac tumors. Mayo Clin Proc 67:957–965, 1992.

CARDIAC SARCOMAS, SPECIFIC HISTOLOGIC TYPES

Angiosarcoma

■ The mean age at presentation of angiosarcoma is 40 years (range 9–80 years).

■ Angiosarcoma shows a male predilection of approximately 2.5:1.

■ Sixty percent or more of angiosarcomas occur in the right atrium.

■ Symptoms are related to hemopericardium with tamponade, pericardial constriction, or right ventricular outflow obstruction.

■ Metastases at the time of presentation are more frequent than in other types of cardiac sarcomas, occurring in 66% to 89% of patients. The usual site of metastasis is the lung, followed by bone, liver, adrenal glands, and spleen.

■ The prognosis for survival is poor (mean survival 3 months to 2 years after diagnosis).

■ Grossly, the tumors are large and multilobular and may resemble melanoma. Typically, the bulk of the tumor is in the right atrium, with extension into the caval veins, tricuspid valve, and pericardium.

■ Angiosarcomas demonstrate vascular channels with atypical endothelial lining cells. Large areas of spindling are often present, and most tumors have areas of necrosis. Extensive sampling is necessary in some cases to find representative areas.

■ Identification of vacuoles containing red blood cells may be helpful.

■ Metastatic foci are often better differentiated and more vasoformative than the primary lesion.

■ Immunohistochemical staining for factor VIII–related antigen is specific but not sensitive; there is characteristic fine granular positivity.

■ Immunohistochemical stains for CD34 and CD21 may be helpful in establishing the diagnosis; in general, a panel of stains is preferred.

■ The differential diagnosis includes undifferentiated spindle cell sarcoma, Kaposi's sarcoma (rare in the absence of immunodeficiency), and hemangioma with papillary endothelial hyperplasia.

Malignant Fibrous Histiocytoma

■ The mean age at presentation of malignant fibrous histiocytoma is 44 years.

■ The most common location is the left atrium, resulting in symptoms of pulmonary vein obstruction, mitral stenosis or regurgitation, and right ventricular failure.

■ Less commonly, the patient may present with peripheral emboli.

- Two-dimensional echocardiography is sensitive in diagnosis of a mass, but the incorrect diagnosis of cardiac myxoma is often made.
- Cerebral aneurysms may result from hematogenous metastases in the brain.
- Grossly, the tumors are sessile or pedunculated and, often, multiple, filling or distending the atrium.
- Histologically, malignant fibrous histiocytomas are similar to their extracardiac counterparts and resemble fibrosarcomas with a greater degree of pleomorphism and histiocyte-like cells.
- Myxoid areas are frequent, and myxoid malignant fibrous histiocytomas as seen in soft tissue are also present in the heart.
- Immunohistochemically, there is usually absence of expression of cytokeratin, desmin, and S-100 protein, and there is positive staining for vimentin. Expression of smooth muscle actin and muscle-specific actin varies.
- The most common diagnostic pitfall is the differential diagnosis with myxoma. Areas of mitotic activity, branching vascular network, and pleomorphism suggest malignant fibrous histiocytoma; in addition, myxoma cells are absent.

Fibrosarcoma

- Cardiac fibrosarcoma is a poorly defined entity that includes myxoid spindle cell sarcoma, so-called fibromyxosarcoma, and so-called myxosarcoma.
- Like other cardiac sarcomas with fibroblastic differentiation (MFH, osteosarcoma, unclassifiable sarcomas), the most common location is the left atrium.
- Long-term prognosis is poor.
- Grossly, fibrosarcomas are soft, polypoid tumors that may fill the atrium or infiltrate ventricles.
- Histologically, fibrosarcomas are cellular tumors with mild to moderate pleomorphism and are composed entirely of spindle cells.
- Unlike in leiomyosarcoma, there are no perinuclear vacuoles, intracytoplasmic glycogen, or intracytoplasmic desmin.
- Unlike in MFH, there are no storiform areas or large, bizarre histiocytic cells.
- "Myxosarcomas" (also called myxofibrosarcoma, fibromyxosarcoma) represent 10% to 20% of primary cardiac sarcomas. These are diffusely myxoid and are composed of spindle cells. Most are best classified as myxoid fibrosarcoma.

Unclassified Sarcoma

- Up to 25% of cardiac sarcomas are not easily classified into extracardiac sarcoma categories and are termed either undifferentiated or unclassifiable.
- The most common location is the left atrium, but any site in the heart, including ventricles and pericardium, may be involved.
- Prognosis for survival is poor, with mean survival measured in months.
- Metastases occur in the lungs and various viscera.
- Histologic patterns include pleomorphic and small round cell varieties, as well as spindle cell sarcomas of myofibroblastic appearance.
- Immunohistochemically, there may be positivity for smooth muscle actin and vimentin. In general, there is an absence of expression of endothelial markers, S-100 protein, desmin, and cytokeratin.

Leiomyosarcoma

- The mean age at presentation of leiomyosarcoma is the fourth decade.
- Most cases occur in the left atrium and may be extensions of sarcomas of pulmonary veins.
- Symptoms are usually the same as with other types of atrial tumors, including dyspnea and congestive failure.
- Budd-Chiari syndrome may occur in patients with right atrial leiomyosarcoma; these tumors may represent extensions of leiomyosarcomas of the inferior vena cava.
- Prognosis for survival is poor, generally measured in months.
- Leiomyosarcomas resemble their extracardiac counterparts; myxoid areas are not uncommon, and epithelioid leiomyosarcomas or areas with epithelioid differentiation occur occasionally.
- Cells form compact fascicles that are often oriented at right angles to one another; fuchsinophilic longitudinal filaments may be seen with Masson trichrome stain.
- Intracytoplasmic glycogen and perinuclear vacuoles are histologic features that aid in the diagnosis.
- Approximately 50% of leiomyosarcomas are desmin positive; thin filaments with focal densities may be seen ultrastructurally, but dense bodies are not considered specific for leiomyosarcoma.

Rhabdomyosarcoma

- The mean age of patients with cardiac rhabdomyosarcoma is approximately 35 years (10–20 years younger than for other sarcomas).
- Rhabdomyosarcomas are relatively uncommon as a subtype of cardiac sarcoma and are generally seen in children and young adults.
- Unlike cardiac sarcomas of fibrous or smooth muscle differentiation, there is no predilection for the left atrium; any cardiac chamber may be involved.
- Virtually all cardiac rhabdomyosarcomas are of the embryonal type.
- Diagnosis depends on the demonstration of rhabdomyoblasts, which may be sparse.
- Rhabdomyoblasts are best located by periodic acid–Schiff (PAS) positivity and confirmation with immunostain for desmin, which is sensitive and helpful in diagnosis, or for myoglobin, which is less sensitive.
- The differential diagnosis includes leiomyosarcoma and undifferentiated or unclassifiable round cell sarcoma.

Osteosarcoma

- Osteosarcoma is defined by the presence of malignant osteoid, which contains atypical osteocytes; often, chondrosarcoma or malignant giant cell tumor is present.

- Osteosarcoma is almost exclusively located in the left atrium.
- Clinically, dyspnea is the most common symptom, and complications include congestive heart failure, recurrent pneumonia, mitral valve obstruction, pulmonary hypertension, and syncope.
- The most common clinical diagnosis is left atrial myxoma.
- Metastases may occur to skin, lymph nodes, thyroid, lung, and thoracotomy incisions.
- Grossly, osteosarcomas are bulky tumors attached to the atrial wall.
- The surface of the tumor may be mucoid or gelatinous, but gritty, firm areas are present within the tumor mass.
- Microscopically, large areas of tumor may resemble fibrosarcoma; diagnostic areas are indistinguishable from osteosarcoma of bone.
- There may be areas indistinguishable from fibrosarcoma, giant cell tumor, and chondrosarcoma.
- Myxoid areas may be prominent, resulting in the incorrect diagnosis of myxoma.
- Immunohistochemically, spindled areas are focally actin positive and vimentin positive; S-100 protein is expressed by chondrosarcomatous areas, if present.

Miscellaneous Histologic Types

- Liposarcomas, synovial sarcomas, neurofibrosarcomas, and malignant Triton tumors are rare as primary cardiac lesions.
- Malignant mesenchymomas have been described in the heart and pulmonary artery. These are composed of two separate types of tissue differentiation, in addition to fibrous tissue (e.g., rhabdomyosarcoma and angiosarcoma).
- Kaposi's sarcoma generally occurs in the heart as multiple masses in immunocompromised patients; it is usually considered a multicentric process.

References

Burke AP, Virmani R. Osteosarcomas of the heart. Am J Surg Pathol 15:289–295, 1991.
Herrmann MA, Shankerman RA, Edwards WD, Shub C, Schaff HV. Primary cardiac angiosarcoma: a clinicopathologic study of six cases. J Thorac Cardiovasc Surg 103:655–664, 1992.
Hui KS, Green LK, Schmidt WA. Primary cardiac rhabdomyosarcoma: definition of a rare entity. Am J Cardiovasc Pathol 2:19–29, 1988.
Janigan DT, Husain A, Robinson NA. Cardiac angiosarcomas. A review and a case report. Cancer 57:852–859, 1986.
Johansson L, Kugelberg J, Thulin L. Myxofibrosarcoma in the left atrium originally presented as a cardiac myxoma with chondroid differentiation. A clinicopathological report. APMIS 97:833–838, 1989.
Karn CM, Socinski MA, Fletcher JA, Corson JM, Craighead JE. Cardiac synovial sarcoma with translocation (X18) associated with asbestos exposure. Cancer 73:74–78, 1994.
Knobel B, Rosman P, Kishon Y, Husar M. Intracardiac primary fibrosarcoma. Case report and literature review. Thorac Cardiovasc Surg 40:227–230, 1992.
Laya MB, Maillard JA, Bewtra C, Levin HS. Malignant fibrous histiocytoma of the heart. A case report and review of the literature. Cancer 59:1026–1031, 1987.
McKenney PA, Moroz K, Haudenschild CC, Shemin RJ, Davidoff R. Malignant mesenchymoma as a primary cardiac tumor. Am Heart J 123:1071–1075, 1992.
Ovcak Z, Masera A, Lamovec J. Malignant fibrous histiocytoma of the heart. Arch Pathol Lab Med 116:872–874, 1992.
Paraf F, Bruneval P, Balaton A, et al. Primary liposarcoma of the heart. Am J Cardiovasc Pathol 3:175–180, 1990.
Siebenmann R, Jenni R, Makek M, Oelz W, James CL, Leong AS. Epithelioid leiomyosarcoma of the left atrium: immunohistochemical and ultrastructural findings. Pathology 21:308–313, 1989.
Terashima K, Aoyama K, Nihei K, et al. Malignant fibrous histiocytoma of the heart. Cancer 52:1919–1926, 1983.

METASTATIC CARDIAC TUMORS

Clinical Findings

- Patients with metastatic tumors in the heart may experience valvular or ventricular outflow obstruction that may be treated palliatively by surgical resection.
- Generally, the cardiac deposits are not isolated lesions.
- Rarely, the cardiac deposits are resected for potential cure and are considered isolated metastases.
- Occasionally, a cardiac metastasis is resected as an incidental finding at open heart surgery for coronary artery disease.
- In series of surgically resected cardiac tumors, metastatic lesions constitute 3% to 17% of all tumor resections and 22% to 61% of malignant tumors.

Pathologic Findings

- Metastatic tumors of all types, including carcinomas, germ cell tumors, sarcomas, melanomas, and endocrine tumors, have been surgically removed from the heart.
- Intracavitary tumors are direct extensions from the venae cavae or pulmonary veins.
- Mural tumors are hematogenous metastases from sarcomas or carcinomas.
- The histologic features of metastatic tumors are similar to those of their corresponding primary tumors.

Differential Diagnosis

- Primary sarcoma and metastatic sarcoma are impossible to differentiate histologically. A metastatic process should always be considered in the case of a right atrial mass.

References

Abraham DP, Reddy V, Gattusa P. Neoplasms metastatic to the heart: review of 3314 consecutive autopsies. Am J Cardiovasc Pathol 3:195–198, 1990.
Labib SB, Schick EC, Isner JM. Obstruction of right ventricular outflow tract caused by intracavitary metastatic disease: analysis of 14 cases. J Am Coll Cardiol 19:1664–1668, 1992.
Lestuzzi C, Biasi S, Nicolosi GL, et al. Secondary neoplastic infiltration of the myocardium diagnosed by two-dimensional echocardiography in seven cases with anatomic confirmation. J Am Coll Cardiol 9:439–445, 1987.
Poole GV Jr, Meredith JW, Breyer RH, Mills SA. Surgical implications in malignant cardiac disease. Ann Thorac Surg 36:484–491, 1983.

LYMPHOMA

Primary cardiac lymphoma is a cardiac mass; regional lymph node involvement may be found, but the bulk of the tumor is intrapericardial.

Incidence and Patient Characteristics

■ Primary lymphomas of the heart are rare; only 50 to 100 cases have been reported.

■ Primary lymphomas of the heart diagnosed by surgical biopsy are especially rare.

■ Fifty percent of cardiac lymphomas occur in patients who are immunosuppressed, either from allografts or acquired immunodeficiency syndrome.

■ In the remainder of patients, the mean age at presentation is 58 years (range 13–80 years).

Pathogenesis

■ Lymphomas in immunosuppressed patients often evolve through a polyclonal, benign lymphoid proliferation (posttransplant lymphoproliferative disorder) that may be histologically difficult to distinguish from severe rejection.

■ Most lymphomas arising in immunocompromised patients contain episomal Epstein-Barr virus DNA, which is believed to be oncogenic.

Clinical Findings

■ Clinical findings include congestive heart failure, chest pain, and complete heart block and other conduction system disturbances.

■ Localization and assessment of response to treatment are facilitated by transesophageal echocardiography, magnetic resonance imaging, and computed tomography.

■ Staging of disease is accomplished by bone marrow biopsy and imaging of mediastinal lymph nodes.

Pathologic Findings

■ Grossly, tumors are firm, white nodules.

■ Most common sites of involvement include the right atrium, atrial septum, and ventricular septum. More than one chamber is involved in more than 75% of cases. Rare lymphomas are confined to the adventitia of a coronary artery.

■ Cardiac lymphomas that have been immunophenotypically characterized have been B-cell lesions.

■ Most cardiac lymphomas are high grade (large cell, large cell immunoblastic, small cell undifferentiated).

References

Brucker EA, Glassy FJ. Primary reticulum cell sarcoma of the heart with review of the literature. Cancer 8:921–931, 1955.

Castelli MJ, Mihalov ML, Posniak HV, Gattuso P. Primary cardiac lymphoma initially diagnosed by routine cytology. Case report and literature review. Acta Cytol 33:335–338, 1989.

Curtsinger CR, Wilson MJ, Yoneda K. Primary cardiac lymphoma. Cancer 64:521–525, 1989.

Gardiner DS, Lindop GBM. Coronary artery aneurysm due to primary cardiac lymphoma. Histopathology 15:537–540, 1989.

Goldfarb A, King CL, Rosenzweig BP, et al. Cardiac lymphoma in the acquired immunodeficiency syndrome. Am Heart J 118:1340–1344, 1989.

Holladay AO, Siegel RJ, Schwartz EA. Cardiac malignant lymphoma in acquired immune deficiency syndrome. Cancer 70:2203–2207, 1992.

Moore JA, DeRan BP, Minor R, Arthur J, Fraker TD. Transesophageal echocardiographic evaluation of intracardiac lymphoma. Am Heart J 124:514–516, 1992.

Rodenburg CJ, Kluin P, Maes A, Paul LC. Malignant lymphoma confined to the heart, 13 years after a cadaver kidney transplant. N Engl J Med 313:122, 1985.

Takagi M, Kugimiya T, Fujii T, et al. Extensive surgery for primary malignant lymphoma of the heart. J Cardiovasc Surg 33:570–572, 1992.

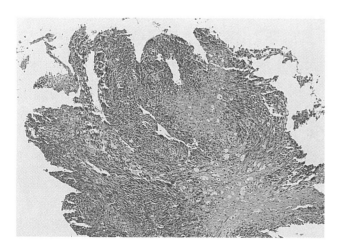

Figure 12–1. Angiosarcoma. Because these tumors usually occur on the right side of the heart, they are accessible to endomyocardial biopsy. This biopsy sample of a tumor was taken from a 45-year-old woman with signs of right-heart failure.

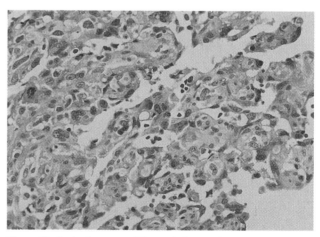

Figure 12–2. Angiosarcoma. Diagnostic features include atypical papillary tufts lined by malignant cells, anastomosing vascular structures, and endothelial cytoplasmic vacuoles containing red blood cells.

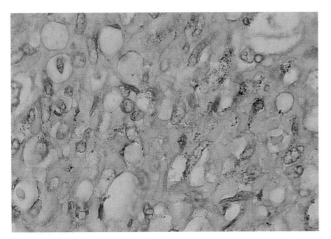

Figure 12–3. Angiosarcoma. An immunohistochemical stain for factor VIII–related antigen may demonstrate characteristic punctate positivity within the cytoplasm.

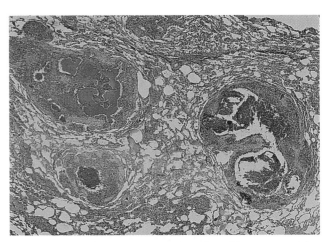

Figure 12–4. Angiosarcoma, metastatic to lung. Metastases are often better differentiated than the primary cardiac lesion.

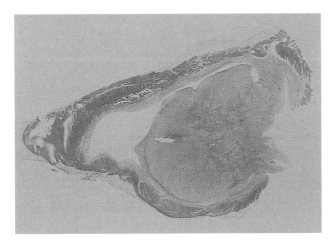

Figure 12–5. Myxoid sarcoma. These tumors are often predominantly intracavitary, mimicking myxoma. This lesion filled the left atrial cavity.

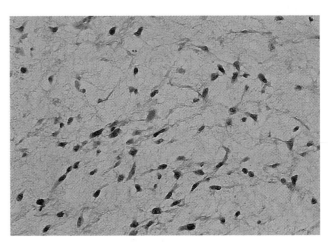

Figure 12–6. Myxoid sarcoma. Some areas of tumor may be deceptively bland and erroneously diagnosed as myxoma. Unlike in myxoma, there are no myxoma cells, and cords and rings are not identified (see Chap. 11). Other areas demonstrate diagnostic features of sarcoma.

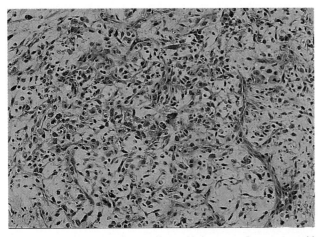

Figure 12–7. Myxoid malignant fibrous histiocytoma. In most myxoid sarcomas, areas of storiform growth and prominent branching vessels are seen, as in this tumor. These features are never present in myxoma.

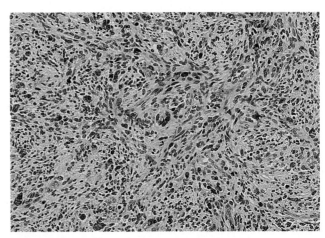

Figure 12–8. This example of cardiac malignant fibrous histiocytoma lacks myxoid stroma and is composed of tightly packed, atypical fibrohistiocytic cells in a storiform pattern.

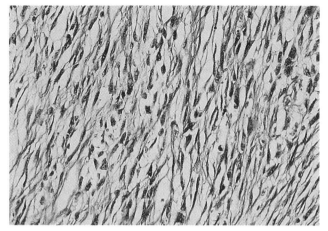

Figure 12–9. Fibrosarcoma. Like malignant fibrous histiocytoma, cardiac fibrosarcomas are generally found in the left atrium. Unlike malignant fibrous histiocytoma, there are no histiocytoid cells, and there is less pleomorphism.

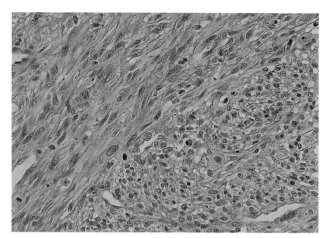

Figure 12–10. Leiomyosarcoma. Cardiac leiomyosarcomas resemble their soft-tissue counterparts: there is abundant cytoplasm, and dense fascicles of cells are often at right angles to one another.

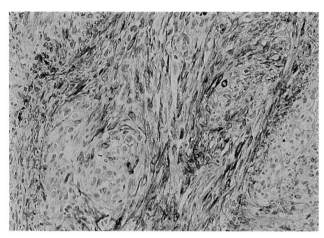

Figure 12–11. Leiomyosarcoma. In more than 50% of these tumors, positivity for desmin is present. This finding in a cellular spindle cell tumor is nearly diagnostic of leiomyosarcoma.

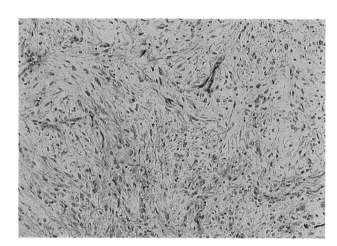

Figure 12–12. Leiomyosarcoma, myxoid area. A different area of tumor illustrated in Figures 12–10 and 12–11 demonstrates myxoid ground substance. Myxoid areas are common in cardiac tumors that project into the atrial or ventricular cavity and may be seen in sarcomas, myxomas, and hemangiomas.

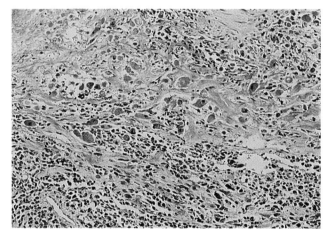

Figure 12–13. Rhabdomyosarcoma. In the heart, rhabdomyosarcomas are of the embryonal type and are seen in children and young adults. There is a mixture of small, undifferentiated round cells and rhabdomyoblasts.

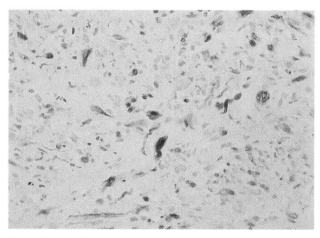

Figure 12–14. Rhabdomyosarcoma. The rhabdomyoblasts stain strongly with desmin (illustrated) as well as myoglobin; the latter is not as sensitive a marker, however.

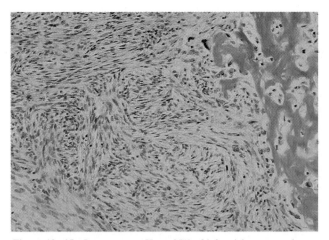

Figure 12–15. Osteosarcoma. Up to 25% of left atrial sarcomas demonstrate areas of osteosarcoma or chondrosarcoma. In this tumor, osteoid is present in the right side of the field, adjacent to a spindle cell tumor resembling fibrosarcoma. Reactive bone may occur in myxoma and fibroma, but it is mature and does not show atypical cells within lacunar spaces.

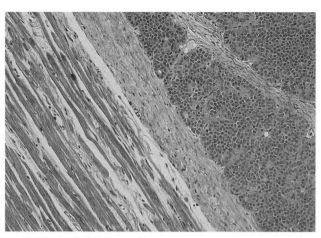

Figure 12–16. Metastatic carcinoid tumor, heart. A wide variety of metastatic lesions may be removed surgically from the ventricles or atria. This lesion, which is typical of a carcinoid tumor histologically, was an incidental finding at open heart surgery for coronary artery disease.

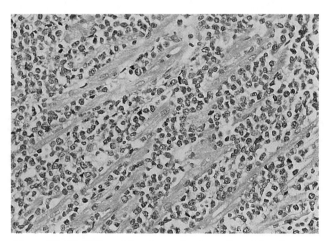

Figure 12–17. Malignant lymphoma. Rarely, malignant lymphoma occurs in the heart as a primary tumor. This undifferentiated small cell lymphoma, which was typed as a B-cell lesion, is seen infiltrating cardiac muscle fibers; the specimen was obtained at cardiac surgery.

SECTION ■ 4

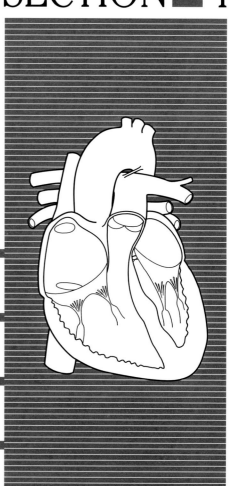

DISEASES OF THE PERICARDIUM

CHAPTER 13

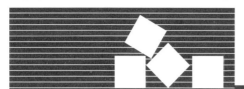

Non-neoplastic Diseases of the Pericardium

Diagnoses made by pericardial biopsy are listed in Table 13–1.

NORMAL PERICARDIUM

Parietal Pericardium

- Outer tough covering
- Composed of broad fibrocollagenous tissue lined by mesothelial cells
- Right and left anterior surfaces are fused with pleura, resulting in a fibrous layer lined on two sides by mesothelium

Visceral Pericardium

- Delicate fibrocollagenous fatty layer overlying epicardial surface
- Lined by mesothelial cells

Pericardial Cavity

- Normally contains 15 to 50 mL of viscous, straw-colored fluid
- Encircled by a continuous mesothelial layer of parietal and visceral pericardium

ACUTE PERICARDITIS

Acute pericarditis is inflammation of the pericardium, resulting in a clinical syndrome characterized by chest pain, pericardial friction rub, and serial electrocardiographic ST-segment changes. Because acute pericarditis is rarely treated with surgery, it is rarely diagnosed in the surgical pathology laboratory.

Causes

- Idiopathic (viral) pericarditis
- Uremia
- Bacterial infection (tuberculous and nontuberculous)
- Acute myocardial infarction
- Postpericardiotomy
- Neoplasms
- Trauma
- Connective tissue diseases

Incidence

- Two percent to 6% of autopsies
- A total of 1/1000 hospital admissions
- Male predominance, uncommon in children

Gross Pathologic Findings

- Dull surface
- Fibrinous adhesions between visceral and parietal pericardium
- Adhesions between sternum and parietal pericardium
- Pericardial effusion

Table 13–1
PERICARDIAL BIOPSIES, EXCLUDING NEOPLASMS AND CYSTS, AFIP* 1970–1993

Diagnosis	Number
Nonspecific (most prominent feature)	
Mesothelial hyperplasia with fibrin deposits	43
Fibrosis	34
Calcification	2
Small vessel vasculitis	2
Cholesterol deposits	2
Granulomatous pericarditis	8
Radiation-induced constrictive pericarditis	4
Collagen vascular disease (clinical)	
Rheumatoid arthritis, nonspecific histology	1
Rheumatoid nodules in pericardial biopsy	1
Lupus erythematosus	1
Scleroderma	1
Hypereosinophilic syndrome	2
Tuberculous pericarditis	2
Amyloidosis	1
Purulent bacterial pericarditis	1
Total	**105**

*Armed Forces Institute of Pathology.

Microscopic Pathologic Findings

- Infiltrate of polymorphonuclear leukocytes and lymphocytes
- Vascular prominence
- Fibrin deposition

Treatment and Course

- Specific treatment includes surgical drainage, antibiotics for bacterial pericarditis, and antineoplastic, and sclerosing agents for neoplastic pericarditis.
- Nonspecific treatment includes nonsteroidal antiinflammatory drugs and, occasionally, steroids.
- Idiopathic, postmyocardial infarct, and postpericardiotomy syndrome are self-limiting.
- Twenty percent to 25% of patients may have recurrent episodes of acute pericarditis, which are treated with prolonged therapy with nonsteroidal antiinflammatory drugs or steroids.
- Complications include effusions, pericardial tamponade, fibrosis, calcification, and constrictive pericarditis.

PERICARDIAL EFFUSIONS

Causes and Effects

- Because pericardial effusions are often a complication of pericarditis, the causes are essentially similar to those of pericarditis.
- The most serious clinical complication is pericardial tamponade, the development of which is dependent on three factors:
  - Total amount of fluid: a normal pericardium can accommodate up to 2 L of pericardial fluid, if accumulated slowly.
  - Rate of fluid accumulation: rapidly accumulated fluid is easily accommodated only up to a volume of 80 to 200 mL; between 350 and 400 mL results in tamponade.
  - Physical characteristics of the pericardium: fibrosis of the pericardium results in a marked decrease in the amount of fluid that can be accommodated.

Pathologic Findings

- Treatment of large pericardial effusions is pericardiectomy or pericardial window.
- Pericardial tissue is generally received in numerous fragments.
- Specific histologic features are those of disease processes that may also result in chronic pericarditis.

Nonspecific Chronic Pericarditis

- Nonspecific chronic pericarditis is the most common diagnosis in pericardial resections for chronic effusions.
- Grossly, the pericardium is a thickened, dull gray, with fibrous tags.
- Occasionally, the pericardium appears grossly normal.
- Microscopically, fibrosis, fibrous adhesions, loss of mesothelial lining, chronic inflammation, and vascularization are seen.
- There is a zonal distribution to the changes, with hemosiderosis predominating in the inner two thirds of the pericardium, with dense fibrosis, inflammation, and vascular thickening predominating in the outer one third.

Pericarditis of Collagen Vascular Diseases

Acute Rheumatic Fever

- Fibrinous, serofibrinous, or, rarely, purulent pericarditis occurs in acute rheumatic fever.
- Chronic calcification and constriction are rare.

Systemic Lupus Erythematosus

- Twenty percent to 42% of patients demonstrate clinical signs and symptoms of pericarditis.
- In autopsy studies, 43% to 100% of patients with systemic lupus erythematosus have evidence of pericardial inflammation.
- Fibrinous, effusive, and constrictive pericarditis may occur.
- Hematoxylin bodies are occasionally found.
- Pericardial tamponade occurs in 10% of cases.
- Constrictive pericarditis is rare.
- Small vessel vasculitis may be present, but this is a nonspecific finding.

Rheumatoid Arthritis

- There is a 50% autopsy incidence of pericarditis and a less than 10% clinical incidence.
- Fibrinous, effusive, or constrictive pericarditis may occur.
- Pathologically, there is fibrous thickening of the parietal and visceral pericardium, with adhesions.
- Necrotizing granulomas with characteristic palisading of histiocytes (rheumatoid nodules) are occasionally identified, and, occasionally, there is a small vessel vasculitis.
- Chronic constrictive pericarditis is more common in men than in women.

Tuberculous Pericarditis

- Grossly, the pericardium is thick, rubbery, hard, or gritty.
- The mesothelial surface is dull with areas of yellowish thickening.
- Necrotizing and non-necrotizing granulomas are present, predominantly in the inner and outer layers.
- There are variable degrees of fibrosis and chronic inflammation, with fibrin deposition.
- Special stains for acid-fast bacilli may demonstrate organisms.
- Calcification of the pericardium may occur.

Sarcoidal Pericarditis

- Sarcoid involves the pericardium in less than 3% of patients at autopsy.

- Occasionally, sarcoid involvement of the pericardium may result in effusions and, less commonly, restrictive pericarditis.
- Histologically, non-necrotizing granulomas, fibrosis, and chronic inflammation may be seen.
- The histologic findings of granulomatous pericarditis raise the differential diagnoses of tuberculosis and foreign body reaction to previous surgery.
- History, the absence of necrotizing granulomas, negative acid-fast stains, and negative polarized microscopy aid in the diagnosis of sarcoid.
- Occasionally, a nonspecific diagnosis of granulomatous pericarditis must be made.

Purulent Pericarditis

- In purulent pericarditis, the pericardium is thick and edematous, with a dull gray mesothelial surface.
- A fibrinous exudate may be grossly evident.
- Histologically, there is cellular fibrosis, acute and chronic inflammation, focal loss and focal hyperplasia of the mesothelial layer, and an organizing fibrinous exudate with granulation tissue.
- Bacteria may be demonstrated by Brown and Brenn or Brown and Hopps stain.

Siderosis of the Pericardium

- Chronic hemorrhagic pericardial effusions may result in marked siderosis of the mesothelial lining cells.
- Pigmented cells in a pericardial biopsy should be evaluated with iron stains to distinguish melanin from iron.

Myxedema

- Pericardial effusions develop in one third of patients with myxedema.
- Effusion may be caused by sodium and water retention, slow lymphatic drainage, and increased capillary permeability.
- Myxedema resolves slowly after treatment with thyroid hormone replacement.

Hypereosinophilic Syndrome

- Pericarditis with effusion is an uncommon complication of hypereosinophilic syndrome.
- There is an overlap of hypereosinophilic syndrome, Churg-Strauss angiitis, eosinophilic gastroenteritis, and hypersensitivity to medications.
- Rarely, a constrictive pericarditis results.
- Histologically, there is an intense infiltrate by eosinophils; classically, there are eosinophilic granulomas.

Cholesterol Pericarditis

- Cholesterol pericarditis is the nonspecific result of pericardial injury, resulting in cholesterol crystal deposition.
- Other changes of chronic, nonspecific pericarditis (e.g., chronic inflammation, fibrosis) are present.
- Hemosiderin deposition is typical and is believed to be secondary to resolving hemorrhage.

- Grossly, cholesterol crystals cause the pericardial fluid in patients with effusions and cholesterol pericarditis to have a "glittering gold" appearance.

CONSTRICTIVE PERICARDITIS

Underlying Conditions

- Idiopathic condition (42%)
- Postradiation therapy (31%)
- Postsurgery (11%)
- Postinfection/tuberculosis (6%)
- Pericarditis of collagen vascular diseases (4%)
- Neoplasm (3%)
- Uremia (2%)
- Sarcoidosis (1%)

Chronic Fibrous Pericarditis

- Chronic fibrous pericarditis is the most common cause (42%) of constrictive pericarditis.
- It is often attributed to remote viral pericarditis.
- Eleven percent to 29% of cases are related to previous trauma, usually surgery.
- Rarely, chronic renal failure with hemodialysis may result in chronic fibrosing pericarditis.
- Histologically, there is destruction of the mesothelial lining with granulation tissue, fibrosis, and adhesions.
- The chronic inflammation is most prominent in the outer two thirds of the pericardium and consists of lymphocytes and plasma cells, with occasional lymphoid follicles.

Chronic Calcific Pericarditis

- Grossly, the pericardium is markedly thickened by dense fibrosis.
- Calcification may diffusely involve the inner pericardial layer and form focal nodules, or there may be a combination of layered and nodular calcific deposits.
- Most cases in the Western world are idiopathic; most remaining cases are the result of tuberculous infection.

Constrictive Tuberculous Pericarditis

- In constrictive tuberculous pericarditis, the pericardium is markedly thickened and rubbery, with appearance of necrotic debris and adhesions.
- Histologically, there is dense scarring, few granulomas, and chronic inflammation.
- The number of granulomas is far fewer than that seen in tuberculous pericarditis with effusions.
- There may be calcification.
- Acid-fast bacilli are rarely identified.
- The specific diagnosis often depends on clinical history.

Radiation-Induced Constrictive Pericarditis

- Radiation-induced constrictive pericarditis most commonly follows radiation treatment for carcinoma of the breast, Hodgkin's disease, and non-Hodgkin's lymphoma.

- Symptoms may occur during treatment, but usually begin months to years later.
- A total of 92% of patients present with effusions within 1 year of radiation therapy. These effusions progress to fibrosis and constriction.
- The latent period between radiation injury and development of constrictive pericarditis appears to be lengthening (4.7 years between 1970 and 1980, 11 years between 1980 and 1985).
- In the acute phase, there is serous, serosanguineous, or hemorrhagic effusion with lymphocytic infiltrate.
- In the chronic phase, fibrous adhesions may extend into the myocardium and there is thickening of blood vessels.
- In the differential diagnosis, recurrent tumor must be distinguished, both clinically and pathologically, from radiation change. Cytologic examination and clinical history are helpful.

References

Blake S, Boner S, Handy P, Dreary I, Flanagan M, Garrett J. Etiology of chronic constrictive pericarditis. Br Heart J 50:273–276, 1983.

Cameron J, Oesterle SN, Baldwin JC, Hancock EW. The etiologic spectrum of constrictive pericarditis. Am Heart J 113:354–360, 1987.

Felman RH, Sutherland DB, Conklin JL, Mitros FA. Eosinophilic cholecystitis, appendiceal inflammation, pericarditis, and cephalosporin-associated eosinophilia. Dig Dis Sci 39:418–422, 1994.

Lui CY, Makoui C. Severe constrictive pericarditis as an unsuspected cause of death in a patient with idiopathic hypereosinophilic syndrome and restrictive cardiomyopathy. Clin Cardiol 11:502–504, 1988.

Mambo NC. Diseases of the pericardium: morphologic study of surgical specimens from 35 patients. Hum Pathol 12:978–987, 1981.

Pesola G, Teirstein AS, Goldman M. Sarcoidosis presenting with pericardial effusion. Sarcoidosis 4:42–44, 1987.

Seifert FC, Miller C, Oesterle SN, Oyer PE, Stinson EB, Shumway NE. Surgical treatment of constrictive pericarditis: analysis of outcome and diagnostic error. Circulation 72(SII):264–272, 1985.

Zelcer AA, LeJemtel TH, Jones J, Stahl J. Pericardial tamponade in sarcoidosis. Can J Cardiol 3:12–13, 1987.

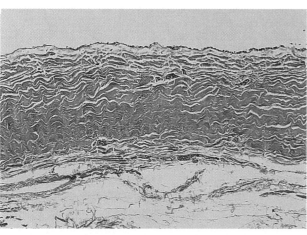

Figure 13–1. Normal pericardium. A section of pericardium was removed at autopsy from a trauma victim with no known pericardial disease. Note the parietal mesothelial layer overlying the fibrous pericardium. The outer portion of pericardium *(bottom)* is composed of loose connective tissue and fat. The visceral pericardium (epicardium) is not illustrated.

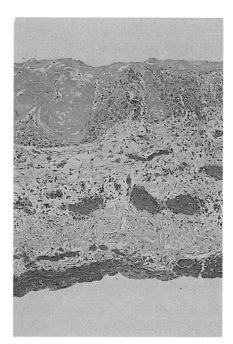

Figure 13–2. Acute pericarditis. There is vascular congestion and a fibrinous exudate with a mesothelial reaction on the parietal pericardial surface. There is no evidence of scarring indicative of chronicity. The histology is nonspecific and compatible with acute pericarditis of diverse causes. The pericardium stripped easily from the epicardial surface.

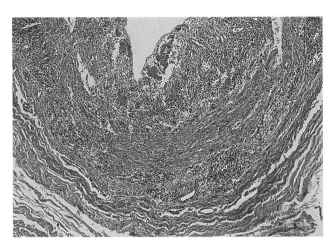

Figure 13–3. Chronic pericarditis. Note the extensive lymphoid infiltration and the mild scarring. There is persistent fibrinous exudate over the mesothelial surface indicative of ongoing inflammation.

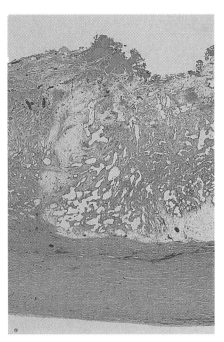

Figure 13–4. Chronic pericarditis with reactive mesothelial hyperplasia. There is pericardial scarring and focal surface fibrin. Note the large area of reactive mesothelial proliferation.

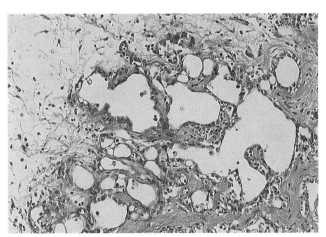

Figure 13–5. Reactive mesothelial hyperplasia. A higher magnification of Figure 13–4 demonstrates irregular cystic structures lined by hyperplastic mesothelial cells.

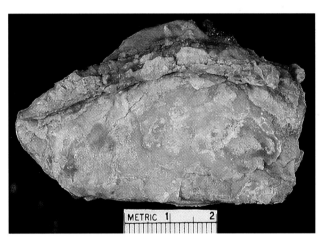

Figure 13–6. Chronic calcific pericarditis. Pericardial stripping was performed in a patient with idiopathic constrictive pericarditis. Note the grossly thickened pericardium with nodules of calcium.

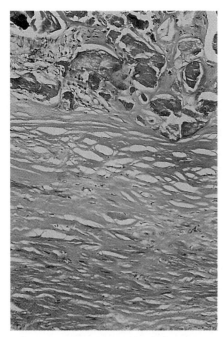

Figure 13–7. Chronic calcific pericarditis. There are irregular calcium deposits, a layer of fibrous tissue, and myocardium. In this surgically resected specimen, the epicardium was densely adherent to the parietal pericardium, and a superficial layer of myocardium was removed.

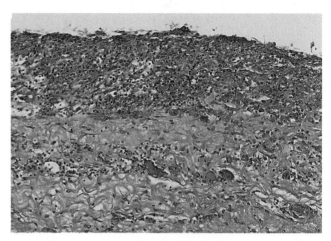

Figure 13–8. Chronic hemorrhagic pericarditis. Blood is resorbed in the pericardial sac by macrophages that contain hemosiderin.

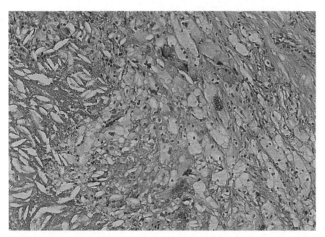

Figure 13–9. Cholesterol pericarditis. Resorption of blood and inflammatory debris results in the accumulation of foam cells and cholesterol clefts in a minority of cases of chronic pericarditis.

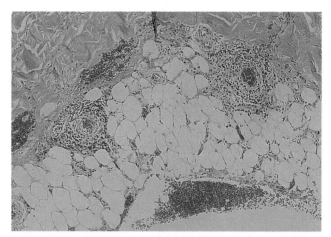

Figure 13–10. Pericarditis, small vessel vasculitis. A lymphocytic perivasculitis may occur in chronic pericarditis. Although not specific, this finding may suggest the diagnosis of collagen vascular disease.

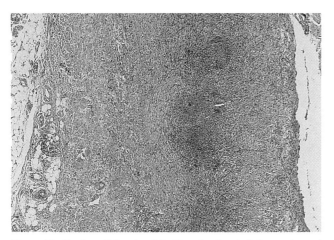

Figure 13–11. Sarcoidal pericarditis. Note the chronic inflammation and granulomas in a patient with known sarcoid and chronic symptomatic pericarditis.

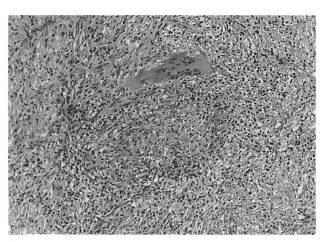

Figure 13–12. Sarcoidal pericarditis. A higher magnification of Figure 13–11 demonstrates non-necrotizing granulomas.

Figure 13–13. Tuberculous pericarditis. There is marked pericardial thickening by necrotizing inflammation.

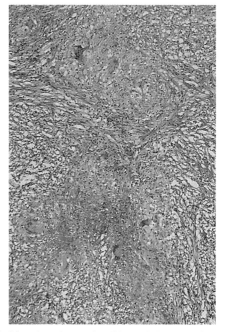

Figure 13–14. Tuberculous pericarditis. A higher magnification of Figure 13–13 demonstrates necrotizing granulomas. Culture was positive for *Mycobacterium tuberculosis,* and special stains for acid-fast bacilli demonstrated rare organisms (not shown).

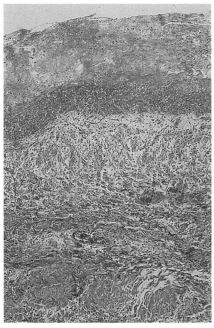

Figure 13–15. Purulent pericarditis. Note the marked fibrin deposits overlying the granulation tissue layer.

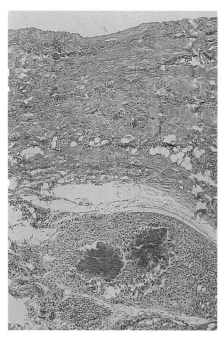

Figure 13–16. Hypereosinophilic syndrome. Note the masses of eosinophilic material external to the thickened parietal pericardium.

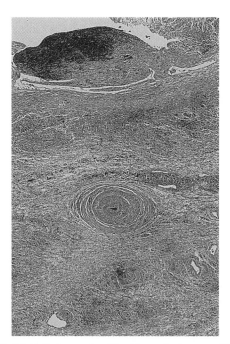

Figure 13–17. Radiation pericarditis. The patient was a 30-year-old man with a history of radiation 7 years prior for mediastinal Hodgkin's disease. Note the fibrosis, hemorrhage, and vascular thickening.

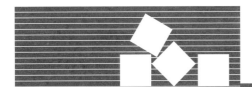

CHAPTER 14

Pericardial Tumors and Cysts

Table 14–1 lists pericardial cysts and tumors diagnosed by pericardial biopsy.

PERICARDIAL (MESOTHELIAL) CYST

A mesothelial cyst (pericardial cyst, coelomic cyst) is a benign cyst lined by mesothelial cells; it may be a closed-off mesothelial diverticulum.

Patient Characteristics and Clinical Findings

- There is no sex predilection.
- Most patients are in their third to fourth decade at the time of detection.
- Pericardial cysts are generally asymptomatic.
- Up to one third of patients have chest pain, dyspnea, atrial tachycardia, or odynophagia.

Gross Pathologic Findings

- Most pericardial cysts are at the right heart border at the right costophrenic angle; other locations are the left heart border and the anterior and posterior mediastinum.
- Cysts are 80% unilocular and occasionally communicate with the pericardial sac (so-called pericardial diverticulum).
- Cysts are 20% multilocular.

Microscopic PatholoFgic Findings

- Cysts are lined by mesothelial cells. Sparse inflammation and fibrosis of the wall are not uncommon, and there is little smooth muscle.
- Xanthomatous changes and reactive mesothelial hyperplasia may occur.

Differential Diagnosis

- Lymphangioma contains smooth muscle bundles and lymphoid aggregates; endothelial cells line some of the cysts, which contain fibrin and a few lymphocytes.
- Duplication (bronchogenic) cysts are in the differential diagnosis.
- Pseudocysts are cysts that are not lined by cellular elements and are generally traumatic or inflammatory in nature.

References

Feigin DS, Fenoglio JJ, McAllister HA, Medwell JE. Pericardial cysts. A radiologic–pathologic correlation and review. Radiology 125:15–20, 1977.

Santoro MJ, Ford LJ, Chen YK, Solinger MR. Odynophagia caused by a pericardial diverticulum. Am J Gastroenterol 88:943–944, 1993.

Table 14–1
PERICARDIAL TUMORS AND CYSTS, DIAGNOSED BY PERICARDIAL BIOPSY, AFIP* 1970–1993

Diagnosis	Number
Metastatic tumor	
Adenocarcinoma	36
Large cell carcinoma	10
Squamous cell carcinoma	3
Small cell carcinoma	1
Undifferentiated tumor	2
Sarcoma	2
Melanoma	1
Mesothelial cyst	14
Malignant mesothelioma	11
Sarcoma, not further classified	9
Angiosarcoma	8
Lymphoma	4
Malignant schwannoma	2
Synovial sarcoma	2
Teratoma (intrapericardial)	2
Benign fibrous tumor	2
Endodermal sinus tumor	1
Hemangioma	1
Paraganglioma	1
Kaposi's sarcoma	1
Thymoma	1
Lymphangioma	1
Total	**115**

*Armed Forces Institute of Pathology.

BRONCHOGENIC CYST (INTRAPERICARDIAL)

Bronchogenic cysts are invaginations of primitive foregut that either form as anomalous structures or result from failure of regression of foregut structures; most have features of bronchial differentiation.

Incidence and Clinical Findings

- Bronchogenic cysts are 10 times less common than mesothelial (pericardial) cysts.
- There is a 2:1 female predominance.
- One third of cases occur in infants; one half of cases are detected only after age 15 years.
- Bronchogenic cysts rarely cause symptoms in adults; in infants, there are typically signs and symptoms of pericardial disease (effusions, tamponade, pericarditis).

Pathologic Findings

- Unlike pericardial cysts, bronchogenic cysts are occasionally partly embedded within myocardium.
- A well-developed muscular layer is present.
- Most bronchogenic cysts have respiratory lining cells (goblet cells, ciliated columnar cells) or cartilage.
- A squamous lining or intestinal mucosa may be present, indicating esophageal or enteric duplication cyst, respectively.
- In some cases, the noncommittal designation of "foregut cyst" is most appropriate.

Differential Diagnosis

- Unlike mesothelial cysts, duplication cysts have a well-developed muscular wall, sometimes with ganglion cells between layers.
- Teratomas, unlike bronchogenic cysts, have three cell types: mesenchymal, neuroectodermal, and epithelial.

References

DiLorenzo M, Collin PP, Vaillancourt R, Durnaceau A. Bronchogenic cysts. J Pediatr Surg 24:988–989, 1989.

Hayashi AH, McLean DR, Peliowski A, Tierney AJ, Finer NN. A rare intrapericardial mass in a neonate. J Pediatr Surg 27:1361–1363, 1992.

MALIGNANT MESOTHELIOMA

Malignant mesothelioma is a neoplasm that demonstrates cytologic, histochemical, and immunohistochemical features of mesothelial cells.

Incidence and Patient Characteristics

- Malignant mesothelioma is a rare tumor when confined to the pericardium; approximately 200 cases have been reported worldwide.
- Most pericardial mesotheliomas are extensions of mesotheliomas that arise in the pleura.
- Pericardial mesotheliomas account for 0.7% of all malignant mesotheliomas.
- The mean age at presentation is 46 years (range 2–78 years).
- There is a 2:1 male predominance.
- Between one fourth and one half of recently reported cases are associated with asbestos exposure.

Clinical Findings

- Dyspnea is the most common presenting symptom.
- Recurrent pericarditis and pericardial tamponade are frequent clinical diagnoses.
- Unexplained persistent effusions with multiple nondiagnostic biopsy results are characteristic.
- Clinical differential diagnosis includes collagen vascular disease and tuberculosis.
- Cardiac compression may result in myocardial infarction or valvular obstruction.

Gross Pathologic Findings

- There is encasement of the heart with relatively little intramyocardial spread.
- Bulky nodules with multiple satellite nodules are common on the diaphragmatic and pleural surfaces.
- Encasement of the great vessels may occur with obstruction of the venae cavae.
- Deep infiltration of the myocardium is unusual.
- The masses are firm and white, with occasional hemorrhagic and cystic areas.

Microscopic Pathologic Findings

- Malignant mesotheliomas are similar to pleural mesotheliomas.
- Most cases are biphasic, demonstrating epithelial (tubular or papillary) and spindle cell (sarcomatoid) areas.
- Periodic acid–Schiff (PAS) staining after treatment with diastase fails to demonstrate intracellular droplets that are characteristic of adenocarcinoma.
- Alcian blue–positive mucin droplets that are sensitive to hyaluronidase may be present.
- Immunostains for B72.3 antigen, carcinoembryonic antigen, BER-EP4, and leu M-1 are generally negative.
- Diffuse immunostain for cytokeratin is strongly positive.
- Use of antibodies against mesothelium-specific antigens is under investigation.

Differential Diagnosis

- Reactive mesothelial hyperplasia does not invade tissues and sheet-like growth is uncommon. Bizarre, pleomorphic, greatly enlarged cells with atypical mitoses are absent.
- Metastatic adenocarcinoma may contain mucin droplets or abortive intracellular glandular structures (PAS stain after diastase and ultrastructure analysis may be helpful). Immunostains may be positive for carcinoembryonic antigen, BER-EP4, B72.3 antigen, and leu M-1.

References

Churg A, Warnock ML, Bensch KG. Malignant mesothelioma arising after direct application of asbestos and fiberglass to the pericardium. Am Rev Respir Dis 118:419–424, 1978.

Coplan NL, Kennish AJ, Burgess NL, Deligdish L, Goldman ME. Pericardial mesothelioma masquerading as a benign pericardial effusion. J Am Coll Cardiol 4:1307–1310, 1984.

Dooley BN, Beckmann C, Hood RH. Primary mesothelioma of the pericardium—successful surgical removal. J Thorac Cardiovasc Surg 55:719–724, 1968.

Fazekas T, Ungi I, Tiszlavicz L. Primary malignant mesothelioma of the pericardium. Am Heart J 124:227–231, 1992.

Hillerdal G. Malignant mesothelioma 1982: review of 4710 published cases. Br J Dis Chest 77:321–343, 1983.

McGuigan L, Fleming A. Pericardial mesothelioma presenting as systemic lupus erythematosus. Ann Rheum Dis 43:515–517, 1984.

Nambiar CA, Tareif HE, Kishore KU, Ravindran J, Banerjee AK. Primary pericardial mesothelioma: one-year event-free survival. Am Heart J 124:802–803, 1992.

Roggli VL. Pericardial mesothelioma after exposure to asbestos (letter). N Engl J Med 304:1045, 1981.

Rose DS, Vigneswaran WT, Bovill BA, Riordan JF, Sapsford RN, Stanbridge RD. Primary pericardial mesothelioma presenting as tuberculous pericarditis. Postgrad Med J 68:137–139, 1992.

Sytman AL, MacAlpin RN. Primary pericardial mesothelioma: report of two cases and review of the literature. Am Heart J 81:760–768, 1971.

PRIMARY PERICARDIAL ANGIOSARCOMA

Incidence and Patient Characteristics

- Primary pericardial angiosarcoma is a rare lesion; fewer than 40 have been reported.
- There is a male predominance, and mean age at presentation is 40 years.

Clinical Findings

- Symptoms include pericardial tamponade, pericarditis, and obstruction of caval or pulmonary veins.
- The differential diagnosis includes metastatic adenocarcinoma, pericardial mesothelioma, and constrictive pericarditis.
- Magnetic resonance imaging (MRI) and computed tomography (CT) scans are helpful in diagnosing mass lesions and extent of infiltration.
- Prognosis is poor, and death from metastatic disease or bulky cardiac tumor occurs in most patients within 2 years of diagnosis.

Pathologic Findings

- Many angiosarcomas of the pericardium demonstrate invasion of the myocardium; the distinction between myocardial and pericardial angiosarcoma may be difficult.
- Histologically, most cases demonstrate well-formed vascular channels with areas of spindle cell growth; epithelioid angiosarcoma of the pericardium has not been reported.
- Immunohistochemically, endothelial markers are present in approximately 50% of cases.
- The most problematic diagnostic pitfall occurs when there is limited sampling on biopsy; mesothelioma may be suspected because of mesothelial hyperplasia, and metastatic carcinoma may also be in the differential diagnosis.
- Adequate sampling with special stains for mucin and immunohistochemical markers for epithelial malignancies are helpful in the differential diagnosis.
- Angiosarcomas of the pericardium may incite a mesothelial reaction; diagnostic areas of atypical vascular structures may be missed if tumor samples are small.

References

McCaughey WT, Dardick I, Barr JR. Angiosarcoma of serous membranes. Arch Pathol Lab Med 107:304–307, 1983.

Poole-Wilson PA, Farnsworth A, Braimbridge MV, Pambakian H. Angiosarcoma of pericardium. Problems in diagnosis and management. Br Heart J 38:240–243, 1976.

OTHER PERICARDIAL SARCOMAS

Incidence and Types

- Other pericardial sarcomas are rarely reported; the incidence is about one half that of pericardial angiosarcoma.
- The majority are spindle cell or pleomorphic sarcomas that are difficult to classify.
- Rare examples of synovial sarcoma and malignant peripheral nerve sheath tumors of the pericardium have been reported.

Differential Diagnosis

- Immunohistochemical positivity for cytokeratin, a biphasic pattern, and a history of asbestos exposure are indicators of mesothelioma rather than pericardial sarcoma.
- PAS with diastase stains may demonstrate intracytoplasmic mucin vacuoles indicative of metastatic carcinoma; immunohistochemical stains demonstrate positivity for cytokeratin and, often, carcinoembryonic antigen, BER-EP4, B72.3 antigen, and other markers of adenocarcinoma.
- Localized fibrous tumors of the pericardium may appear to be malignant and are forms of pericardial fibrosarcoma.

References

Fukuda T, Ishikawa H, Ohnishi Y, et al. Malignant spindle cell tumor of the pericardium. Evidence of sarcomatous mesothelioma with aberrant antigen expression. Acta Pathol Jpn 39:750–754, 1989.

Lazoglu AH, DaSilva MM, Iwahara M, et al. Primary pericardial sarcoma. Am Heart J 127:553–558, 1994.

Witkin GB, Miettinen M, Rosai J. A biphasic tumor of the mediastinum with features of synovial sarcoma. Am J Surg Pathol 13:490–499, 1989.

LOCALIZED FIBROUS TUMOR

Localized fibrous tumor is a benign neoplasm of submesothelial fibrocytes occurring in serosal cavities (localized fibrous tumor); 90% occur on the pleural surfaces, 10% on pericardial or peritoneal surfaces.

Clinical Findings

- Pericardial effusions have a mass effect on cardiac structures.
- Ten percent of cases may recur.

Gross Pathologic Findings

- Localized fibrous tumors are well-demarcated, firm masses, with attachment to pericardium.
- The pericardial attachment may be a pedicle or broad base, or there may be diffuse encasement of the myocardium, especially in aggressive lesions.

Histologic Findings

- Dense collagen and benign-appearing fibroblasts are present in indolent tumors.
- There may be a vascular pattern, imparting a hemangiopericytoid appearance.
- By immunohistochemistry and ultrastructure analysis, the tumor cells are fibroblasts and not mesothelial cells; they are negative for keratin and do not have intercellular junctions or microvilli characteristic of mesothelial cells.
- Rarely, atypical cellular areas are present, with occasional mitoses; these tumors have a propensity for recurrence and are a form of low-grade fibrosarcoma.

References

Weidner N. Solitary fibrous tumor of the mediastinum. Ultrastruct Pathol 15:489–492, 1991.
Witkin GB, Rosai J. Solitary fibrous tumor of the mediastinum. Report of 14 cases. Am J Surg Pathol 13:547–557, 1989.

MISCELLANEOUS TUMORS OF THE PERICARDIUM

Thymoma

- Thymic rests may rarely give rise to intrapericardial thymoma.
- In a pericardial biopsy, locally infiltrative thymoma arising in a normally situated thymus gland is more common than primary intrapericardial thymoma.
- Patients with intrapericardial thymomas are often women who present with dyspnea or chest pain.
- Treatment is generally surgical, although chemotherapy may result in tumor regression in inoperable cases.
- Histologic features are similar to those of thymomas arising in normally situated thymus glands, with epithelial thymomas predominating.

Germ Cell Tumors

- Seventy-five percent of patients with germ cell tumors are children younger than 15 years, but adults are also affected.
- Teratoma may be diagnosed in utero.
- Female:male ratio is 2:1.
- Symptoms in infants include respiratory distress, pericardial tamponade, and cyanosis.

- Adult teratomas are often incidental radiographic findings.
- Pathologically, intrapericardial teratomas are generally located on the right side of the heart, displacing the ventricular septum to the left and posteriorly.
- Often, there is a pedicle attaching the tumor to a great vessel, with blood supply directly from the aorta.
- Histologically, most tumors are benign teratomas, with elements of all germ cell layers, especially cartilage, neuroglial tissue, smooth muscle, mucous glands, intestine, pancreas, respiratory mucosa, ependyma, and bone.
- A myxoid stroma is often present.
- Rarely, other germ cell elements may be present, including embryonal carcinoma, squamous cell carcinoma, and choriocarcinoma.
- Pure endodermal sinus tumor (yolk sac tumor, infantile embryonal carcinoma) may occur.

Paraganglioma

- Paragangliomas are rare cardiac tumors that are usually on the epicardial surface near the base of the heart.
- Most patients are young adults (age range 15–60 years).
- Fifty percent of patients have hypertension and evidence of catecholamine secretion by tumor (functioning paragangliomas, or "pheochromocytomas").
- Chromaffin reactivity does not correlate well with functional activity.
- Histologically and immunohistochemically, intrapericardial paragangliomas are similar to extracardiac paragangliomas.
- Most intrapericardial paragangliomas are benign, although malignant examples with recurrence have been reported.

Other Miscellaneous Tumors

- Primary benign neoplasms, such as hemangiomas, leiomyomas, lymphangiomas, and benign neural tumors, have rarely been reported in the pericardium. Lymphomas of the pericardium are usually extensions of mediastinal lymphomas, but may be exclusively found in the pericardial sac.

METASTATIC TUMORS

Clinical Findings

- Dyspnea, cardiac arrhythmias, and pericardial tamponade are the most common symptoms of metastatic tumors.
- In additional to pericardial effusion, pleural effusions are often present; bloody effusions are typical.
- Electrocardiographic findings characteristically include low-voltage QRS.
- Echocardiography is a sensitive tool in diagnosis, revealing effusions and ventricular dyskinesia.
- More than one half of malignant pericardial biopsies occur in patients in whom the diagnosis of malignancy has not yet been made clinically.

■ Not all pericardial effusions in cancer patients are malignant:

- Small, asymptomatic effusions are usually idiopathic.
- Fifty percent of symptomatic effusions are malignant in patients with known carcinoma.
- The clinical differential diagnosis of pericardial effusion in cancer patients includes radiation pericarditis and drug toxicity.

Pathologic Findings

■ Most tumors metastatic to the pericardium are carcinomas; the most common primary sites are lung and breast.

■ When there is no prior clinical diagnosis of malignancy, the most common diagnosis (90%) is carcinoma of the lung.

■ Other metastatic tumors found in pericardial biopsies include lymphoma, melanoma, sarcoma, and thymoma.

■ In children, the most common pericardial tumors are non-Hodgkin's lymphoma, neuroblastoma, sarcoma, nephroblastoma, and hepatoblastoma.

■ Histologic features are those of the primary tumor; the most common histologic types are adenocarcinomas and large cell carcinomas.

■ Squamous cell carcinomas are unusual, and small cell carcinomas are rare in pericardial biopsies.

■ In carcinoma, there are typically detached cell clusters and a fibrinous, hemorrhagic exudate.

Differential Diagnosis

■ Mesothelioma or reactive mesothelial hyperplasia is an unlikely diagnosis if certain stains are positive: PAS with diastase (mucin vacuoles), carcinoembryonic antigen, B72.3 antigen, BER-EP4, and leu M-1.

■ A site-specific diagnosis cannot be made with certainty; large cell or squamous carcinomas are almost always of lung primary tumor; carcinomas of the breast involve the pericardium, generally after the primary tumor is diagnosed.

■ Although there is some site specificity of carcinomas that express cytokeratins 7 and 18, these markers do not differentiate between carcinomas of the breast and lung, which commonly metastasize to the pericardium.

■ Many "breast-specific antigens" have been proposed, although none has been a reliable carcinoma marker for mammary origin of disease.

■ Recently, gross cystic disease fluid protein-15 has been shown to be a relatively specific marker for breast carcinoma, but this remains to be established.

References

Adenle AD, Edwards JE. Clinical and pathologic features of metastatic neoplasms of the pericardium. Chest 81:116–119, 1982.

Frisman DM, McCarthy WF, Schleiff P, Buckner S-B, Nocito JD, O'Leary T. Immunocytochemistry in the differential diagnosis of effusions: use of logistic regression to select a panel of antibodies to distinguish adenocarcinomas from mesothelial proliferation. Mod Pathol 6:179–184, 1993.

Loire R, Hellal H. Neoplastic pericarditis. Study by thoracotomy and biopsy in 80 cases. Presse Med 22:244–248, 1993.

Mukai K, Shinkai T, Tominaga K, Shimosato Y. The incidence of secondary tumors of the heart and pericardium: a 10-year study. Jpn J Clin Oncol 18:195–201, 1988.

Ramaekers F, van Niekerk C, Poels LG, Schaafsma E, Huysmans A, Vooijs PG. Use of monoclonal antibodies to keratin 7 in the differential diagnosis of adenocarcinomas. Am J Pathol 136:641–645, 1990.

Wick MR, Lillemoe TJ, Copland GT, Swanson PE, Manivel JC, Kiang DT. Gross cystic disease fluid protein-15 as a marker for breast cancer: immunohistochemical analysis of 690 human neoplasms and comparison with alpha-lactalbumin. Hum Pathol 94:18–26, 1989.

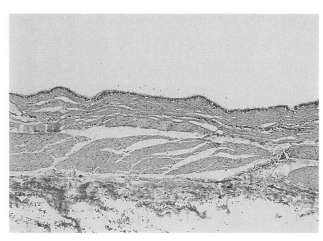

Figure 14–1. Bronchogenic cyst, pericardium. Note the well-developed smooth muscle layer and the single-cell lining.

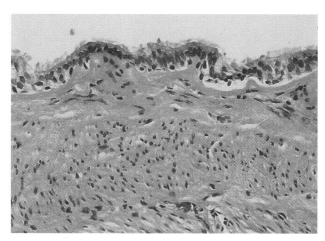

Figure 14–2. Bronchogenic cyst, pericardium. A higher magnification of Figure 14–1 demonstrates muscular coat and ciliated cuboidal lining.

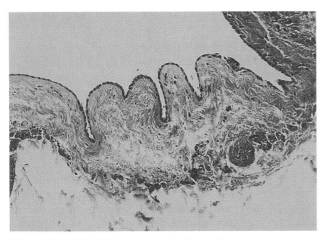

Figure 14–3. Mesothelial cyst, pericardium. Also known simply as "pericardial cysts," these cysts lack a muscular wall; there is a simple cuboidal lining typical of mesothelial cells.

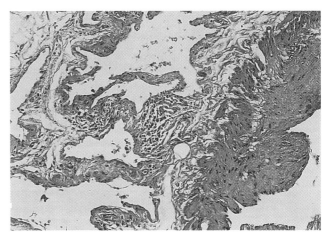

Figure 14–4. Lymphangioma, pericardium. Note the endothelium-lined channels, smooth muscle bundles, and absence of a well-formed muscle layer.

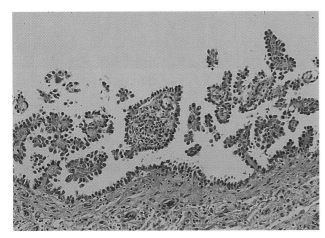

Figure 14–5. Mesothelial hyperplasia, pericardium. In contrast to malignant proliferations, the surface lining tends to be a single layer, there are no detached cell clusters containing many cells, and there is relatively little pleomorphism.

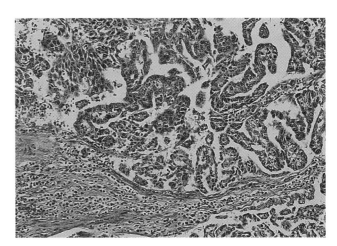

Figure 14–6. Malignant mesothelioma, pericardium, papillary type. There is cellular atypia and decreased cohesion in papillary structures; compare these structures with the benign papillary structures in Figure 14–5.

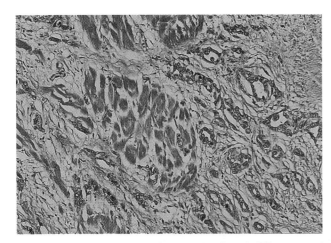

Figure 14–7. Malignant mesothelioma, pericardium. A different area of the tumor illustrated in Figure 14–6 demonstrates an infiltrating, tubular component. Metastatic adenocarcinoma is in the differential diagnosis.

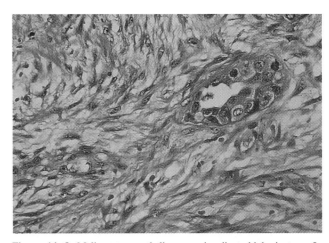

Figure 14–8. Malignant mesothelioma, pericardium, biphasic type. In this tumor, there was a biphasic pattern of glands and spindled cells. Included in the differential diagnosis is desmoplastic carcinoma, arising in the lung or pleura.

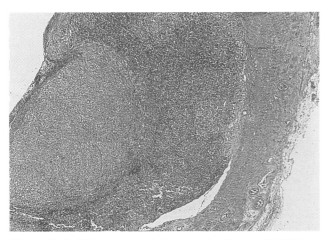

Figure 14–9. Malignant mesothelioma, pericardium, epithelial type. There is diffuse thickening of the pericardium by a cellular infiltrate.

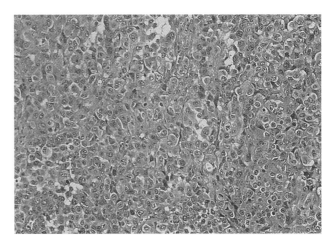

Figure 14–10. Malignant mesothelioma, pericardium, epithelial type. A higher magnification of Figure 14–9 demonstrates sheets of epithelial cells. A metastatic carcinoma must be ruled out by history and by lack of expression of adenocarcinoma markers, such as carcinoembryonic antigen, B72.3 antigen, and BER-EP4.

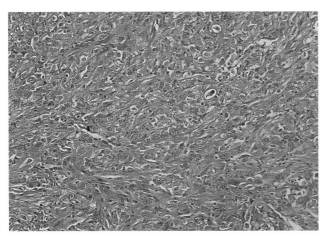

Figure 14–11. Malignant mesothelioma, sarcomatoid type. Some mesotheliomas are relatively undifferentiated. If a tumor encasing the pericardium resembles a sarcoma, mesothelioma should be considered.

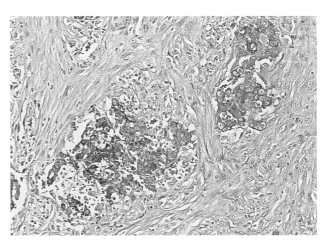

Figure 14–12. Mesothelioma, sarcomatoid type. An area of tumor illustrated in Figure 14–11 demonstrates focal strong expression of cytokeratin, revealing epithelioid areas that were not apparent on routine stains. The spindle cell component of biphasic mesothelioma expresses this marker to a variable degree.

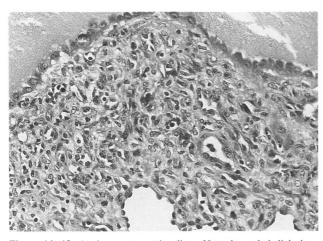

Figure 14–13. Angiosarcoma, pericardium. Note the endothelial channels lined by atypical cells and the overlying reactive mesothelial layer.

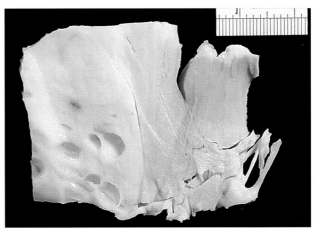

Figure 14–14. Localized fibrous tumor, pericardium. Note the sharp demarcation between tumor and myocardium.

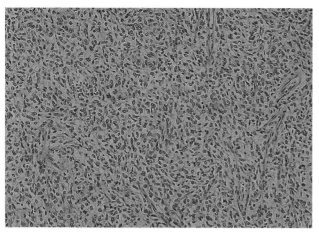

Figure 14–15. Localized fibrous tumor, pericardium. A histologic section of the tumor illustrated in Figure 14–14 demonstrates a proliferation of bland, fibroblastic cells.

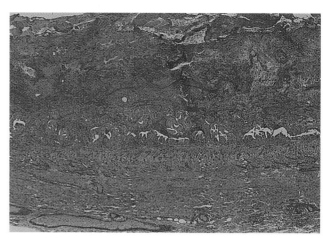

Figure 14–16. Metastatic carcinoma, pericardium. Note the fibrinous, bloody exudate mixed with malignant cells close to the pericardial surface.

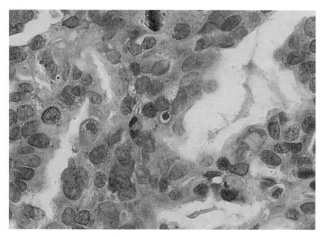

Figure 14–17. Metastatic adenocarcinoma, pericardium. This periodic acid–Schiff stain demonstrates an intracytoplasmic mucin vacuole with central globule.

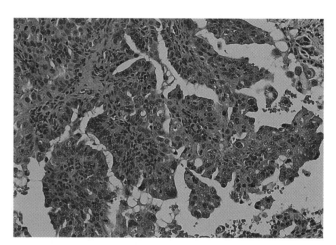

Figure 14–18. Metastatic carcinoma, pericardium. In this tumor, intracytoplasmic vacuoles were not observed; included in the differential diagnosis was malignant mesothelioma.

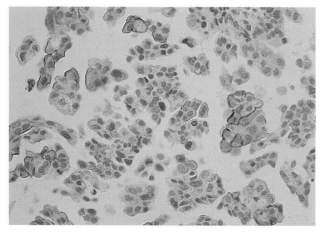

Figure 14–19. Metastatic carcinoma, pericardium. This immunohistochemical stain of a higher magnification of the tumor shown in Figure 14–18 demonstrates membrane positivity for B72.3 antigen; this antigen is rarely expressed by mesothelial proliferations.

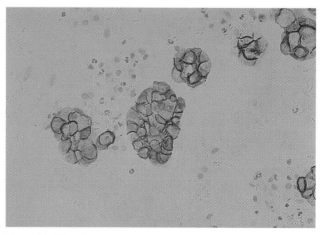

Figure 14–20. Metastatic carcinoma, pericardium. Membrane positivity for BER-EP4, like positivity for B72.3 antigen and carcinoembryonic antigen, is suggestive of carcinoma and is helpful in excluding mesothelioma from the differential diagnosis.

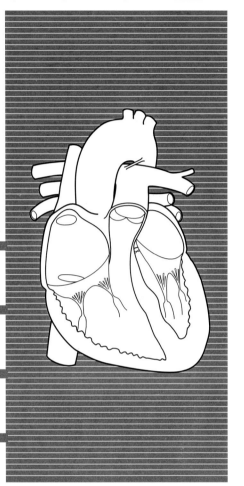

SECTION ■ 5

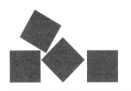

DISEASES OF THE GREAT VESSELS AND PULMONARY CIRCULATION

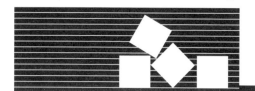

CHAPTER 15

Aorta: Overview and Noninflammatory Diseases

OVERVIEW OF AORTIC DISEASES

Aneurysms

- Most aortic resections are performed for the presence of aneurysms or dissections (Table 15–1).
- Aneurysms may be resected to prevent rupture or after rupture has commenced.
- Aneurysms and dissections may be caused by a variety of underlying pathologic processes, many of which are poorly understood and which have nonspecific histologic findings.

Stenoses

- Aortic resections in infants, children, and young adults are generally performed for congenital coarctations, which occur at the level of the ductus arteriosus.
- Takayasu's disease may result in stenoses (see Chap. 16), and when it occurs it usually involves the descending thoracic aorta.
- Rare causes of aortic narrowing include isolated aortic thrombosis in patients with hypercoagulable states (see Chap. 24), aortic intimal sarcoma (see Chap. 18), and embolism from cardiac myxoma (see Chap. 11).

Classification of Aortic Aneurysms

- Aortic aneurysms are generally classified by shape (saccular, fusiform); as true (lined by attenuated media) or false (lined by adjacent fibrous tissue); and as dissecting or nondissecting.
- The shape of an aneurysm has little bearing on the etiologic type, although there are important surgical implications. Fusiform aneurysms are repaired by bypass grafts, and small saccular aneurysms by patch repair.
- False aneurysms are usually the result of a healed traumatic injury but may also be the result of a healed dissection.
- Dissecting aneurysms may be the result of a variety of processes, and not all dissections are aneurysmal.

Aneurysms of the Ascending Thoracic Aorta

- Annuloaortic ectasia (50%)
- Aortitis (20%) (syphilitic and noninfectious; see Chap. 16).
- Marfan syndrome (5%–10%)
- Dissections (15%); may complicate Marfan syndrome, annuloaortic ectasia, and, rarely, aortitis

Table 15–1
SURGICAL AORTIC RESECTIONS,
NONINFLAMMATORY DISEASES, AFIP*
FILES 1970–1993

Diagnosis	Thoracic Aorta		Abdominal Aorta	Totals
	Ascending	*Descending*		
Atherosclerotic aneurysm	0	2	20	22
Annuloaortic ectasia				
Marfan syndrome	4	1	0	5
Bicuspid aortic valve	4	0	0	4
Etiology unknown	5	1	0	6
Dissection				
Bicuspid aortic valve	2	0	0	2
Marfan syndrome	1	0	1	2
Etiology unknown	1	6	1	8
Coarctation	0	6	0	6
Traumatic aneurysm	0	3	1	4
Intimal sarcoma	0	1	3	4
Occlusive thrombus	0	0	1	1
Fibromuscular dysplasia	0	0	1	1
Amyloid tumor	0	0	1	1
Penetrating ulcer	0	1	0	1
Totals	**17**	**21**	**29**	**67**

*Armed Forces Institute of Pathology.

121

- Atherosclerosis (5%)
- Aneurysms of the sinus of Valsalva (1%)
- Ehlers-Danlos syndrome, osteogenesis imperfecta, pseudoxanthoma elasticum, and cutis laxa (1%) (diagnosis made by clinical history)

Aneurysms of the Transverse or Descending Thoracic Aorta

- Dissections (approximately 50%)
- Atherosclerosis (30%)
- Noninfectious aortitis (5%–15%)
- Medial degeneration, with or without Marfan syndrome (5%)
- Syphilis and other infections (<5%)

Aneurysms of the Abdominal Aorta

- Atherosclerosis (90%)
- Inflammatory aneurysm (5%–10%)
- Tuberculous aneurysm (1%)
- Medial degeneration (1%)
- Syphilitic, mycotic aneurysm (<1%)

ANNULOAORTIC ECTASIA

Annuloaortic ectasia is the idiopathic noninflammatory dilatation of the aortic root that invariably results in aortic regurgitation; aortic root diameter generally exceeds 5 cm.

Background

- The term "annuloaortic ectasia" was first coined by Ellis and colleagues in 1961 to indicate noninflammatory aortic root dilatation. The term is generally used to indicate idiopathic aortic root dilatation.
- The term "cystic medial necrosis" was first applied by Erdheim to the histologic changes seen in patients with annuloaortic ectasia with spontaneous rupture.
- Mild to moderate aortic root dilatation may also occur as a consequence of hypertension and advanced age and in long-term survivors of congenital heart disease, such as tetralogy of Fallot.

Relationship to Marfan Syndrome

- The major distinction between annuloaortic ectasia and classic Marfan syndrome is the lack of skeletal and ocular features in the former (see Chap. 24).
- The mean age at the occurrence of dissecting aneurysm is 30 years in classic Marfan syndrome, but the age of patients with annuloaortic ectasia and dissections ranges from 40 to 70 years (mean 50 years).
- A basic defect in fibrillin synthesis, which underlies Marfan syndrome, has yet to be established for patients with annuloaortic ectasia.
- Marfan syndrome is inherited in an autosomal dominant pattern; only occasional cases of annuloaortic ectasia have been shown to have an autosomal dominant inheritance.
- There is an association between bicuspid aortic valve and annuloaortic ectasia, reflected in the increased incidence of dissection; patients with Marfan syndrome do not have an increased risk for bicuspid aortic valve.
- Aortic root dilatation in patients with stenotic bicuspid valves is probably a poststenotic hemodynamic phenomenon and is especially prominent in patients with hypertension.

Clinical Findings

- There is a male predominance (male:female ratio 2–8:1); most patients are in their fourth to sixth decade.
- Mean aortic root diameter is 7.6 cm (range 4.8–15 cm).
- Aortic regurgitation, often with sudden exacerbation, is sometimes precipitated by dissection.
- Annuloaortic ectasia accounts for a large proportion of patients who undergo aortic valve replacement for pure aortic regurgitation (see Chap. 6) and of patients who undergo valve replacement with composite aortic grafting.
- Eleven percent to 25% of patients who require aortic resection with or without aortic valve replacement show evidence of dissection.
- Aortic rupture without dissection is an infrequent complication.

Pathologic Findings

- "Cystic medial necrosis" was the term initially used by Erdheim in patients with annuloaortic ectasia and aortic rupture without dissection. The term denotes large pools or lakes of mucin with loss of elastic fibers.
- The term "medial degeneration" is preferred and embraces any degenerative aortic change in which there is loss of elastic fibers with variable degrees of proteoglycan deposition.
- Medionecrosis denotes areas devoid of smooth muscle nuclei with apposition of elastic lamellae; true necrosis is absent.
- Neither medial degeneration nor medionecrosis is a specific pathologic change, but rather they are secondary phenomena reflecting advanced age, hypertension-induced medial weakening, or genetic defects in connective tissue synthesis.
- Severe medial degeneration is generally seen in patients with Marfan syndrome or annuloaortic ectasia with aortic rupture; hypertension- and age-induced medial degeneration is generally mild or moderate.
- Aortae from patients with Marfan syndrome may have minimal medial degeneration, making this histologic feature unreliable in making a specific diagnosis.
- Changes of chronic dissection may be present.

Treatment

- In patients with Marfan syndrome, elective repair is recommended when the aortic root diameter exceeds 6 cm; criteria for valve replacement in patients with annuloaortic ectasia (without Marfan syndrome) have not been established.
- The most common repair is by composite graft (pros-

thetic valve and aortic tube graft); coronary arteries are transected and implanted in the graft.

References

Kouchoukos NT; Wareing TH; Murphy SF; Perrillo JB. Sixteen-year experience with aortic root replacement. Results of 172 operations. Ann Surg 214:308–318, 1991.
Roberts WC, Honig HS. The spectrum of cardiovascular disease in the Marfan syndrome: a clinico-morphologic study of 18 necropsy patients and comparison to 151 previously reported necropsy patients. Am Heart J 104:115–135, 1982.
Savunen T, Aho HJ. Annulo-aortic ectasia: light and electron microscopic changes in aortic media. Virchows Arch A 407:279–288, 1985.

ANEURYSM OF THE SINUS OF VALSALVA

An aneurysm of the sinus of Valsalva is a dilatation of one or more sinuses of Valsalva resulting from congenital, degenerative, or inflammatory processes.

Etiology

■ Congenital (approximately two thirds of surgically resected cases), including a small proportion of patients with Marfan syndrome
■ Infectious endocarditis (approximately one third of surgically resected cases)
■ Syphilis

Clinical Findings

■ There is a male:female ratio of 4:1.
■ Age at presentation is in the second to fourth decade.
■ Rupture results in sudden onset of chest pain, shortness of breath, congestive heart failure, wide pulse pressure, and murmur and thrill. Aneurysms rupture into the right ventricle or atrium in 92% of cases; left ventricle or atrium, 3% of cases; pericardium, pulmonary artery, and superior vena cava, 5% of cases.
■ There is association with ventricular septal defect (approximately 20% of cases), coarctation of the aorta, and bicuspid aortic valve.
■ Aortic regurgitation occurs in one third of patients.
■ Mitral regurgitation is present in those patients with ventricular septal defect.
■ Obstruction of right ventricular outflow tract, conduction disturbances, and coronary occlusion occur rarely.
■ Some cases are discovered in asymptomatic patients.

Pathologic Findings

■ Sites of involvement are right sinus (70%), noncoronary sinus (29%), and left sinus (<1%).
■ Surgical treatment consists of valve replacement or repair with autologous pericardium, and multiple pieces of tissue are usually sent for pathologic evaluation.
■ In congenital cases, the specimen consists of membranous tissue with little elastic tissue.
■ Acute and organizing inflammation is present in cases due to infectious endocarditis; culture and special stains for microorganisms are indicated.

References

Chu S-H, Hong C-R, How S-S, et al. Ruptured aneurysms of the sinus of Valsalva in Oriental patients. J Thorac Cardiovasc Surg 99:288–298, 1990.
Heggtveit HA. Nonatherosclerotic disease of the aorta. In Silver MD (ed). Cardiovascular Pathology, 2nd ed. New York, Churchill Livingstone, 1991, pp 307–340.
Mayer ED, Ruffmann K, Saggau W, et al. Ruptured aneurysm of the sinus of Valsalva. Ann Thorac Surg 42:81–85, 1986.

AORTIC DISSECTIONS

Aortic dissection is the separation of the aortic media in a course parallel to the direction of blood flow and is almost always accompanied by a transverse intimal and medial tear.

Classification

■ Classification is by site of intimal tear; these are classified into three major groups by DeBakey:
  • Type I (54%): intimal tear in the ascending aorta, with dissection extending to the descending aorta
  • Type II (21%): intimal tear in the ascending aorta, dissection limited to the ascending aorta
  • Type III (25%): intimal tear in the descending or transverse aorta, usually in the distal arch or proximal descending aorta
    • Type IIIa (9%): dissection extends retrograde into the ascending aorta
    • Type IIIb (16%): dissection confined to the transverse arch or descending aorta
■ Type III dissections may be further divided into those with an intimal tear in the transverse aorta (approximately 7% of total), those in the descending thoracic aorta, and those in the abdominal aorta (rare).

Patient Characteristics

■ There is a male predominance (male:female ratio 2–3:1).
■ The rate of occurrence among blacks is higher than in whites.
■ The age range is 14 to 94 years (mean 55–60 years).
■ Patients with type I and II dissections are younger than those with type III dissections, reflecting the higher frequency of underlying congenital diseases in proximal dissections.

Clinical Findings

■ Severe chest pain occurs in 90% of patients.
■ Pain is usually described as "tearing," "ripping," or "stabbing." Pain migrates to the back in 70% of patients.
■ Disturbances of consciousness and vasovagal manifestations are common.

Risk Factors

■ Hypertension is present in 70% of all cases and is most prevalent in type III cases.

▪ Unicuspid or bicuspid aortic valve is frequently seen in types I and II cases:

- Forty percent of aortic valves in types I and II dissections are bicuspid or unicuspid and are usually stenotic.
- Patients with unicuspid or bicuspid aortic valves are younger (mean 35–55 years) than patients with tricuspid aortic valves.
- The risk of aortic dissection in patients with bicuspid aortic valves is 9 times that of patients with normal aortic valves; for unicuspid aortic valves, 18 times greater.
- Aortic stenosis from noncongenital causes is not associated with an increased risk of aortic dissection.

▪ Marfan syndrome predisposes the patient to aortic dissection (types I and II).

- One third of patients have aortic dissections at a young age, unaccompanied by hypertension.
- An additional one third of patients have proximal aortic aneurysms.

▪ Twenty-five percent of dissections in women occur during pregnancy, but a firm association has not been established.
▪ Coarctation of the aorta is associated with aortic dissection but may not be independent of the association with bicuspid aortic valve and hypertension.
▪ Turner's syndrome is associated with dissection, bicuspid aortic valve, and coarctation of the aorta.
▪ Hereditary factors are important, primarily in types I and II dissections; these are manifestations of Marfan syndrome, partial forms of Marfan syndrome, or familial non-Marfan aortic dissections. Familial type III dissections are rare.
▪ Aortic dissections in weight lifters have been described, suggesting that strenuous isometric exercise may precipitate aortic intimal damage.
▪ Blunt trauma may result in intimal tears and aortic dissections; the tears are usually near the ligamentum arteriosum.
▪ Iatrogenic dissections result from arterial cannulation, aortotomy, or aortic cross-clamping.
▪ Atherosclerosis does not predispose the patient to medial weakness. When atherosclerosis is present in aortae with dissection, the planes of dissection are usually limited (see Penetrating Atherosclerotic Ulcer).
▪ Vasculitis (Takayasu's aortitis, giant cell aortitis) and fibromuscular dysplasia rarely result in aortic dissections (see Chap. 16).

Gross Pathologic Findings

▪ An intimal tear is present in virtually all cases of aortic dissection and is generally transverse.
▪ The intimal tear is usually 1 to 2 cm above the sinotubular junction in types I and II, usually involving the right lateral aortic wall and no more than one third to one half of the circumference.
▪ The dissection results in a false lumen, lined by a thin outer wall and the intact media, which is about four times as thick (dissection is usually in the outer half of the aortic circumference).
▪ The dissection in types I and II generally extends along the greater curvature of the aorta, involving the arch vessels.
▪ Proximal extension of the dissection may involve the coronary circulation, usually the right coronary artery, and may result in ischemic symptoms.
▪ The thin outer wall results in a high frequency of rupture and relatively low frequency of reentry intimal tears.
▪ Moderate to severe atherosclerosis is present in approximately 10% of cases.
▪ Multiple dissections are rare, may involve aorta and other muscular arteries, and may be related to smooth muscle cell vacuolar degeneration.

Microscopic Pathologic Findings

▪ Medial degeneration is characterized by loss and fragmentation of elastic lamellae, loss of smooth muscle cells, and accumulation of basophilic ground substance.
▪ Medial degeneration is variable. Severe degeneration with pooling of proteoglycans is suggestive of Marfan syndrome and is present in 20% of cases.
▪ Medionecrosis, or laminar medial necrosis, refers to loss of smooth muscle cells with resultant close apposition of intervening elastic laminae; it is present in 10% of aortic dissections.
▪ The histologic assessment of dissections is generally *not* important, except to rule out unusual causes, such as vasculitis and fibromuscular dysplasia.

Transverse Arch Tears

▪ Transverse arch tears are a subset of type III dissections with tears in the aortic arch, accounting for 7% of all dissections.
▪ There is equal frequency of anterograde and retrograde dissections.
▪ Rupture generally occurs into the pericardium or left hemothorax, resulting in rapid death.
▪ Most patients have systemic hypertension.

Descending Thoracic Arch Tears

▪ There is a higher frequency of healed tears (approximately 40%) than dissections in the ascending aorta (6%) or transverse arch (< 1%).
▪ Aneurysms of the false channel occur in 20% of cases.
▪ Cause of death is rupture of false channel in 65% of cases, renal failure in 15% of cases, and unrelated causes in 20% of cases.
▪ Systemic hypertension is present in 83% of cases.

Treatment

▪ Treatment is surgical repair with graft placement for types I and II.
▪ Treatment is medical therapy with beta-blockers and vasodilators for type III, with surgery performed for dissection extension, rupture, or compromise of flow to major branches of the descending aorta.

- Death occurs within 30 days in up to 20% of cases.
- The highest mortality rate is in patients requiring arch replacement and coronary bypass grafting and in patients with congestive heart failure and diabetes mellitus.

References

de Virgilio C, Nelson RJ, Milliken J, et al. Ascending aortic dissection in weight lifters with cystic medial degeneration. Ann Thorac Surg 49:638–642, 1990.
Edwards WD, Leaf DS, Edwards JE. Dissecting aortic aneurysm associated with congenital bicuspid aortic valve. Circulation 57:1022–1025, 1978.
Gatalica Z, Gibas Z, Martinez-Hernandez A. Dissecting aortic aneurysm as a complication of generalized fibromuscular dysplasia. Hum Pathol 23:586–588, 1992.
Larson EW, Edwards WD. Risk factors for aortic dissection: a necropsy study of 161 cases. Am J Cardiol 53:849–855, 1984.
Nicod P, Bloor C, Godfrey M, et al. Familial aortic dissecting aneurysm. J Am Coll Cardiol 13:811–819, 1989.
Roberts CS, Roberts WC. Aortic dissection with the entrance tear in the abdominal aorta. Am Heart J 121:1834–1835, 1991.
Roberts CS, Roberts WC. Aortic dissection with the entrance tear in the descending thoracic aorta. Ann Surg 213:356–368, 1991.
Roberts CS, Roberts WC. Dissection of the aorta associated with congenital malformation of the aortic valve. J Am Coll Cardiol 17:712–716, 1991.
Schlatmann TJM, Becker AE. Pathogenesis of dissecting aneurysm of aorta. Comparative histopathologic study of significance of medial changes. Am J Cardiol 39:21–26, 1977.
Wilson SK, Hutchins GM. Aortic dissecting aneurysms. Causative factors in 204 subjects. Arch Pathol Lab Med 106:175–180, 1982.

TRAUMATIC PSEUDO ANEURYSMS

A traumatic pseudoaneurysm is an aneurysm lined by scar tissue overlying a traumatic aortic laceration. Pseudoaneurysms at surgical graft anastomoses are discussed in Chapter 9.

Clinical Findings

- Although most traumatic lacerations of the aorta result in sudden death, some heal and may not be diagnosed for years.
- The mean age of occurrence is 15 to 25 years.
- Most patients have a history of some trauma, although 60% do not have a history of apparent thoracic trauma.
- Approximately 50% of chronic dissections are asymptomatic.
- Symptoms include chest and back pain, and hypotension related to leakage or rupture.

Pathologic Findings

- Most traumatic pseudoaneurysms are located at the aortic isthmus, near the ligamentum arteriosum.
- A minority are located at other sites, including the distal thoracic aorta, ascending aorta, or abdominal aorta.
- Grossly, an intimal tear, which is generally transverse, is found.
- The intimal tear is partial in 50% of cases and circumferential in 50% of cases.
- The lining of the aneurysm is organized hematoma and fibrous tissue.

- There is a sharp demarcation between the normal media and the fibrous lining of the pseudoaneurysm.
- Complications include rupture into the pleural space or fistulas to the esophagus.

Treatment

- Surgical bypass is the treatment of choice, generally with a Dacron graft.

References

Jensen BT. Fourteen years' survival with an untreated traumatic rupture of the thoracal aorta. Am J Forensic Med Pathol 9:58–59, 1988.
Prat A, Warembourg H Jr, Watel A, et al. Chronic traumatic aneurysms of the descending thoracic aorta (19 cases). J Cardiovasc Surg (Torino) 27:268–272, 1986.
Swanson SA, Gaffey MA. Traumatic false aneurysm of descending aorta with aortoesophageal fistula. J Forensic Sci 33:816–822, 1988.

ATHEROSCLEROTIC ANEURYSMS

Atherosclerotic aneurysms are segmental dilatation of the aorta with superimposed atherosclerosis and no underlying inflammatory disease.

Pathogenesis

- Several facts challenge the atherosclerotic origin of abdominal aortic aneurysms and suggest a multifactorial or heterogeneous disease:
  - Aneurysms have not been produced in animals fed high-cholesterol diets.
  - There is a familial nature to atherosclerotic aneurysms independent of familial lipid diseases.
  - Increased collagenase and elastase activity has been found within aneurysms, as has a deficiency of metalloprotease inhibitors.
  - There is an association with alpha-1-antitrypsin deficiency.
  - There is an increased incidence of acromegaly in patients with abdominal aortic aneurysms compared with control subjects.
- Possible reasons for the propensity for atherosclerotic aneurysms to recur in the abdominal aorta include increased aortic pressure, pulse wave reflected at aortic bifurcation, and preferential age-related weakening at the abdominal site.
- Genetic predisposition is possibly X-linked, autosomal, or multifactorial.

Patient Characteristics and Epidemiology

- There is a male predominance (male:female ratio 3–8:1), which increases for popliteal and femoral artery aneurysms.
- Whites are more frequently affected than blacks.
- Incidence increases with age: 6% prevalence in sixth decade, 14% prevalence in ninth decade.
- Autopsy incidence is 1.8% to 6.6%.
- Recently, incidence has increased (sevenfold increase between 1951 and 1980 in a Minnesota population).

There has been a more than twofold increase in symptomatic abdominal aortic aneurysms.

■ Increase in incidence is partly due to improved diagnostic capability and aging of the population.
■ Risk factors include cigarette smoking and hypertension, but many patients have neither risk factor.

Clinical Findings

■ Patients are usually asymptomatic.
■ Patients may experience vague abdominal discomfort or lower back pain.
■ A pulsating abdominal mass is palpable if the aneurysm is larger than 4.5 cm.
■ Ultrasound examination is most reliable for screening and monitoring growth; computed topography is also useful.
■ The rate of growth is estimated to be 0.2 to 0.5 cm per year.
■ Symptoms of rupture include abdominal or back pain, hypotension, and a tender abdominal mass; the only symptom may be hypovolemic shock.

Complications

■ Complications include rupture, infection, and embolization.
■ Rupture occurs most commonly into the retroperitoneal space; aneurysms may also bleed into the pleural space, gastrointestinal tract, inferior vena cava, or left renal vein.
■ Aneurysms of less than 5 cm have a minimal risk of rupture over 5 years.
■ Aneurysms of greater than 5 cm have a 25% risk of rupture over 5 years.
■ Presence of chronic obstructive lung disease is a better predictor of aneurysm rupture than is smoking.
■ Secondary bacterial infection is a rare complication; organisms include salmonella, staphylococcus, *Escherichia coli,* and bacteroides. The source of infection is not always apparent and may involve arterial or venous catheters.
■ Embolism of thrombus may result in occlusion of lower limbs.

Gross Findings

■ Most atherosclerotic aneurysms are single.
■ The most common site of occurrence is the infrarenal aorta above the iliac bifurcation.
■ Fusiform (cylindric) aneurysms are most common.
■ Fusiform aneurysms affect the entire circumference of the aorta and may extend into the iliac arteries distally, or proximally to the celiac trunk or even the thoracic aorta.
■ Saccular aneurysms are sharply demarcated, affect a portion of the aortic circumference, and may communicate with the aortic lumen via a narrow neck.
■ Saccular aneurysms are more likely than fusiform aneurysms to occur in the thoracic aorta.
■ All aneurysms show laminated yellow-brown thrombus.
■ The caliber of the lumen generally approximates that of the adjoining aorta in fusiform aneurysms.

■ Often, the surgeon leaves the aneurysm in place while performing a bypass; the pathologist receives luminal thrombus and/or fragment of aortic wall in one or multiple pieces.

Histologic Findings

■ The aorta adjacent to aneurysms generally shows severe atherosclerosis.
■ Atherosclerosis extends a variable distance into the aneurysms, showing destruction of elastic lamellae by gradual attenuation with smooth muscle cell atrophy.
■ Elastic stains are helpful in showing loss of media and increase in collagen.
■ Calcification and bony metaplasia are common.
■ There is luminal thrombus, with little organization.
■ Old leaks indicative of previous rupture are identified by hemosiderin-laden macrophages in adventitial infiltrates.

Treatment

■ Surgical treatment of fusiform aneurysms consists of bypass with Dacron or polytetrafluoroethylene (Gore-Tex) tube grafting, with inclusion of prosthesis and oversewing with aneurysmal tissue.
■ Woven Dacron tube graft placement with inclusion technique often yields relatively little tissue for the surgical pathologist. Tissue consists of that obtained at anastomotic and thrombus sites.
■ In patients with significant iliac stenosis or aneurysms, bifurcating graft is used between the aorta and iliac arteries.
■ Saccular aneurysms may be repaired by a Dacron patch if less than 50% of the aortic circumference is involved.
■ Survival depends on the initial risk of the patient:

  • High-risk patients (>75 years of age, presence of other life-threatening medical conditions, aneurysm >6 cm): operative mortality 40%, 5-year survival 10%
  • Low-risk patients (aneurysm >4.5 cm and <6 cm, no other significant medical conditions): 4% operative mortality with 55% 5-year survival, similar to age-matched controls

References

Bengtsson H, Nilsson P, Bergqvist D. Natural history of abdominal aortic aneurysm detected by screening. Br J Surg 80:718–720, 1993.
d'Amati G, Silver MD. Atherosclerosis of the aorta and its complications. In Silver MD (ed). *Cardiovascular Pathology,* 2nd ed. New York, Churchill Livingstone, 1991, pp 267–340.
Reilly JM, Tilson MD. Incidence and etiology of abdominal aortic aneurysms. Surg Clin North Am 69;705–717, 1989.

PENETRATING ATHEROSCLEROTIC ULCER

A penetrating atherosclerotic ulcer is an atherosclerotic lesion with ulceration that penetrates the internal elastic lamina and allows hematoma formation within the aortic wall.

Clinical Findings

■ Mean age of onset is 55 to 75 years.

■ Elderly hypertensive patients with severe atherosclerosis are usually affected.

■ There is a sudden onset of severe chest or back pain.

■ The patient may also present with distal embolization, or there may be incidental findings on chest radiograph.

■ Penetrating atherosclerotic ulcer clinically mimics classic aortic dissection but has imaging features that are distinct.

■ Chest radiograph shows diffuse or, less commonly, focal enlargement of the descending thoracic aorta.

■ Contrast-enhanced computed tomography is the primary imaging modality, which shows intramural hematoma, focal ulcer, displaced intimal calcification, and a thick or enhancing aortic wall in the absence of a double lumen as seen in dissection.

Pathologic Findings

■ The descending thoracic aorta is most often involved, but the ascending aorta may also be involved.

■ There is a discrete ulcer crater with atherosclerotic plaque and mural hemorrhage; dissection is limited to 1 to 2 cm or less.

Complications

■ Progression to saccular pseudoaneurysm (via rupture) or fusiform aneurysm can occur.

■ Extended aortic dissection, aortic rupture, and embolization are uncommon.

Treatment

■ The rate of progression of penetrating ulcers is controversial, as is the need for surgical rather than medical therapy.

■ Conservative treatment consists primarily of antihypertensive medications.

■ Resection of only a conservative segment of the proximal descending aorta suffices for classic dissection in the upper descending thoracic aorta, but the penetrating aortic ulcer requires graft replacement in the area of the ulcer and intramural hematoma.

References

Cooke JP, Kazmier FJ, Orszulak TA. The penetrating aortic ulcer: pathologic manifestations, diagnosis, and management. Mayo Clin Proc 63:718–725, 1988.

Harris JA, Bis KG, Glover JL, Bendick PJ, Shetty A, Brown OW. Penetrating atherosclerotic ulcers of the aorta. J Vasc Surg 19:90–98, 1994.

Hussain S, Glover JL, Bree R, Bendick PJ. Penetrating atherosclerotic ulcers of the thoracic aorta. J Vasc Surg 9:710–717, 1989.

Kazerooni EA, Bree RL, Williams DM. Penetrating atherosclerotic ulcers of the descending thoracic aorta: evaluation with CT and distinction from aortic dissection. Radiology 183:759–765, 1992.

Stanson AW, Kazmier FJ, Hollier LH, et al. Penetrating atherosclerotic ulcers of the thoracic aorta: natural history and clinicopathologic correlations. Ann Vasc Surg 1:15–23, 1986.

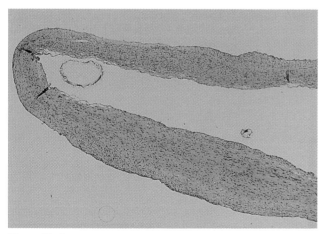

Figure 15–1. Aneurysm, sinus of Valsalva, Movat pentachrome stain. A 35-year-old woman with congestive heart failure had a right aortic sinus of Valsalva aneurysm, which was surgically removed. Note the thin, elongated section of aortic sinus.

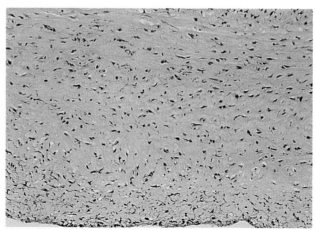

Figure 15–2. A higher magnification of Figure 15–1 demonstrates smooth muscle proliferation in a proteoglycan matrix; no elastic fibers are identified.

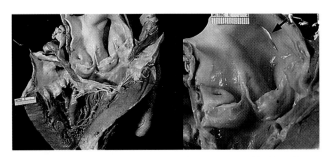

Figure 15–3. Marfan syndrome, annuloaortic ectasia with dissection. A 23-year-old man died suddenly. At autopsy, there were classic features of Marfan syndrome. Note the annuloaortic ectasia of the ascending aorta, with a longitudinal tear (arrow).

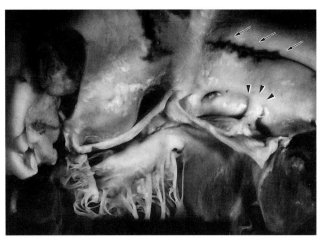

Figure 15–4. Aortic dissection, bicuspid aortic valve. A 55-year-old white woman with a history of systemic hypertension was found to have a bicuspid aortic valve with annuloaortic ectasia 9 years before the sudden onset of chest pain. Angiography demonstrated an acute dissection, but the patient died before surgical repair could be attempted. The pericardium contained 400 mL of blood, and there was a transverse tear of the ascending aorta *(arrows)* with dissection extending to involve the arch vessels. The heart has been opened through the left ventricular outflow, exposing a bicuspid aortic valve with a raphe *(arrowheads)* in the right cusp. The valve was mildly calcific and incompetent; the heart weighed 620 g.

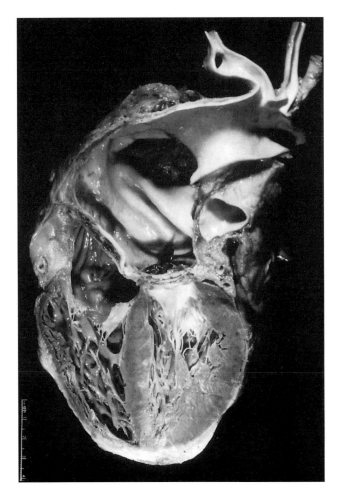

Figure 15–5. Dissecting aneurysm, postsurgical. A 59-year-old man had a history of chronic hypertension and aortic valve replacement 8 years before his death. Postoperatively, the patient experienced complications of ascending aortic aneurysm, which, despite partial resection, recurred. The patient experienced sudden chest pain immediately before death and died from dissection of the aneurysm. At autopsy, the ascending aortic aneurysm involved the root of the aorta, which is thin walled. Note the transverse intimal tear indicative of dissection.

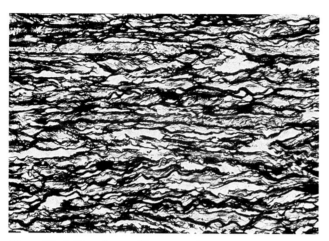

Figure 15–6. Normal aorta, Movat pentachrome stain. Histologic section of the medial wall of the ascending aorta shows parallel elastic lamellae with intervening smooth muscle cells, collagen, and some proteoglycan.

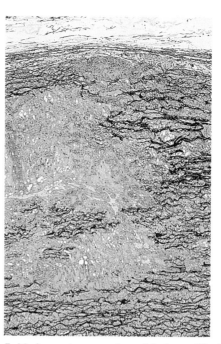

Figure 15–7. Marfan syndrome, cystic medial change. Histologic section of the aorta from a patient with aortic dissection secondary to Marfan syndrome. There is marked loss of elastic lamellae and focal extensive proteoglycan deposition.

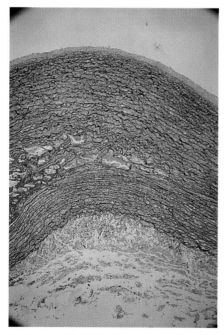

Figure 15–8. Marfan syndrome, acute dissection. Histologic section of the aorta demonstrates acute dissection. Note the minimal increase in proteoglycans consistent with mild cystic medial change.

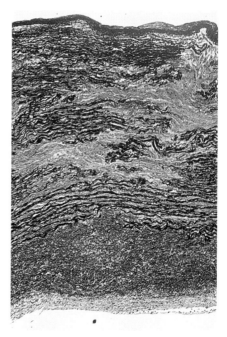

Figure 15–9. Marfan syndrome, chronic dissection and medial degeneration. Note the loss of elastic fibers without proteoglycan deposition. The intima is seen at the top of the figure, and the organized lining of the false lumen is the relatively homogeneous area at the bottom of the photomicrograph.

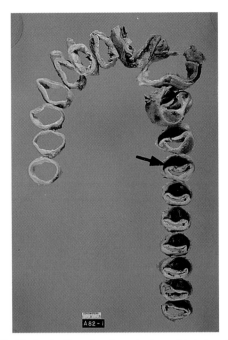

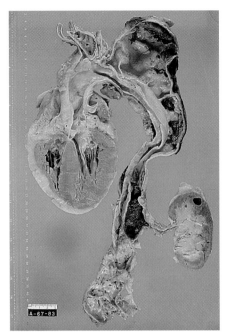

Figure 15–10. Aortic dissection, hypertension related, type III. A 64-year-old man with a history of smoking, diabetes, peripheral vascular disease, and hypertension died suddenly. At autopsy, there was extensive left hemothorax and an acute dissection *(arrow)* of the descending thoracic aorta, which was sectioned at 1- to 1.5-cm intervals. Note the acute posterior dissection, commencing distal to the left subclavian artery and extending into the descending thoracic aorta. A healed dissection in the anterior wall is present at the level of the subclavian artery, extending only 3 cm distally.

Figure 15–11. Aortic dissection, hypertension related, type III. A 71-year-old man with systemic hypertension died of rupture of a dissecting saccular aneurysm into the left pleural cavity. A healed dissection is present in the descending thoracic aorta, extending just distal to the left renal artery. There is organizing thrombus in the large aneurysm near the left subclavian artery and a thrombus in the dissection to the left of the kidney.

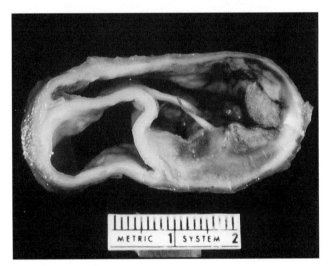

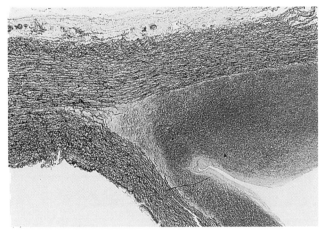

Figure 15–12. Chronic dissection. A transverse section of the aorta shows a false and a true lumen. The false lumen is the larger and the luminal surface shows organizing thrombus. Note the presence of a fibrous tag. The true lumen (to the left) is smaller with a smooth surface.

Figure 15–13. Chronic dissection. A histologic section shows a true lumen (to the left) and a false lumen (to the right) with organization of the false lumen.

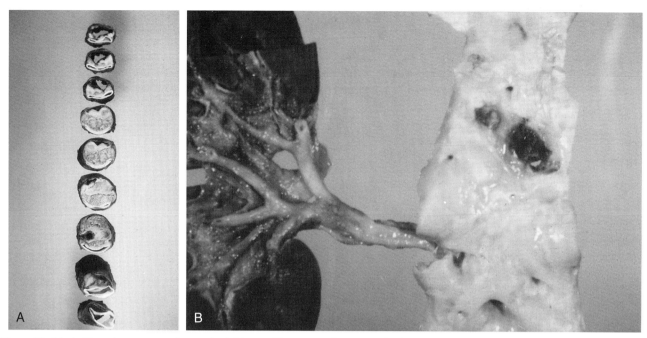

Figure 15–14. *A,* Dissecting aneurysm, iatrogenic. A 64-year-old woman underwent repair of atrial septal defect and replacement of tricuspid and mitral valves. Intraoperative shock necessitated placement of an intra-aortic balloon; death occurred 30 days postoperatively. At autopsy, a thoracic aortic dissection was noted. Note the multiple transverse sections of aorta. The false lumen is largely filled by thrombus. *B,* The intimal tear is proximal to the renal artery at the site of an ulcerated atheroma.

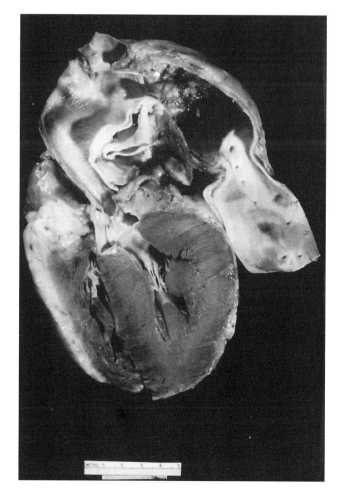

Figure 15–15. Traumatic aneurysm. Heart and attached ascending, transverse, and descending thoracic aorta from a young woman with a history of chest trauma 5 years before her death show a localized aneurysm in the descending thoracic aorta near the ligamentum arteriosus.

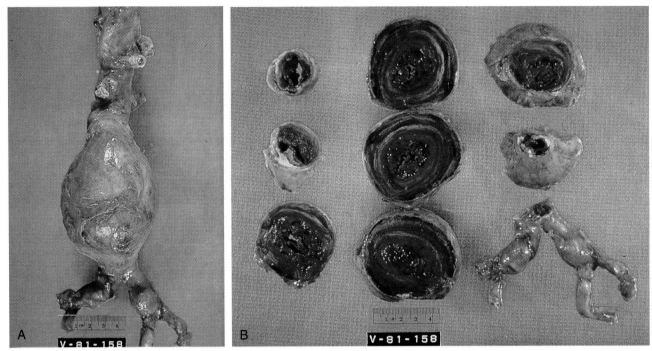

Figure 15–16. *A,* Atherosclerotic aneurysm. A 67-year-old man died of multiple cerebrovascular accidents with ischemic cardiomyopathy. At autopsy, there were an incidental infrarenal abdominal aortic fusiform aneurysm and an aneurysm in both common iliac arteries. *B,* The abdominal aorta is cut transversely without prior fixation at 1- to 1.5-cm intervals. Note the small lumen with multiple circumferential layers of thrombus. There was severe atherosclerosis of the rest of the thoracic aorta, and multiple atheroemboli were noted in most organs.

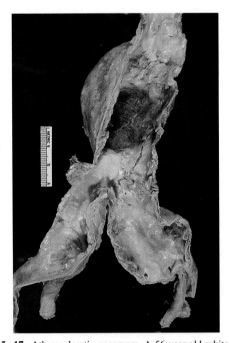

Figure 15–17. Atherosclerotic aneurysm. A 56-year-old white man had heterozygous type II hyperlipidemia and a long history of coronary artery disease; he died 1 hour after the onset of chest pain. A longitudinally opened saccular abdominal aortic aneurysm (ventral aspect) shows luminal thrombus and aneurysms of the common iliac arteries with extensive atherosclerotic plaquing and calcification.

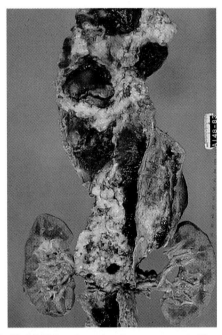

Figure 15–18. Multiple atherosclerotic aneurysms. A 75-year-old man had aortofemoral bypass graft surgery for peripheral vascular disease. Risk factors included smoking and hypertension. An incidental tortuous, dilated aorta was found. One year later, the patient had severe chest pain and fatal cardiac arrest. At autopsy, a right hemothorax from a ruptured thoracic aneurysm was found. The longitudinally opened descending thoracic aorta and a portion of infrarenal abdominal aorta show five saccular aneurysms and extensive atherosclerosis. The lumina of the saccular aneurysms are filled with thrombus. The largest aneurysm was ruptured *(right, above renal arteries).*

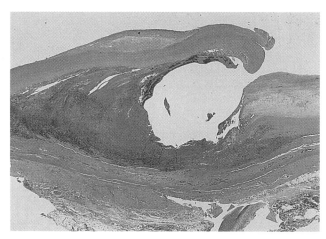

Figure 15–19. Atherosclerotic penetrating ulcer. A 75-year-old man had severe back pain. A computed tomography scan demonstrated a penetrating ulcer on the anterior wall of the aorta with a flap indicating local dissection. Note the extensive atherosclerotic ulceration and erosion of the ulcer with organizing thrombus.

CHAPTER 16

Inflammatory Diseases of the Aorta

CLASSIFICATION

- There is overlap in the gross and microscopic findings of the different aortitis syndromes, especially in the late stages of disease.
- Clinical and radiologic information are often crucial in diagnosis.
- Grossly, a "tree bark" appearance occurs secondary to obliteration of the vasa vasorum and medial necrosis and is seen in syphilitic and noninfectious aortitis.
- Certain aortitides may be unclassifiable because either there is unclear history or there are nonspecific pathologic findings.
- Table 16–1 lists types of inflammatory diseases treated with surgical aortic resection.

TAKAYASU'S AORTITIS

Takayasu's aortitis is also called aortic arch syndrome, pulseless disease, occlusive thromboaortopathy, and young female arteritis.

Clinical Manifestations

Patient Characteristics

- Takayasu's aortitis affects women more frequently than men at a ratio of 8:1.
- The highest incidence is in Asian and African patients, but there is worldwide distribution.
- The age range at onset is 3.5 to 66 years (mean 20–50 years).

Early Phase

- The early phase is characterized by malaise, weakness, fever, night sweats, arthralgias, arthritis, myalgias, weight loss, pleuritic pain, and anorexia.
- The early phase precedes the occlusive phase by weeks to months.

Late Phase

- Late phase symptoms are related to the aorta and arch vessels as follows:

  - Absent pulses (96%)
  - Bruits (94%)
  - Hypertension (74%)
  - Heart failure (28%)
  - Retinopathy (25%); associated with carotid artery involvement

- Involvement of the aortic root and aortic valve occurs in 10% to 20% of patients and leads to aortic insufficiency.
- Coronary ostial stenosis occurs in 10% to 15% of patients and leads to angina or myocardial infarction.
- Aneurysmal dilatations are reported in 10% to 30% of patients. Complications include pulsatile masses, em-

Table 16–1
SURGICAL AORTIC RESECTIONS,
INFLAMMATORY DISEASES, AFIP*
1970–1993

| Diagnosis | Thoracic Aorta | | Abdominal Aorta | Totals |
	Ascending	Descending		
Takayasu's disease	4	5	2	11
Inflammatory abdominal aneurysm	0	0	11	11
Nonspecific aortitis	8	0	0	8
Giant cell/granulomatous aortitis	4	1	2	7
Syphilis	2	0	1	3
Reiter's syndrome	1	0	0	1
Staphylococcal aneurysm	0	1	0	1
Total	**19**	**7**	**16**	**42**

*Armed Forces Institute of Pathology.

134

bolism from mural thrombus, and rupture of aneurysm, leading to hemothorax.

Types of Takayasu's Disease

- In type I, the aortic arch and arch vessels are involved.
- In type II, the descending thoracic aorta and abdominal aorta are involved.
- Type III is a combination of types I and II.
- Type IV has the features of type I, II, or III plus involvement of pulmonary arteries.

Laboratory Abnormalities

- Elevated erythrocyte sedimentation rate
- Low-grade leukocytosis
- Mild, normocytic, normochromic anemia (early systemic phase)
- Elevated serum IgG and IgM
- Association with HLA-B5, Bw52, and Dw12 antigens

Pathologic Findings

Early Phase

- There is vascular edema and florid infiltration by lymphocytes, plasma cells, occasional giant cells, and histiocytes.
- The inflammatory process is marked in the outer two thirds of the media, with extension into the adventitia.
- Cuffing, intimal proliferation, and obliteration of the vasa vasorum occur, without fibrinoid necrosis.
- There is patchy coagulative necrosis of media with surrounding histiocytes and occasional giant cells.
- Intima is normal.

Late Phase

- Grossly, there are segmental or diffuse narrowings, generally of the arch vessels, descending thoracic aorta, and less commonly abdominal aorta.
- Aneurysms occur in 10% to 30% and are generally in the ascending aorta; occasionally there may be diffuse ectasia of the entire aorta.
- Gross appearance resembles tree bark.
- Histologically, there is marked fibrointimal proliferation and adventitial thickening.
- Intimal proliferation of smooth muscle cells in a myxoid, proteoglycan-rich background leads to stenotic lesions of the arch vessels at their origin.
- There is medial destruction and replacement by fibrous tissue.
- Arteries involved and their frequency in the United States include the following:

  - Aorta (80%–100%)
  - Subclavian (90%)
  - Carotid (45%)
  - Vertebral (25%)
  - Renal (20%)

Treatment and Course

- Survival rate is 97% over 5 to 7 years in patients without complications and 57% in patients with complications.

- Slow natural progression is the rule.
- Treatment includes corticosteroid therapy or cyclophosphamide therapy in the acute phase of the disease.
- Surgical bypass may be necessary for chronic obstructive lesions or aneurysm repair.

References

Hall S, Barr W, Lie JT, Stanson AW, Kazimier FJ. Takayasu's arteritis. A study of 32 North American patients. Medicine 64:89–99, 1985.

Ishikawa K. Patterns of symptoms and prognosis in occlusive thromboaortopathy (Takayasu's disease). J Am Coll Cardiol 8:1041–1046, 1986.

Lupi-Herrera E, Sanchez-Torres G, Marcushamer J, Mispireta J, Horowitz S, Vela JE. Takayasu's arteritis. Clinical study of 107 cases. Am Heart J 93:94–103, 1977.

Rose AG, Sinclar-Smith CC. Takayasu's arteritis: a study of 16 autopsy cases. Arch Pathol Lab Med 107:231–237, 1980.

Subramanyan R, Roy J, Balakrishnan KG. Natural history of aortoarteritis (Takayasu's disease). Circulation 80:429–437, 1989.

Virmani R, Lande A, McAllister HA Jr. Pathologic aspects of Takayasu's arteritis. In Lande A, Berkman YM, McAllister HA (eds). *Aortitis: Clinical, Pathologic and Radiographic Aspects*. New York, Raven Press, 1986, pp 55–79.

GIANT CELL ARTERITIS

Patient Characteristics

- Giant cell arteritis is rare in patients younger than 50 years of age.
- There is a female predominance (female:male ratio 2–4:1).
- The highest frequency recorded is in Denmark.
- In U.S. upper Midwest, prevalence was 133 per 100,000 individuals older than 50 years of age in 1975; annual incidence in the same population was 17 per 100,000.
- The disease is rare in Asians and blacks.

Clinical Features of Aortic Involvement

- Aortic involvement occurs in approximately 10% to 15% of severe cases of giant cell arteritis.
- Generally, patients have symptoms of polymyalgia rheumatica (see Chap. 20), including fatigue, fever, headaches, jaw claudication, loss of vision, and scalp tenderness.
- Aortic arch syndrome is typical of aortic involvement and includes the following features:

  - Upper and lower extremity claudication
  - Paresthesias
  - Raynaud's phenomenon
  - Abdominal angina
  - Transient ischemic attacks

- Subclavian steal syndrome occurs in patients with proximal carotid disease.
- Less common complications include

  - Aortic aneurysms
  - Aortic dissection
  - Aortic valve insufficiency

- Renal artery involvement does not occur.

Radiologic and Laboratory Findings

- Similar to giant cell arteritis without aortic involvement (see Chap. 20), there are an elevated erythrocyte sedimentation rate, elevated acute phase reactants, hypergammaglobulinemia, and increased serum C3 and C4 levels.
- Angiographically, there are long, smooth, tapering stenoses with intervening normal or slightly dilated areas.
- Angiographically, there is an absence of ulcerated plaques of atherosclerosis, and involvement of the subclavian, axillary, and brachial arteries, as seen in Takayasu's disease, occurs often.

Gross Pathologic Findings

- In symptomatic patients, aneurysms of the thoracic and rarely abdominal aorta may result in dissections or rupture.
- The "tree bark" appearance is similar to that of other inflammatory disease of the aorta.
- The gross features are distinguishable from Takayasu's in that there is less intimal thickening and adventitial scarring.

Microscopic Pathologic Findings

- Features are nonspecific, necessitating clinicopathologic correlation.
- Panarteritis involves all three layers of the aorta.
- Inflammatory infiltrate consists of lymphocytes, plasma cells, histiocytes, and giant cells in areas of elastic lamellar disruption and fragmentation.
- Inflammation is most pronounced in the inner one half of the aorta.
- The finding of a large number of giant cells is helpful, but it is not a prerequisite for the diagnosis.
- Intimal fibrosis is present, but usually not to the degree that is seen in Takayasu's aortitis.
- Dissection may rarely occur.

References

Evans JM. Bowles CA, Bjornsson J, Mullany CJ, Hunder GG. Thoracic aortic aneurysm and rupture in giant cell aortitis. A descriptive study of 41 cases. Arthritis Rheum 37:1539–1547, 1994.
Klein RG, Hunder GG, Stanson AW, Sheps SG. Large artery involvement in giant cell (temporal) arteritis. Ann Intern Med 83:806–812, 1975.
Salisbury RS, Hazelman B. Successful treatment of dissecting aortic aneurysm due to giant cell arteritis. Ann Rheum Dis 40:507–508, 1981.

RHEUMATOID AORTITIS

- Rheumatoid aortitis occurs in only 5% of patients with rheumatoid arthritis and is less common than myocardial or valvular involvement.
- The mean duration of symptoms of rheumatoid arthritis is 10 years.
- There is no sex predilection.

Symptoms

- Aneurysms may occur in the thoracic or abdominal aorta and may be detected incidentally, or they may rupture or cause aortic insufficiency.
- Congestive heart failure may occur from a combination of valvular disease, myocardial disease, and aortic disease.

Pathologic Findings

- The aortic wall is grossly thickened and dilated.
- Areas of dilatation may result in fusiform aneurysms of either the thoracic or abdominal aorta.
- Histologically, inflammation consists of lymphocytes, plasma cells, and histiocytes, with or without rheumatoid nodules.
- Inflammation typically involves the media and adventitia.
- Although perivascular cuffing is present, endarteritis obliterans is not typical as is seen in syphilitic aortitis or Takayasu's aortitis.
- Medial destruction results in replacement of smooth muscle cells and elastic fibers by collagen.

References

Gravallese EM, Carson JM, Coblyn JS, Pinkus GS, Weinblatt ME. Rheumatoid aortitis: a rarely recognized but clinically significant entity. Medicine 68:95–106, 1989.
Reimer KA, Rodgers R, Oyasu R. Rheumatoid arthritis with rheumatoid heart disease and granulomatous aortitis. JAMA 235:2510–2512, 1976.

SERONEGATIVE SPONDYLOARTHROPATHIES

Seronegative spondyloarthropathy is an idiopathic inflammatory disease characterized by progressive bilateral sacroiliitis, peripheral arthritis, and uveal inflammation. There is an association with HLA-B27 antigen, previous bacterial infections, and inflammatory bowel disease. Seronegative spondyloarthropathies include ankylosing spondylitis, Reiter's syndrome, and psoriatic arthritis; there is a possible relationship with Behçet's disease. Synonyms and related terms include seronegative arthritis, ankylosing spondylitis, HLA-B27 disease, and hereditary multifocal relapsing inflammation (HEMRI).

Ankylosing Spondylitis

- Ankylosing spondylitis includes bilateral sacroiliitis (>90%), peripheral arthritis (75%), and uveitis (10%–20%).
- There is a male predominance of 9:1. Most patients are between 15 and 40 years of age.
- There is an association with previous exposure to *Klebsiella*.
- Ninety-five percent of patients and 50% of first-degree relatives possess HLA-B27 antigen, providing evidence of a genetic linkage.

- Aortic disease occurs in 1% to 10% of patients and is related to the duration of the disease and severity of peripheral joint disease.
- A major cardiovascular complication is aortic insufficiency, which results from dilatation of the proximal aorta and scarring of the aortic valve.
- Heart block may result from inflammation extending into the ventricular septum and conduction tissues.
- Unlike rheumatoid aortitis, aortitis of ankylosing spondylitis may rarely precede the arthritic symptoms.
- Cardiac and aortic disease occur in up to 30% of patients with more than 10 years of joint symptoms; these include aortic insufficiency, pericardial effusions, and cardiac conduction disturbances (atrioventricular block).

Reiter's Syndrome

- In Reiter's syndrome, a triad of nongonococcal urethritis, conjunctivitis, and sacroiliitis follow a bout of nongonococcal urethritis or bacillary dysentery.
- There is a strong association with HLA-B27.
- Disease may be precipitated by exposure to *Chlamydia*.
- Aortitis occurs in 2% to 5% of patients and may be accompanied by coronary ostial stenosis.

Psoriatic Arthritis

- In psoriatic arthritis, there is a weaker association with HLA-B27 or uveitis, as compared with that of Reiter's syndrome or ankylosing spondylitis.
- There is a male predominance.
- Aortic disease is rare; less than 3% of patients have aortic regurgitation.
- The incidence of mitral valve prolapse may be increased compared with that of the normal population.

Pathologic Findings

- Seronegative spondyloarthropathies preferentially involve the proximal ascending aorta (sinuses of Valsalva and proximal several centimeters of the ascending tubular aorta).
- Thickening of the aortic valve and anterior leaflet of the mitral valve results in a characteristic "bump" in ankylosing spondylitis.
- Histologically, perivascular inflammation of the vasa vasorum, endarteritis obliterans, and inflammation of the aortic valve occur; inflammation consists of chronic inflammatory cells and scattered neutrophils.
- Coronary ostial stenosis may occur.
- Chronically, there is fibrosis of the adventitia, media, and intima as well as focal calcification.
- Inflammation may extend into the conduction system, including the atrioventricular node and bundle of His.

References

Ansell BM, Bywaters EGL, Doniach I. The aortic lesion of ankylosing spondylitis. Br Heart J 20:507–515, 1958.

Brewerton DA, James DC. Histocompatibility antigen (HLA-B27) and disease. Semin Arthritis Rheum 4:191–207, 1975.

Bulkley BH, Roberts WC. Ankylosing spondylitis and aortic regurgitation. Description of the characteristic cardiovascular lesion from study of eight necropsy patients. Circulation 48:1014–1027, 1973.

Hoogland TY, Alexander DP, Patterson RH, Nashel DJ. Coronary artery stenosis in Reiter's syndrome: a complication of aortitis. J Rheumatol 21:757–759, 1994.

Paulus HE, Pearson CM, Pitts W Jr. Aortic insufficiency in five patients with Reiter's syndrome. A detailed clinical and pathologic study. Am J Med 53:464–472, 1972.

BEHÇET'S DISEASE

Behçet's disease is a recurrent, idiopathic inflammatory illness characterized by aphthous stomatitis, genital ulceration, and uveitis (see Chap. 20).

Patient Characteristics

- Behçet's disease is most common in patients from the Mediterranean region, Middle East, and Japan.
- Most patients are middle aged, and there is a slight male predominance.

Aortitis of Behçet's Disease

- In the active stage, there is chronic inflammatory infiltrate in media and adventitia with cuffing of vasa vasorum; rare giant cells occur.
- In the late stage, there is fibrous thickening of media and adventitia with endarteritis obliterans.

References

Chajek T, Fainara J. Behçet's disease: report of 41 cases and a review of the literature. Medicine (Baltimore) 54:179–196, 1975.

Hamza M. Large artery involvement in Behçet's disease. J Rheumatol 14:554–559, 1987.

Matsumoto T, Uekusa T, Fukuda Y. Vasculo-Behçet's disease: a pathologic study of eight cases. Hum Pathol 22:45–51, 1991.

INFLAMMATORY ANEURYSMS OF THE ABDOMINAL AORTA

- Inflammatory aneurysms of the abdominal aorta was first described by Walker and colleagues in 1972 as a variant of abdominal atherosclerotic aneurysm.
- The incidence is 5% to 10% of all operated abdominal aortic aneurysms.
- There is a male predominance (male:female ratio 9:1).
- The mean age of patients is 62 to 69 years.
- There is a possible relation to idiopathic sclerosing mesenteritis (idiopathic retroperitoneal fibrosis).

Clinical and Laboratory Findings

- Chronic abdominal and back pain often lasts several weeks.
- Weight loss occurs in 10% to 20% of patients.
- A triad of pain, weight loss, and medial deviation of ureters occurs.
- Seven percent to 33% of patients are asymptomatic.
- Symptoms caused by inflammation and ureteral obstruction may be confused with rupture.

■ Elevated erythrocyte sedimentation rate is frequent.
■ Computed tomography and ultrasound show soft-tissue density surrounding the atherosclerotic aneurysm.
■ Displacement and obstruction of ureters, duodenum, jejunoileum, mesentery, sigmoid colon, renal arteries and veins, and inferior vena cava may occur.

Pathologic Findings

■ Atherosclerotic plaque lines the luminal surface.
■ Attenuated media is partly or totally replaced by scar.
■ Adventitial and periadventitial fibrosis occur, as does inflammation with entrapped lymphoid aggregates and lymph nodes, areas of fat with fat necrosis, nerves, and ganglia.
■ Inflammatory infiltrate consists of lymphocytes, plasma cells, and macrophages.
■ The histologic appearance is reminiscent of sclerosing mesenteritis (idiopathic retroperitoneal fibrosis).

Complications and Treatment

■ Inflammatory aneurysms rupture less frequently than atherosclerotic aneurysms.
■ Treatment with steroids is sometimes beneficial.

References

Curci JJ. Modes of presentation and management of inflammatory aneurysms of the abdominal aorta. J Am Coll Surg 178:573–580, 1994.
Feiner HD, Raghavendra BN, Phelps R, Rooney L. Inflammatory abdominal aortic aneurysm: report of six cases. Hum Pathol 15:454–459, 1984.
Rose AG, Dent DM. Inflammatory variant of abdominal atherosclerotic aneurysm. Arch Pathol Lab Med 105:409–413, 1981.
Walker DI, Bloor K, Williams G, Gillie I. Inflammatory aneurysms of the abdominal aorta. Br J Surg 59:609–614, 1972.

SYPHILITIC AORTITIS

■ Syphilitic aortitis caused 1% of all cardiovascular deaths in adults between 1950 and 1965 in the United States.
■ The current incidence is much lower, but there may be a resurgence with the increase in cases of acquired immunodeficiency syndrome.
■ The latent period between primary syphilis and syphilitic aortitis is 5 to 40 years (typically 10–25 years).
■ Syphilitic heart disease is a constellation of

• Syphilitic aortitis
• Syphilitic aortic aneurysm
• Syphilitic aortic valvulitis
• Syphilitic coronary ostial stenosis

■ In syphilitic heart disease, ostial stenosis, aneurysm, or aortic regurgitation occurs in 66% of patients.
■ Asymptomatic aortitis is the most prevalent form of syphilitic cardiovascular involvement and may be suspected by a rough systolic ejection murmur, radiographic dilatation of the proximal aorta, and linear calcification of the ascending aorta.

Complications

■ Aortic insufficiency
■ Aneurysm rupture, thrombosis, or bony erosion
■ Superior vena cava syndrome
■ Rarely, dissections

Gross Pathologic Findings

■ There is involvement of the proximal aorta without extension beyond the renal arteries.
■ There is a "tree bark" appearance, with intervening areas of intimal thickening that are white and shiny.
■ In late stages, characteristic lesions may be obscured by atherosclerosis.
■ Aneurysms are saccular or fusiform as follows:

• Ascending aorta (46%)
• Transverse arch (24%)
• Sinus of Valsalva (10%)
• Upper abdominal aorta (7%)
• Descending thoracic aorta (5%)
• Descending aortic arch (5%)
• Multiple sites (4%)

Microscopic Pathologic Findings

■ Perivascular lymphocytes and plasma cells appear around the vasa vasorum, with endarteritis.
■ Inflammation extends into the media, resulting in a gross "tree bark" appearance.
■ Inflammation extends into the aorta root, resulting in dilatation of the aortic root and aortic regurgitation.
■ Areas of acute necrosis of the aortic wall, with neutrophilic infiltrates (microgummas), may contain treponemes, as demonstrated by Warthin-Starry stain.

Laboratory Diagnosis

■ Only 10% to 30% of patients have a history of syphilis or other manifestations of tertiary syphilis, emphasizing the need for serologic diagnosis.
■ Nontreponemal tests (Venereal Disease Research Laboratory, other serologic tests for syphilis) may be positive in as few as 40% of patients and lack specificity.
■ Treponemal tests (*Treponema pallidum* immobilization, fluorescent treponemal antibody absorption) are reactive in more than 90% of cases.
■ In elderly patients with tertiary syphilis, there may be false-negative serology.
■ Because of the lack of specificity of histologic findings, the diagnosis of syphilitic aortitis should not be made in the absence of serologic confirmation.
■ Some cases of inflammatory aortitis remain idiopathic because of limitations in histologic findings and serologic tests.

References

Heggtveit HA. Syphilitic aortitis. A clinicopathologic autopsy study of 100 cases, 1950–1960. Circulation 29:346–355, 1964.
Jackman JD, Radolf JD. Cardiovascular syphilis. Am J Med 87:425–433, 1989.

MISCELLANEOUS AORTITIS

Tuberculous Aortitis

- Tuberculous aortitis involves the thoracic and abdominal aortae with equal frequency.
- Tuberculous aortitis results from the contiguous spread of the tuberculous process from a tuberculoma in the lung or periaortic lymph node, or from an adjacent empyema or osteomyelitis.
- Pathologic features include necrotizing granulomas involving the adventitia and media.
- Complications include rupture and aneurysm.

Sarcoid Aortitis

- Although sarcoid granulomas frequently involve the adventitia of small and medium-sized arteries of the heart and lungs, aortic involvement is rare.
- Sarcoid aortitis is usually limited to the adventitia.
- Reported sites of involvement are the abdominal and descending thoracic aortae and the pulmonary, subclavian, and iliac arteries.

Pyogenic Aortitis

- Pyogenic aortitis was originally described by Osler as a "mycotic aneurysm."
- The term "infected aneurysm" is preferred, to avoid confusion with a fungal infection.

- There is a predilection for areas of congenital anomalies (coarctation) and previous surgery (graft anastomoses). It may occur in structurally normal aortae, especially in patients prone to endocarditis (e.g., drug abusers).
- Ulcerated atherosclerotic plaques may rarely become infected.
- Radiologically, there is marked soft-tissue swelling around the aneurysm.
- Routes of invasion of the aorta by organisms are as follows:

  - Implantation on intimal surface
  - Infection via the vasa vasorum
  - Direct extension from contiguous extravascular site
  - Traumatic inoculation of contaminated material

- Histologically, there is medial destruction with microabscess formation.
- Differential diagnosis includes atherosclerosis with inflammation (which is common) and inflammatory aneurysm.
- Organisms implicated include salmonella, streptococci, staphylococci, and gonococci.

Reference

Worrell JT, Buja LM, Reynolds RC. Pneumococcal aortitis with rupture of the aorta. Am J Clin Pathol 89:565–568, 1988.

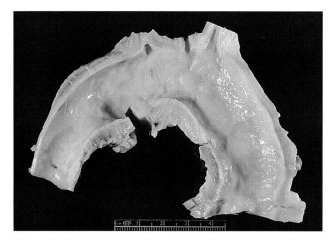

Figure 16–1. Takayasu's aortitis, stenotic lesions. A 51-year-old white woman had severe congestive heart failure. Physical examination revealed aortic incompetence and pericarditis. Coronary angiography showed bilateral ostial stenosis. At autopsy, there was marked thickening of the ascending aorta, the arch vessels, and a portion of the descending thoracic aorta. Note the normal thickness of the wall of the distal thoracic aorta.

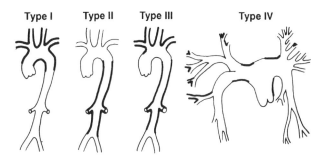

Figure 16–2. Classification of Takayasu's arteritis as modified by Lupi-Herrera and colleagues (1977). Type I: Disease is limited to the aortic arch and its branches. Type II: Lesions affect the descending thoracic and abdominal aortae without involving the arch. Type III. Extensive lesions involve the arch and the thoracic and abdominal aortae. Type IV: The features of types I, II, and III are present as is pulmonary artery involvement. Thickened lines represent areas of inflammation.

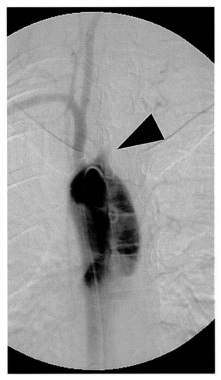

Figure 16–3. Takayasu's aortitis, stenotic lesion. Angiogram from a 21-year-old woman with a carotid bruit and stroke. Note the occlusion of the brachiocephalic artery near its origin.

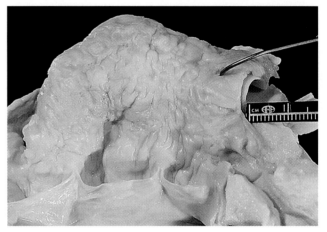

Figure 16–4. Takayasu's aortitis, aneurysm formation. Note the "tree bark" appearance and dilatation of the ascending aorta.

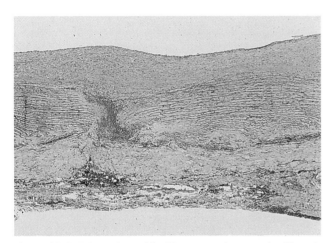

Figure 16–5. Takayasu's aortitis, Movat pentachrome stain. There is marked thickening of the adventitia (yellow) and intima (green). Note the focal disruption of the media.

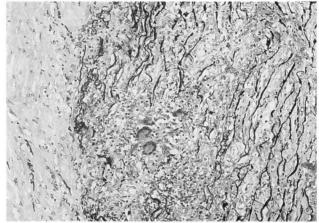

Figure 16–6. Takayasu's aortitis. A higher magnification of Figure 16–5 demonstrates destruction of medial elastic lamellae and a chronic inflammatory infiltrate with giant cells.

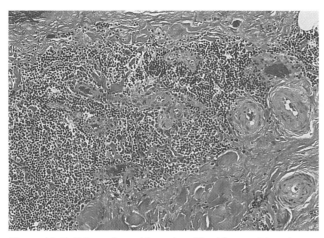

Figure 16–7. Takayasu's aortitis, endarteritis obliterans. There is scarring and inflammation of the adventitia.

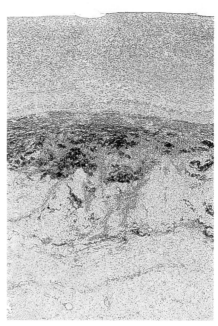

Figure 16–8. Takayasu's aortitis, healed lesion. There is marked disorganization and destruction of elastic fibers in the media. Note the marked intimal and adventitial thickening.

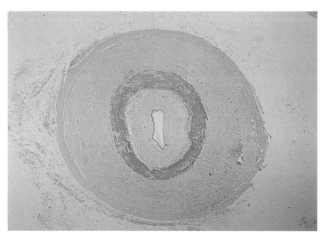

Figure 16–9. Takayasu's arteritis, arch vessel, elastic van Gieson's stain. Histologic section shows focal mild loss of elastic tissue of media and marked fibrosis of the intima and adventitia without inflammation (healed lesion).

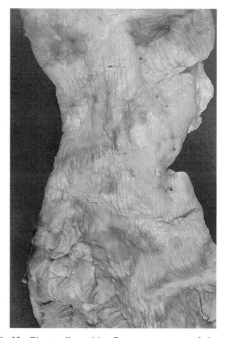

Figure 16–10. Giant cell aortitis. Gross appearance of the aorta in a 74-year-old woman. Note the wrinkling "tree bark" appearance and the mild focal atherosclerosis.

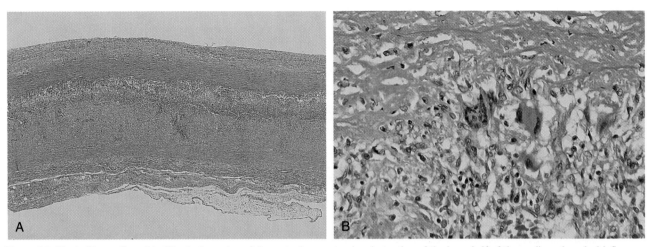

Figure 16–11. *A,* Giant cell aortitis. Histologic section of the aorta shows extensive destruction of the inner half of the media and marked inflammation. *B,* Higher magnification demonstrates necrosis of the media with surrounding lymphocytic infiltrate with macrophages and giant cells.

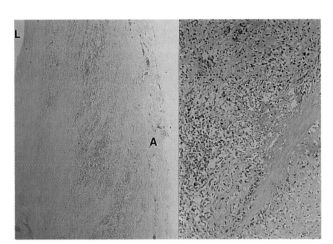

Figure 16–12. Rheumatoid arthritis. A 57-year-old woman with long-standing rheumatoid arthritis, myocardial infarction, and congestive heart failure died of cardiac complications. At autopsy, there were rheumatoid nodules in the aortic, mitral, and tricuspid valves, the left ventricle, the coronary arteries, and the aorta. Note the rheumatoid nodule in the adventitial medial interface. A, adventitia; L, lumen.

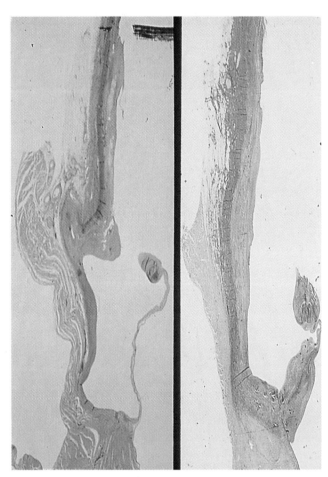

Figure 16–13. Ankylosing spondylitis, elastic van Gieson's stain. Aortic valve from a normal heart *(left)* and from a patient with ankylosing spondylitis *(right).* Note the thickened aorta, sinus of Valsalva, and base of the aortic valve *(right).* (Courtesy Dr. William C. Roberts.)

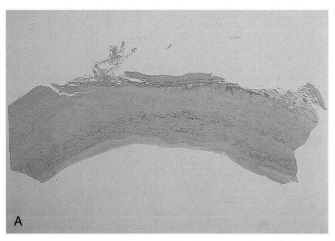 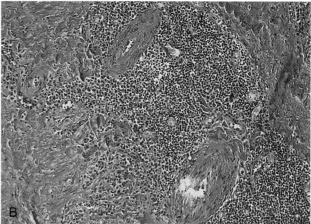

Figure 16–14. *A,* Ankylosing spondylitis. Low-power view of the ascending aorta. Note the extensive inflammation in the media and adventitia. *B,* Higher magnification shows extensive lymphoplasmacytic infiltrate around the vasa vasorum.

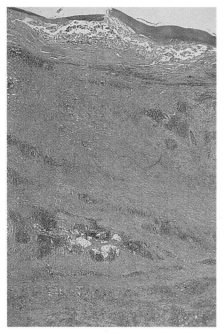 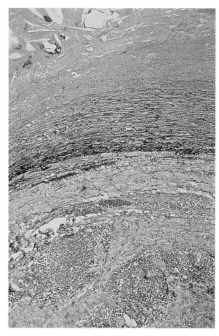

Figure 16–15. Inflammatory aneurysm. A 49-year-old man had an abdominal aortic aneurysm. The intimal surface is at the top of the field. Note the lymphoid aggregates and dense scarring of the adventitia.

Figure 16–16. Inflammatory aneurysm. A 54-year-old man had excision of an abdominal aortic aneurysm. Note the intimal atherosclerosis, focal destruction of media, and marked adventitial fibrosis and lymphoid nodules.

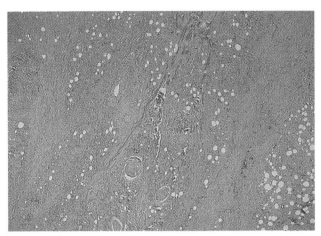

Figure 16–17. Inflammatory aneurysm. Note the entrapped fat and nerves within the scarred, inflammatory process.

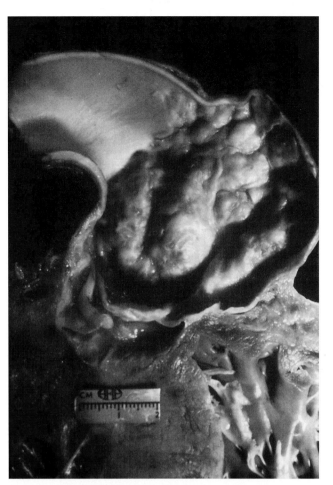

Figure 16–18. Syphilitic aortic aneurysm. Localized aneurysm of the ascending aorta with dilatation of the sinus of Valsalva is shown from a 58-year-old man with a history of syphilis. Note the wrinkling of the intima and thickening of the aortic valve's free margins.

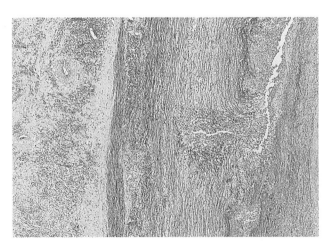

Figure 16–19. Syphilitic aneurysm, Movat pentachrome stain. The histology is nonspecific and demonstrates adventitial inflammation and scarring, and focal disruption of the media.

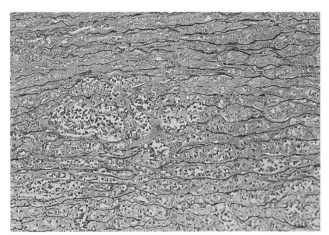

Figure 16–20. Syphilitic aneurysm. A higher magnification of Figure 16–19 shows medial acute and chronic inflammation with focal disruption of elastic lamellae as well as focal necrosis.

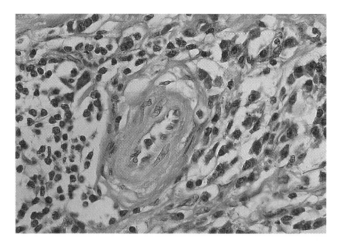

Figure 16–21. Syphilitic aneurysms, adventitial perivascular inflammation. The infiltrates are composed of plasma cells and lymphocytes. The histology is nonspecific, and similar infiltrates, as well as endarteritis obliterans, may be seen in the aortitis of Takayasu's disease and Behçet's disease.

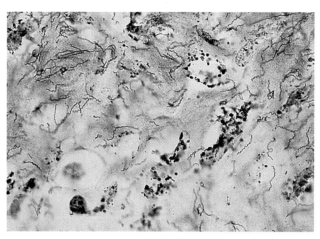

Figure 16–22. Syphilitic aneurysm, treponemal organisms. In rare cases of syphilitic aneurysms, the organisms of *Treponema pallidum* may be identified. This photomicrograph was taken from a section stained by Warthin-Starry silver technique from the same case illustrated in Figures 16–19 and 16–20.

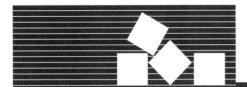

CHAPTER 17

Pulmonary Hypertension

EVALUATION OF LUNG BIOPSY SAMPLES FOR PULMONARY HYPERTENSION

- Elastic stains (e.g., Movat pentachrome, elastic van Gieson's) should be used for evaluation of vessels.
- The distinction between arteries and veins may be difficult; serial sections with elastic stains may be necessary.
- In general, pulmonary arteries travel with bronchi and are normally approximately the same diameter.
- Veins travel with lymphatics in the septa.
- Normal arteries have a distinct demarcation between adventitia and media. This demarcation is less distinct in veins, which typically possess numerous layers of adventitial elastic tissue separating bundles of smooth muscle cells.
- There are several causes for nonspecific thickening of arteries and veins, which do not indicate pulmonary hypertension, as follows:

  - Fibrosis and hyalinization of venous and arterial intima may occur as an age-related change.
  - Medial hypertrophy and intimal thickening may occur in areas of pulmonary scarring and are localized phenomena not reflective of pulmonary hypertension.

- Lung vessels should be evaluated in areas of relatively normal lung parenchyma.
- Major causes of pulmonary hypertension are listed in Table 17–1.
- Grading of pulmonary hypertensive changes is useful in patients with congenital heart disease (Table 17–2).

IDIOPATHIC PRIMARY PULMONARY HYPERTENSION

Idiopathic primary pulmonary hypertension is increased pulmonary arterial pressure (>25 mm Hg mean, resting) in the absence of heart disease, pulmonary outflow obstruction, and embolic disease. Synonyms include plexi-

form arteriopathy and unexplained pulmonary hypertension.

Clinical Findings

- There is a female predominance (mean age at presentation 20–30 years).
- Presenting symptoms include progressive dyspnea, syncope, and sudden death.

Table 17–1
MAJOR CAUSES OF PULMONARY HYPERTENSION

Condition	Etiology	Pathologic Finding
Precapillary lesions		
Congenital heart disease and left–right shunts	Increased pulmonary flow Chronic vasoconstriction	Spectrum of plexiform arteriopathy*
Primary pulmonary hypertension	Idiopathic disease Portal hypertension Autoantibodies/connective tissue diseases	Spectrum of plexiform arteriopathy*
Embolic disease	Thromboemboli Fat emboli Foreign deposits, drug abuse Embolic carcinoma	Medial thickening Organizing thrombi, fat, talc, or carcinoma
Hypoxia	Severe chronic obstructive pulmonary disease High altitude disease	Muscularization of arterioles
Pulmonary fibrosis	Various interstitial lung diseases	Medial and intimal thickening
Postcapillary lesions		
Left ventricular inflow obstruction or increased end-diastolic pressure	Mitral stenosis Left ventricular failure Sclerosing mediastinitis Left atrial myxoma	Pulmonary congestion Medial hypertrophy, arteries Venous thickening
Veno-occlusive disease	Idiopathic disease	Venous thickening with organized thrombi
Granulomas	Sarcoidosis Idiopathic disease	Granulomas in veins

*Includes medial hypertrophy, intimal proliferation, and plexiform/dilatation lesions with focal arteritis.

Table 17–2
GRADING OF PULMONARY
HYPERTENSION IN PATIENTS WITH
CONGENITAL HEART DISEASE

*Heath/Edwards**
  1 Medial thickening
  2 Cellular intimal thickening
  3 Intimal fibrosis
  4 Plexiform lesions
  5 Dilatation lesions/hemosiderosis
  6 Arteritis
*Yamaki/Wagenvoort**
  1 No intimal changes
  2 Cellular intimal thickening
  3 Intimal fibrosis and fibroelastosis
  4 Partial or total medial destruction
*Rabinovitch, et al.**
  1 Muscularization of acinar arterioles
  2 Medial thickening
  3 Increase in arterial–alveolar ratio
*Roberts**
  1 Medial thickening
  2 Intimal thickening
  3 Plexiform lesions/arteritis
*Mark**
  1 Medial thickening
  2 Cellular intimal thickening
  3 Intimal fibroelastosis
  4 Plexiform lesions

*References

Heath D, Edwards JE. The pathology of hypertensive pulmonary vascular disease. A description of six grades of structural changes in the pulmonary arteries with special reference to congenital cardiac septal defects. Circulation 18:533–547, 1958.

Yamaki S, Wagenvoort CA. Plexogenic pulmonary arteriopathy: significance of medial thickness with respect to advanced pulmonary vascular lesions. Am J Pathol 105:70–75, 1981.

Rabinovitch M, Haworth SG, Vance Z, et al. Early pulmonary vascular changes in congenital heart disease studied in biopsy tissue. Hum Pathol 11:499–508, 1980.

Roberts WC. A simple histologic classification of pulmonary arterial hypertension. Am J Cardiol 58:385–386, 1986.

Mark EJ. Vascular disease. In *Lung Biopsy Interpretation.* Baltimore, Williams & Wilkins, 1984, pp 131–150.

- Angiographically, pulmonary emboli obstructing larger vessels are absent; there is tapering or pruning of distal pulmonary arteries.
- Biopsy is occasionally performed to exclude secondary causes or to exclude venous obstruction.
- A significant proportion of patients have elevated serum autoantibodies or overt collagen vascular disease.
- Types of collagen vascular disease that have been associated with pulmonary hypertension with plexiform lesions include mixed connective tissue disease, scleroderma, systemic lupus erythematosus, and rheumatoid arthritis.
- There is an increased risk for the development of plexiform arteriopathy in patients with portacaval shunting due to cirrhosis, LeVeen shunts, or other hepatic diseases.

Gross Pathologic Findings

- Right ventricular hypertrophy
- Dilatation and atherosclerosis of the pulmonary trunk
- Rarely, rupture or dissection of the pulmonary trunk, causing sudden death

Microscopic Pathologic Findings

- The diagnostic lesion is the "plexiform lesion." There is focal loss of internal elastic laminae with proliferation of endothelial channels across the dilated pulmonary arterial wall.
- "Dilatation lesions" often surround plexiform lesions. These are dilated capillaries that extend into pulmonary parenchyma.
- Necrotizing arteritis may occur and is considered to be the precursor to plexiform lesions.
- Nonspecific findings include medial hypertrophy, intimal proliferation, and small vessel thrombi.
- Occasionally, only nonspecific findings are present in the absence of plexiform lesions. In such cases, cardiac disease should be carefully excluded before making the diagnosis of primary pulmonary hypertension.
- Three histologic subsets of idiopathic pulmonary hypertension have been described: the plexiform type, the thrombotic type, and the medial type.
- In thrombotic pulmonary hypertension, there are thrombi in different stages of organization, primarily in arterioles, and plexiform lesions are absent.
- In the medial type of primary pulmonary hypertension, histologic changes are limited to medial hypertrophy and intimal proliferation.
- The intimal proliferation may be cellular or acellular (fibrotic). Some of the intimal proliferation, especially eccentric lesions, are presumed to be secondary to organized thrombi, which can occur in all types of pulmonary hypertension.

Differential Diagnosis

- Organized thrombi may occasionally be mistaken for plexiform lesions; however, the intima is intact, and these do not occur at small arterial branch points as do plexiform lesions.
- Chronic pulmonary thromboembolism from the right side of the heart or peripheral veins may be difficult to histologically distinguish from primary pulmonary hypertension. There is a lack of plexiform lesions, and larger arteries demonstrate emboli with recanalization.
- Patients with clinically typical primary pulmonary hypertension may occasionally at lung biopsy show only small vessel thrombosis; this has been classified as the thrombotic form of primary pulmonary hypertension.
- Intra-arterial thrombi with organization may occur in pulmonary hypertension associated with hemoglobinopathies (sickle cell disease, hemoglobin SC disease).
- Congenital heart disease with shunts may cause pulmonary hypertension with changes identical to idiopathic pulmonary hypertension, including plexiform lesions; therefore, there must be clinical exclusion of heart disease, especially previously undetected atrial or ventricular septal defects.

- Nonspecific hyalinization of veins and, to a lesser extent, of small arteries should not be interpreted as pulmonary hypertension.
- Pulmonary fibrosis and restrictive lung disease may result in arterial thickening and pulmonary hypertension, but plexiform lesions are absent.

References

Bjornsson J, Edwards WD. Primary pulmonary hypertension: a histopathologic study of 80 cases. Mayo Clin Proc 60:16–25, 1985.

Burke AP, Farb A, Virmani R. The pathology of primary pulmonary hypertension. Mod Pathol 4:269–282, 1991.

Pietra GG, Edwards WD, Kay JM, et al. Histopathology of primary pulmonary hypertension. A qualitative and quantitative study of pulmonary blood vessels from 68 patients in the National Heart, Lung, and Blood Institute, Primary Pulmonary Hypertension Registry. Circulation 80:1198–1206, 1989.

Rich S, Dantzker DR, Ayers SM, et al. Primary pulmonary hypertension: a national prospective study. Ann Intern Med 107:216–223, 1987.

Wagenvoort CA, Wagenvoort N: Primary pulmonary hypertension: a pathologic study of the lung vessels in 156 clinical diagnosed cases. Circulation 42:1163–1184, 1970.

PULMONARY HYPERTENSION SECONDARY TO CONGENITAL HEART DISEASE

Patients with congenital heart disease with left to right shunts have increased pulmonary arterial pressure that results from chronic increased pulmonary flow. Increased pressure is followed by progressive elevation in pulmonary vascular resistance, resulting eventually in a bidirectional shunt or reversal of the shunt (right to left).

Clinical Findings

- Any condition with significant left to right shunting, especially at the level of the ventricles or great vessels, may result in pulmonary hypertension if left untreated.
- The recognition of chronic pulmonary hypertension preoperatively is critical before operative repairs are made. If significant pulmonary hypertension is present preoperatively, right-sided heart failure may occur after surgery.
- Large ventricular septal defects, atrioventricular canal defects, truncus arteriosus, transposition of the great arteries, large atrial septal defects, persistent patent ductus arteriosus, among others, are associated with progressive pulmonary hypertension.
- There is a relatively small risk of developing pulmonary hypertension in tetralogy of Fallot because there is right ventricular outflow obstruction.
- Lung biopsy is occasionally performed preoperatively to assess the degree of pulmonary hypertensive changes before corrective surgery is attempted.

Gross Pathologic Findings

- Pulmonary artery dilatation, atherosclerosis
- Right ventricular hypertrophy

Microscopic Pathologic Findings

- Essentially, changes are identical to those seen in idiopathic pulmonary hypertension; however, the changes are progressive, and several grading systems exist for staging biopsies before surgery:
  - Earliest changes: medial hypertrophy (2 times medial thickness divided by vessel diameter is greater than 0.15); no intimal proliferation or plexiform lesions
  - Intermediate changes: intimal cellular proliferation, often eccentric, along with medial hypertrophy
  - Late changes: concentric acellular intimal proliferation with elastosis; plexiform and dilatation lesions; arteritis
- Quantitative techniques have been applied to the frozen-section analysis of lung biopsy disease.
- The quantitative grading scheme is based on the abnormal extension of muscle into small arteries, medial hypertrophy (percentage of wall thickness), and alveolar:arterial ratio.

Differential Diagnosis

- In the setting of lung biopsy in a patient with known congenital heart disease and increased pulmonary lung flow, there are few entities in the differential diagnosis.
- Diagnostic problems may occur in grading; the type of intimal proliferation affects the grade in some schemes, and it may be difficult to characterize.
- Diagnostic problems may occur because of sampling; a biopsy may show minimal hypertensive changes, and autopsy may reveal high-grade lesions.

References

Heath D, Edwards JE. The pathology of hypertensive pulmonary vascular disease. A description of six grades of structural changes in the pulmonary arteries with special reference to congenital cardiac septal defects. Circulation 18:533–547, 1958.

Rabinovitch M, Keane JF, Norwood W, et al. Vascular structure in lung tissue correlated with pulmonary hemodynamic findings after repair of congenital heart defects. Circulation 69:655–667, 1984.

Virmani R, Roberts WC. Pulmonary arteries in congenital heart disease: a structure–function analysis. In Roberts WC (ed). *Advances in Congenital Heart Disease.* Philadelphia, FA Davis, 1987, pp 77–131.

Wagenvoort CA. Lung biopsy specimens in the evaluation of pulmonary vascular disease. Chest 77:614–625, 1980.

CHRONIC HYPOXIC LUNG DISEASE AND PULMONARY HYPERTENSION

Chronic hypoxia results in vasoconstriction and pulmonary hypertension.

Clinical Findings

- The most common cause of chronic hypoxia is chronic obstructive lung disease, which results from a decrease in the effective cross-sectional area of the pulmonary vascular bed as well as from a decrease in the anatomic vascular bed.
- Residents at high altitudes have chronic low levels of

pulmonary hypertension manifested by increased pulmonary arterial pressures measured at arteriography and by right ventricular hypertrophy.

Pathologic Findings

■ Right ventricular hypertrophy
■ Muscularization of pulmonary arterioles; generally normal larger vessels

EMBOLIC DISEASE AND PULMONARY HYPERTENSION

Recurrent Thromboembolism

■ Deep venous thrombosis or right cardiac thrombi with embolization may cause chronic pulmonary hypertension.
■ Generally, large vessels with acute and organizing thrombi are involved.
■ Thrombectomies of pulmonary arteries may relieve obstruction.
■ The differential diagnosis includes rare pulmonary artery sarcomas, which represent less than 0.5% of pulmonary endarterectomies for presumed embolic pulmonary hypertension.

Carcinoma Emboli

■ Metastatic deposits occasionally involve arterioles and capillaries, instead of lymphatics; if extensive, they cause chronic pulmonary hypertension.
■ Tumor types include adenocarcinomas of breast, prostate, kidney, lung, liver, and stomach and choriocarcinoma.

Foreign Body and Fat Emboli

■ A granulomatous intravascular reaction may occur in intravenous drug abusers; talc and other fillers are common foreign materials.
■ Talc is present in 94% of lungs in intravenous drug abusers; in a small percentage of patients, pulmonary hypertension may develop secondary to granulomatous obliteration of vessels.
■ Fat emboli may occur as a result of infarcts of bone marrow or after orthopedic surgery. There is dilatation of arterioles and capillaries; fat is demonstrated by fat stain on frozen sections.

References

Arnett EN, Battle WE, Russo JV, Roberts WC. Intravenous injection of talc-containing drugs intended for oral use. A cause of pulmonary granulomatosis and pulmonary hypertension. Am J Med 60:711–718, 1976.

Fuster V, Steele PM, Edwards WD, Gersh BJ, McGoon MD, Frye RL. Primary pulmonary hypertension: natural history and the importance of thrombosis. Circulation 70:580–587, 1984.

Jamieson SW, Auger WR, Fedullo PF, et al. Experience and results with 150 pulmonary thromboendarterectomy operations over a 29-month period. J Thorac Cardiovasc Surg 106:116–126, 1993.

Palevsky HI, Weiss DW. Pulmonary hypertension secondary to chronic thromboembolism. J Nucl Med 31:1–9, 1990.

PARENCHYMAL/INTERSTITIAL LUNG DISEASES AND PULMONARY HYPERTENSION

■ Chronic obstructive lung disease, connective tissue disease, sarcoid lung disease, interstitial fibrosis, pulmonary schistosomiasis, and pulmonary amyloidosis may cause pulmonary hypertension.
■ Small arteries and arterioles show medial hypertrophy and intimal thickening.
■ Larger arteries demonstrate secondary medial hypertrophy and acellular intimal thickening in areas of interstitial fibrosis.
■ The major mechanism for the development of hypertension in chronic obstructive lung disease is hypoxia-induced vasoconstriction.
■ Sarcoid granulomas may directly obstruct veins, simulating veno-occlusive disease (see Veno-occlusive Disease).
■ Connective tissue disease (lupus erythematosus, mixed connective tissue disease, scleroderma) may be associated with plexiform arteriopathy.
■ Takayasu's disease (type IV) may involve the pulmonary arteries, and pulmonary hypertension may be the presenting feature. In Takayasu's disease, elastic pulmonary arteries are infiltrated by giant cells and granulomas, with sparing of muscular arteries and arterioles.

VENO-OCCLUSIVE DISEASE

Pulmonary veno-occlusive disease is an idiopathic sclerosis of pulmonary veins resulting in postcapillary pulmonary hypertension; it is often considered a form of primary pulmonary hypertension.

Clinical Findings

■ Adolescents and young adults are primarily affected.
■ There is an equal male to female ratio, unlike in idiopathic arterial pulmonary hypertension.
■ There is some association with use of chemotherapeutic agents.

Pathologic Findings

■ Sclerosis of pulmonary veins, with recanalization
■ Edema, and later fibrosis, of interlobular septa
■ Secondary changes of pulmonary congestion (hemosiderin-laden macrophages, osteoliths)
■ Thickened arteries, presumably as a secondary mechanism, showing medial hypertrophy and intimal proliferation
■ Absent plexiform lesions
■ Surrounding of interlobular septa by capillary proliferation (capillary hemangiomatosis) in some cases
■ Capillary hemangiomatosis occasionally considered a separate entity (most cases are associated with typical venous changes of veno-occlusive disease)

Differential Diagnosis

- Considered in the differential diagnosis is pulmonary hypertension caused by secondary impedance of pulmonary venous drainage; occasionally, lung biopsy is performed before left-sided cardiac diseases have been adequately excluded.

References

Carrington CB, Liebow AA. Pulmonary veno-occlusive disease. Hum Pathol 1:322–324, 1970.

Crissman JD, Koss M, Carson RP. Pulmonary veno-occlusive disease secondary to granulomatous venulitis. Am J Surg Pathol 4:93–99, 1980.

Faber CN, Yousem SA, Dauber JH, Griffith BP, Hardesty RL, Paradis IL. Pulmonary capillary hemangiomatosis. A report of three cases and a review of the literature. Am Rev Respir Dis 140:808–813, 1989.

Hoffstein V, Ranganathan N, Mullen JB. Sarcoidosis simulating pulmonary veno-occlusive disease. Am Rev Respir Dis 134:809–811, 1986.

Wagenvoort CA, Wagenvoort N. The pathology of pulmonary veno-occlusive disease. Virchows Arch A Pathol Anat Histopathol 364:69–79, 1974.

OTHER CAUSES OF PULMONARY HYPERTENSION SECONDARY TO IMPEDANCE OF PULMONARY VENOUS DRAINAGE

Underlying Causes

- Mitral stenosis or regurgitation
- Left atrial myxoma
- Myocardial ischemia/infarction
- Cardiomyopathy
- Congenital pulmonary vein stenosis
- Fibrosing mediastinitis

Pathologic Findings

- Congested, heavy lungs
- Hemosiderin-laden macrophages, occasionally with iron deposition in septa and blood vessel walls
- Septal fibrosis
- Intra-alveolar microlithiasis and ossification
- Medial and intimal thickening of muscular arteries and veins
- Absence of plexiform lesions

Pathophysiology

- Pulmonary hypertension is due to the increase in resistance of pulmonary venous drainage and backward transmission of the elevated left atrial pressure.
- Patients develop pulmonary vasoconstriction and anatomic changes in pulmonary arterioles and small muscular arteries.
- Right-sided heart failure results in distended neck veins, hepatomegaly, and ascites.

Reference

Farb A, Burke AP, Virmani R. Pulmonary hypertension caused by chronic left heart failure, obstruction of pulmonary venous return, and parenchymal lung disease. In Saldana (ed). *Pathology of Pulmonary Diseases.* Philadelphia, JB Lippincott, 1994, pp 203–216.

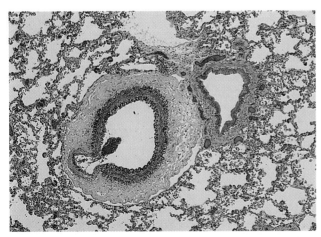

Figure 17–1. Pulmonary artery, Movat pentachrome stain. Pulmonary arteries that accompany bronchioles are muscular arteries with distinct external and internal elastic laminae. Twice the medial thickness should not exceed 15% of the vessel diameter; in this case of congenital heart disease, there was mild pulmonary hypertension and medial hypertrophy.

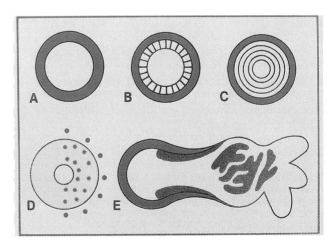

Figure 17–2. Morphologic stages of pulmonary hypertension. *A,* shows medial hypertrophy; *B,* medial hypertrophy with cellular intimal proliferation; *C,* medial hypertrophy with concentric, layered intimal proliferation with elastosis; *D,* arteritis with destruction of the media; *E,* plexiform lesion. (From Wagenvoort CA, Wagenvoort N. *Pathology of Pulmonary Hypertension.* New York, Copyright © 1977. Reprinted by permission of John Wiley & Sons, Inc.)

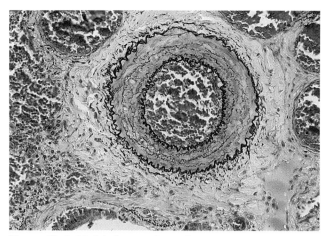

Figure 17–3. Medial hypertrophy, pulmonary artery, Movat pentachrome stain. Twice the medial thickness is nearly 50% of the vessel diameter, indicating marked medial hypertrophy. In this case of primary pulmonary hypertension, plexiform lesions were identified in other lung sections.

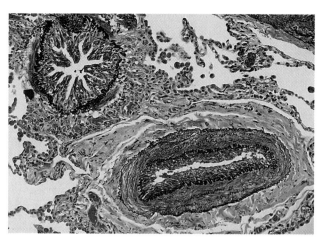

Figure 17–4. Medial hypertrophy with intimal proliferation, pulmonary artery, Movat pentachrome stain. Note the layer of thickened intima on the luminal aspect of the internal elastic lamina.

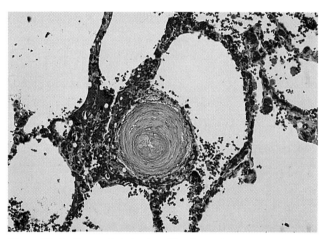

Figure 17–5. Concentric intimal proliferation, pulmonary arteriole, Movat pentachrome stain. Note several layers of intimal proliferation; this finding is indicative of severe pulmonary hypertension that is usually nonreversible.

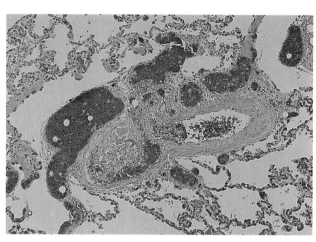

Figure 17–6. Plexiform/dilatation lesion, Movat pentachrome stain. Note the markedly dilated capillaries surrounding a thickened pulmonary artery and adjacent plexiform lesion.

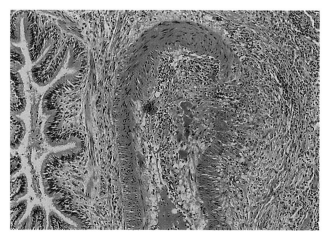

Figure 17–7. Arteritis. Inflammatory destruction of a segment of the arterial wall is believed to precede the formation of plexiform lesions. In most cases of pulmonary hypertension, this phase is not found.

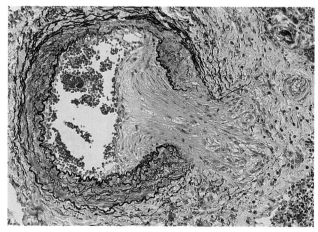

Figure 17–8. Plexiform lesion, Movat pentachrome stain. There is focal destruction of the arterial wall with a proliferation of capillaries into the adventitia. Plexiform lesions are seen in primary pulmonary hypertension and pulmonary hypertension secondary to congenital heart disease.

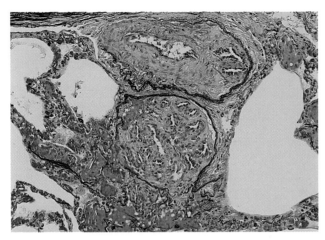

Figure 17–9. Plexiform lesion, Movat pentachrome stain. Level of sectioning may separate the bulk of the plexiform lesion *(bottom)* from the parent artery *(top)*. Note the strong resemblance to a glomerulus, hence the synonym "glomeruloid lesion" for plexiform lesion.

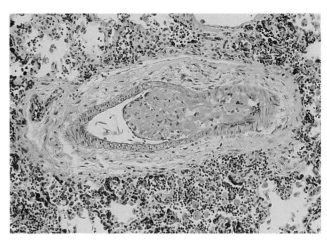

Figure 17–10. Organizing thrombus, Movat pentachrome stain. Thrombi within peripheral arteries are not unusual in cases of pulmonary hypertension and may be in situ lesions that do not represent embolism.

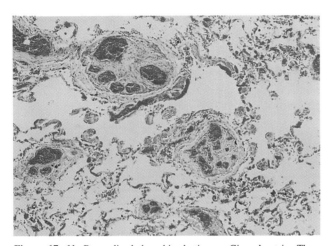

Figure 17–11. Recanalized thrombi, elastic van Gieson's stain. There are numerous recanalized peripheral arteries in this field. In contrast to plexiform lesions, the internal elastic laminae are intact.

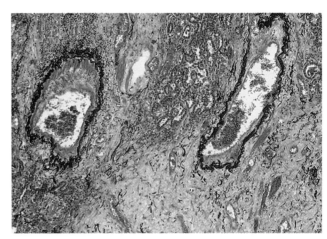

Figure 17–12. Nonspecific thickening, pulmonary arteries, Movat pentachrome stain. Intimal thickening can occur in areas of pulmonary scarring and is not indicative of a generalized process reflecting pulmonary hypertension.

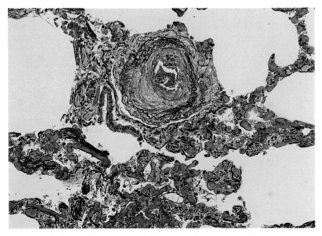

Figure 17–13. Scleroderma. There is thickening with fibroelastosis of pulmonary arteries; occasionally, plexogenic arteriopathy may also occur in patients with collagen vascular disease.

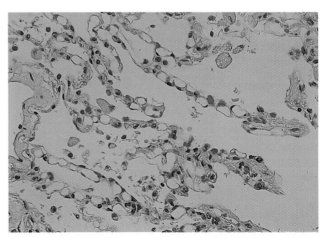

Figure 17–14. Fat embolism. There is diffuse vacuolization of capillaries. The patient, who had sickle cell disease, had sudden respiratory failure after bone infarction.

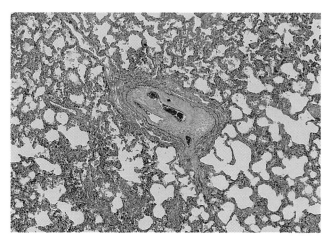

Figure 17–15. Veno-occlusive disease, Movat pentachrome stain. A pulmonary vein, which is located in a lobular septum, is greatly thickened.

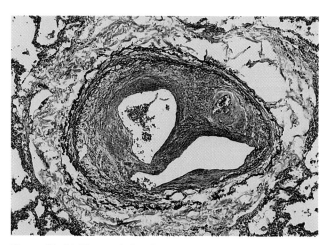

Figure 17–16. Veno-occlusive disease, elastic van Gieson's stain. Recanalization of pulmonary veins is typical in veno-occlusive disease and rarely seen in other conditions.

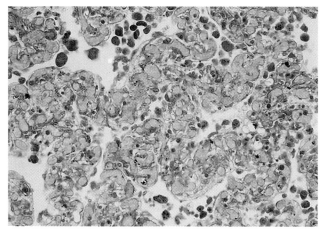

Figure 17–17. Veno-occlusive disease, Masson trichrome stain. There are secondary changes of capillary congestion and hemosiderosis.

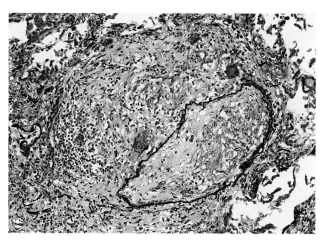

Figure 17–18. Sarcoidosis obstructing pulmonary vein, Movat pentachrome stain. Occasionally, sarcoid granulomas may infiltrate pulmonary veins, clinically mimicking veno-occlusive disease.

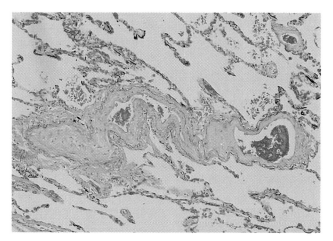

Figure 17–19. Nonspecific hyalinization, pulmonary veins, Movat pentachrome stain. In this elderly patient with emphysema, there is hyalinized thickening of venous intima, a relatively common age-related degenerative change.

CHAPTER 18

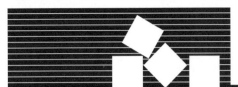

Tumors of Great Vessels

SARCOMAS OF THE AORTA

Sarcoma of the aorta is a malignant mesenchymal neoplasm with origin from aortic intimal cells (intimal sarcoma), medial cells, or aortic adventitia; most are predominantly luminal and are, therefore, of presumed intimal origin.

Clinical Findings

- Only approximately 100 cases have been reported.
- Usually middle-aged persons are affected, and there is no clear sex predilection
- Mean age of occurrence is 62 years.
- Symptoms are related to embolization to lower extremities and mesenteric arteries (claudication, abdominal angina).
- Other symptoms include back pain, shock from rupture of aneurysm formed by the tumor, and malignant hypertension.
- Occasionally, the tumor is the unexpected cause of aortic aneurysm.
- The prognosis is usually poor, although rare long survivors have been reported.
- Metastatic sites include bone, peritoneum, liver, and mesenteric lymph nodes.

Gross Pathologic Findings

- The surgical pathologist often receives the initial specimen as an embolic implant in the mesenteric arteries or arteries of the lower extremities.
- Most aortic sarcomas are predominantly intraluminal (intimal).
- Occasionally, there is thinning and aneurysm formation, resulting in clinical diagnosis of atherosclerotic aneurysm.
- Common sites include the abdominal aorta between the celiac artery and the iliac bifurcation and the descending thoracic aorta.
- Several cases of aortic sarcomas arising at the site of a synthetic aortic graft anastomosis have been reported.

Histologic Findings

- Intimal sarcomas have a variety of histologic appearances. Most are spindle cell sarcomas demonstrating myofibroblastic differentiation, expressing smooth muscle and muscle-specific actin and vimentin.
- The luminal surface of intimal sarcoma is often stratified into a cellular layer, which overlies a second layer of dense fibrous tissue.
- Epithelioid and myxoid areas may be present, and foci, especially in areas of extraluminal growth, may resemble malignant fibrous histiocytoma (MFH).
- Other histologic variants of intimal sarcomas are angiosarcoma, epithelioid angiosarcoma, leiomyosarcoma, and myxoid chondrosarcoma.
- Mural aortic sarcomas without extensive luminal growth are rare; these usually resemble MFH or leiomyosarcoma.

Differential Diagnosis

- Embolic myxoma may be confused with aortic sarcomas that have a myxoid matrix; however, myxoma cells are absent in sarcoma, and an echocardiogram does not demonstrate an atrial mass.
- Metastatic tumors arising in soft tissue or viscera rarely embolize and lodge in the aorta; therefore, a luminal aortic tumor is generally a primary aortic sarcoma or primary cardiac tumor.

References

Burke AP, Virmani R. Sarcomas of the great vessels. Cancer 69:387–395, 1993.

Fenoglio JJ Jr, Virmani R. Primary malignant tumors of the great vessels. In Waller B (ed). *Pathology of the Heart and Great Vessels,* vol 12. New York, Churchill Livingstone, 1988, pp 429–438.

Tejada E, Becker GJ, Waller BF. Malignant myxoid emboli as the presenting feature of primary sarcoma of the aorta (myxoid malignant fibrous histiocytoma): a case report and review of the literature. Clin Cardiol 14:425–430, 1991.

Weinberg DS, Maini BS. Primary sarcoma of the aorta associated with a vascular prosthesis: a case report. Cancer 15:398–401, 1980.

Wright EP, Glick AD, Virmani R, Page DL. Aortic intimal sarcoma with embolic metastases. Am J Surg Pathol 9:890–897, 1985.

AORTIC BODY PARAGANGLIOMAS

Aortic body paragangliomas are neoplasms of the dispersed paraganglia located predominantly near the ligamentum arteriosum (aorticopulmonary paragangliomas) and at the inferior mesenteric artery (organ of Zuckerkandl).

Clinical Findings

∎ Carotid body paragangliomas, which are more common than aortic paragangliomas, have been associated with chronic hypoxia and high-altitude living; this association has not been made with aortic paragangliomas.

Histologic Findings

∎ Histologic findings are identical to those of extra-aortic paragangliomas, that is, there are nested bland ovoid cells, abundant finely granular cytoplasm, positivity for chromogranin and enkephalins and negativity for cytokeratin.

Reference

Lack EE, Stillinger RA, Colvin DB, Groves RM, Burnette DG. Aortic–pulmonary paraganglioma: report of a case with ultrastructural study and review of the literature. Cancer 43:269–278, 1979.

SARCOMAS OF THE PULMONARY ARTERY

Sarcomas of the pulmonary artery are malignant mesenchymal neoplasms, presumably derived from intimal myofibroblasts.

Incidence and Clinical Findings

∎ Approximately 150 cases have been reported.
∎ Mean age at presentation is 41 years, and there is no clear sex predilection.
∎ Symptoms are similar to those of recurrent pulmonary emboli.
∎ The diagnosis is rarely considered early in the course of disease.
∎ The diagnosis is occasionally made at endarterectomy, but is often made first at autopsy.
∎ Metastases to the kidney, brain, lymph nodes, and skin have been reported.
∎ Survival of more than 2 years without metastases or treatment is common, but few patients live 5 years after diagnosis.

Gross Pathologic Findings

∎ Mucoid clots and gritty areas corresponding to osteosarcoma may be found.
∎ Sites of attachment to the artery are often multiple or difficult to define.
∎ Tumors typically extend to multiple sites, including the pulmonary trunk (80%), left pulmonary artery (58%), right pulmonary artery (57%), both pulmonary arteries (37%), pulmonary valve (29%), and right ventricle (8%).
∎ Distal luminal extension is common. There is occasional involvement of pulmonary parenchyma.

Histologic Findings

∎ More than 50% of cases are spindle cell sarcomas of presumed myofibroblastic derivation that resemble the majority of aortic sarcomas
∎ Other histologic types include leiomyosarcoma (20%), chondrosarcoma or osteosarcoma (7%), angiosarcoma (7%), rhabdomyosarcoma (6%), malignant mesenchymoma (6%), malignant fibrous histiocytoma (3%), and liposarcoma (1%).
∎ With current classifications of soft-tissue sarcomas, more cases are being diagnosed as malignant fibrous histiocytoma.
∎ Myxoid, osteosarcomatous, and chondrosarcomatous areas are more common than in aortic intimal sarcomas.

References

Kruger I, Borowski A, Horst M, de Vivie ER, Theissen P, Gross-Fengels W. Symptoms, diagnosis and therapy of primary sarcomas of the pulmonary artery. Thorac Cardiovasc Surg 38:91–95, 1990.
Nonomura A, Kurumaya H, Kono J, et al. Primary pulmonary artery sarcoma. Report of two autopsy cases studied by immunohistochemistry and electron microscopy, and review of 110 cases reported in the literature. Acta Pathol Jpn 38:883–896, 1988.

LEIOMYOSARCOMAS OF THE INFERIOR VENA CAVA

Leiomyosarcomas of the inferior vena cava are malignant mesenchymal tumors of smooth muscle differentiation that arise within the wall of the inferior vena cava or other great vein.

Incidence and Clinical Features

∎ Leiomyosarcomas of the inferior vena cava are somewhat more common than sarcomas of the aorta and pulmonary artery; more than 150 cases have been reported.
∎ Most patients are women (female:male ratio 4.5:1).
∎ Mean age at presentation is approximately 54 years.
∎ Presenting symptoms are related to Budd-Chiari syndrome (hepatic vein extension), pain, inferior vena caval syndrome, recurring pulmonary emboli, and metastatic tumor.
∎ Mean survival is 3 years.
∎ Metastases occurs to lungs, kidneys, pleura, chest wall, liver, and bones.

Gross Pathologic Findings

∎ Thirty-four percent of cases are infrarenal, 42% arise in the midportion of the inferior vena cava, and 24% arise between the liver and heart.
∎ Tumors are firmly attached to the inferior vena cava and are discrete, firm, whorled masses that extend into the retroperitoneum.

■ More than 75% of masses are attached to the vessel wall, and the remainder are primarily intraluminal.

Microscopic Findings

■ Most sarcomas of the inferior vena cava are relatively well differentiated leiomyosarcomas that are composed of fascicles of spindle cells oriented at acute angles to one another. The cells possess blunt-ended nuclei, occasional cytoplasmic perinuclear vacuoles, and fuchsinophilic intracytoplasmic fibers.

■ Intracytoplasmic desmin is identified by immunohistochemistry in about half of cases.

■ Tumor giant cells are occasionally present.

Reference

Mingoli A, Feldhaus RJ, Cavallaro A, Stipa S. Leiomyosarcoma of the inferior vena cava: analysis and search of world literature on 141 patients and report of three new cases. J Vasc Surg 14:688–699, 1991.

LEIOMYOMAS OF VEINS

■ Leiomyomas of large veins, such as the inferior vena cava or hepatic veins, are rare.

■ Leiomyomas of large veins are pathologically and clinically similar to intravascular leiomyomatosis, except that origin in the uterus is not found.

■ Leiomyomas of small veins are generally painful, subcutaneous masses.

References

Norris HJ, Parmley T. Mesenchymal tumors of the uterus. V. Intravenous leiomyomatosis. A clinical and pathologic study of 14 cases. Cancer 36:2164–2178, 1975.

Payan MJ, Xerri L, Choux R, et al. Giant leiomyoma of the inferior vena cava. Ann Pathol 9:44–46, 1989.

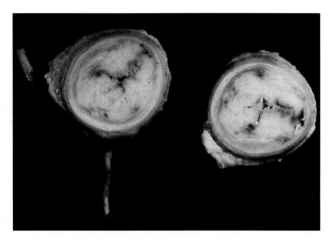

Figure 18–1. Aortic sarcoma. Two segments of abdominal aorta are seen transected, filled with necrotic tumor.

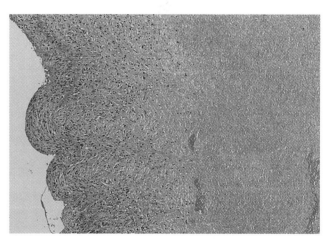

Figure 18–2. Aortic sarcoma. The luminal surface *(left)* is cellular, relative to the hyalinized portion of tumor *(right)*.

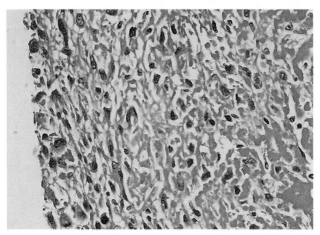

Figure 18–3. Aortic sarcoma. A higher magnification of the luminal surface of the tumor shown in Figure 18–2 demonstrates atypical spindle cells in a background of fibrin.

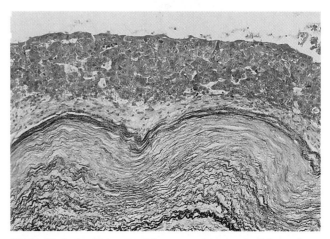

Figure 18–4. Aortic sarcoma, Movat pentachrome stain. A layer of malignant epithelioid cells coats the intima. Elastic fibers are shown as black.

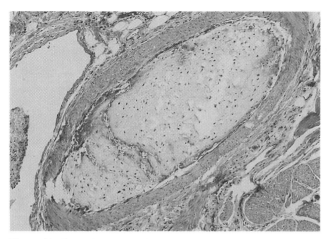

Figure 18–5. Aortic sarcoma. Occasionally, there may be myxoid chondrosarcomatous areas, as in this embolus in a peripheral artery.

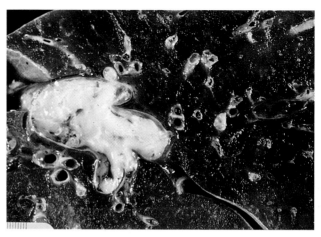

Figure 18–6. Pulmonary artery sarcoma. The tumor resembles a mucoid clot, filling the pulmonary artery.

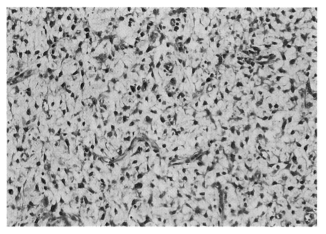

Figure 18–7. Pulmonary artery sarcoma. These tumors are typically myxoid.

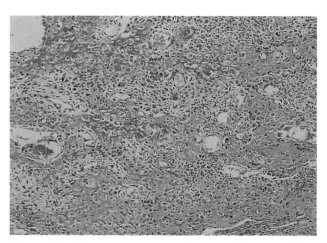

Figure 18–8. Pulmonary artery sarcoma. There are often areas of chondrosarcoma and osteosarcoma.

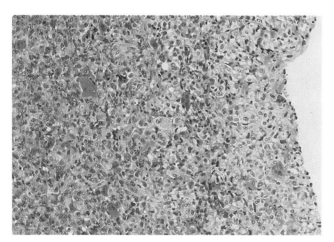

Figure 18–9. Pulmonary artery sarcoma. Pleomorphic areas with giant cells may be present.

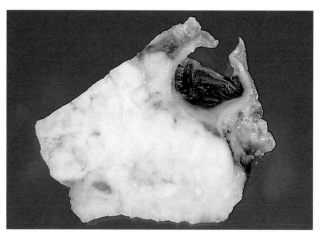

Figure 18–10. Leiomyosarcoma, inferior vena cava. A portion of the vena cava is seen in transverse section, as is the tumor, which is white and fleshy, and which, in contrast to aortic and pulmonary artery sarcomas, does not fill the lumen.

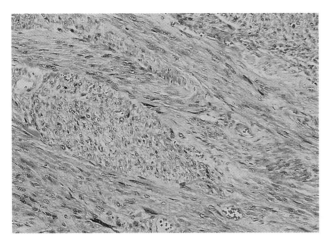

Figure 18–11. Leiomyosarcoma, inferior vena cava. Histologically, there are fascicles of spindle cells with abundant cytoplasm, typical of leiomyosarcoma.

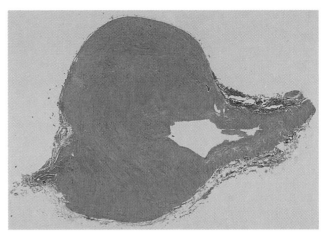

Figure 18–12. Leiomyoma, vein. Note the bulging mass attached to the vein walls.

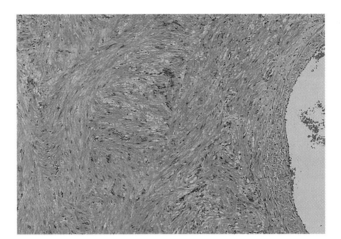

Figure 18–13. Leiomyoma, vein. A higher magnification of leiomyoma shown in Figure 18–12 demonstrates leiomyoma adjacent to the vein lumen.

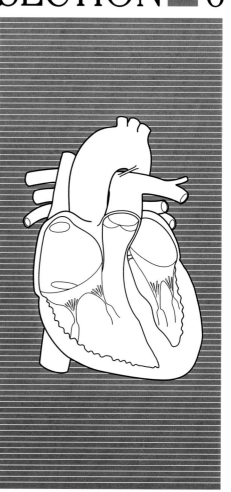

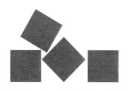

DISEASES OF
PERIPHERAL
VESSELS

CHAPTER 19

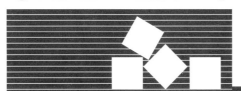

Approach to Blood Vessels and Overview of Vasculitis

SPECIMEN PROCESSING

Fixation

- Decalcification procedures should be used, if necessary, after fixation and before sectioning.
- Decalcification procedures that are slow-acting should be used, and the tissue should be monitored every 10 to 24 hours.

Sectioning

- Tangential sections of vessels should be avoided. Cross sections should be made at right angles.
- For the diagnosis of fibromuscular dysplasia, longitudinal sections are preferred.
- In vasculitis, adequate sectioning is necessary. For example, in temporal artery biopsies, because the disease is focal, complete exhaustion of the block is recommended with step sections.

Special Stains

- Elastic stain demonstrates internal elastic lamina, external elastic lamina, and intimal and adventitial fibroelastosis. Elastic stains are essential for the identification of arteries and veins and of destructive processes that specifically damage the elastic laminae. Elastic stains are used in staging of pulmonary hypertension.
- Acid mucopolysaccharide stain (stain for proteoglycans) shows deposition of ground substance in reactive lesions (e.g., fibrointimal proliferation), myxoid tumors, and "cystic medial necrosis."
- Trichrome stain identifies smooth muscle in media, neointima, and fibrous tissue.
- Movat pentachrome stain is an invaluable tool that combines the three stains listed above. It is helpful in the diagnosis of vasculitis, pulmonary hypertension, dissections, fibromuscular dysplasia, and atherectomy by clearly delineating elastic laminae, elastosis, scarring

or destruction of media, cystic medial change, and intimal fibromuscular proliferation.

CLASSIFICATION OF VASCULITIS

Background

- Vasculitic syndromes are inflammatory processes without a clear underlying etiology.
- The histologic findings are often nonspecific.
- In many patients, a pathologic diagnosis cannot be rendered without considering clinical presentation and laboratory findings.
- Clinically, patients with vasculitis are generally managed by rheumatologists, nephrologists, and dermatologists; each subspecialty has its preferred terms and classification system based on variations encountered in the different organs, which may differ from terms used by pathologists.

Table 19–1
PATHOLOGIC CLASSIFICATION OF
PRIMARY VASCULITIC SYNDROMES

Vasculitis of elastic arteries
   Takayasu's disease
   Giant cell arteritis
Vasculitis of muscular arteries
   Polyarteritis nodosa
   Giant cell arteritis
Vasculitis with extravascular granulomas
   Wegener's granulomatosis
   Allergic angiitis and granulomatosis of Churg-Strauss
Inflammatory thromboses, muscular arteries and veins
   Thromboangiitis obliterans (Buerger's disease)
Small vessel vasculitis
   Hypersensitivity vasculitis

Systemic Vasculitic Syndromes

■ Vasculitic syndromes are listed in Table 19–1 and are diagnosed, in part, based on systemic clinical symptoms, or clinical criteria.
■ The diagnostic contribution of biopsy may be limited by specimen sampling, sample size, stage of disease, and previous treatment.

Etiologic Classification

■ A practical etiologic classification of vasculitic syndromes is not yet established.
■ Antineutrophil cytoplasmic antibodies may be an etiologic factor in Wegener's granulomatosis, microscopic polyarteritis, nonimmune complex–related (pauci-immune) crescentic glomerulonephritis, some forms of pulmonary capillaritis, and, possibly, Kawasaki disease.
■ Vasculitis associated with antigen–antibody complexes include drug-induced hypersensitivity vasculitis, vasculitis of collagen vascular disease, and cases of polyarteritis associated with hepatitis B antigenemia.
■ The immune basis of some well-defined pathologic entities (Buerger's disease, giant cell arteritis, Takayasu's aortitis) is yet to be elucidated.

Secondary Vasculitis

■ Secondary vasculitis includes a variety of entities, including those with a specific etiology, such as infections, connective tissue diseases, radiation vasculitis, and vasculitis that accompanies a disease process that primarily involves other organs. Some diseases, such as Behçet's disease, Kawasaki disease, and Takayasu's aortitis, have been considered primary vasculitides, although inflammation is not localized to vessels, especially in the acute phases of illness (Table 19–2).
■ Infectious vasculitis denotes the presence of inflammation and infectious organisms within a vessel wall. Certain organisms, such as aspergillus species, pseudomonas species, and *Treponema pallidum,* have a propensity for invading blood vessels. The aortic de-

Table 19–2
CLASSIFICATION OF SECONDARY VASCULITIDES

Underlying Disease	Type of Vasculitis
Collagen vascular disease*	Small-vessel vasculitis, polyarteritis
Kawasaki disease**	Coronary polyarteritis
Henoch-Schönlein purpura	Small vessel vasculitis
Malignancy	Small vessel vasculitis, polyarteritis
Cryoglobulinemia	Small vessel vasculitis
Hypocomplementemic vasculitis	Small vessel vasculitis
Behçet's disease**	Various arterial and venous vasculitides with venous thrombosis
Miscellaneous	Transplant vasculitis, pulmonary and malignant systemic hypertension, AIDS-related vasculitis, radiation vasculitis

*Rheumatoid arthritis, lupus erythematosus, Sjögren's syndrome, dermatomyositis, scleroderma, mixed connective tissue disease, relapsing polychondritis.
**Alternatively considered a primary vasculitic syndrome.

Table 19–3
LOCALIZED VASCULITIS

Type of Vasculitis	Organ Site
Isolated polyarteritis	Skin Gastrointestinal tract Genitourinary tract Breast
Localized Wegener's granulomatosis	Lung
Giant cell phlebitis	Right colon Mesentery Skin
Giant cell arteritis	Central nervous system Breast Spermatic cord Miscellaneous sites

struction in syphilitic aortitis is mediated partly through immune mechanisms. In general, there is extensive extravascular acute inflammation in addition to vasculitis. Syphilitic vasculitis has a propensity for occurring in the thoracic aorta. In patients with bacterial sepsis, there can be generalized perivascular microabscesses, generally found at autopsy. Infections can involve aortic aneurysms, coarctation, and vascular prostheses.

Localized Vasculitis

■ Often, symptoms may result from a localized vasculitis in patients without apparent systemic disease (Table 19–3; see Chap. 21).

Vasculitis Look-alikes

■ The term vasculitis should be avoided when inflammation of vessels is secondary to other factors.
■ Vessels adjacent to abscesses or acutely ulcerated mucosa may become infiltrated by acute inflammatory cells and even show fibrinoid necrosis.
■ Infarction may result in acute inflammation of veins, and later arteries, with subsequent chronic inflammatory infiltrates in vessel walls.
■ Acute margination of neutrophils occurs rapidly in surgical trauma and may simulate a vasculitis.
■ Atherosclerotic plaques may be infiltrated by a large number of chronic, even acute, inflammatory cells; such changes should not be overinterpreted as vasculitis.
■ T-cell lymphomas and other lymphoproliferative processes may invade blood vessels, mimicking vasculitis.
■ Clinically, several conditions can mimic vasculitic syndromes. These include embolic myxoma, neurofibromatosis, cholesterol atheroembolism, endocarditis emboli, arterial dysplasia, radiation-induced arteriopathy, and chronic ergotism.

References

Brasile L, Kremer JM, Clarke JL, Cerilli J. Identification of an autoantibody to vascular endothelial cell–specific antigens in patients with systemic vasculitis. Am J Med 87:74–80, 1989.
Calabrese LH. Vasculitis and infection with the human immunodeficiency virus. Rheum Dis Clin North Am 17:131–147, 1991.

Churg J. Nomenclature of vasculitic syndromes: a historical perspective. Am J Kidney Dis 18:148–153, 1991.

Churg J, Churg A. Idiopathic and secondary vasculitis: a review. Mod Pathol 2:144–160, 1989.

Jorizzo JL. Classification of vasculitis. J Invest Dermatol 100:106S–110S, 1993.

Lie JT. Illustrated histopathologic classification criteria for selected vasculitis syndromes. American College of Rheumatology Subcommittee on Classification of Vasculitis. Arthritis Rheum 33:1074–1087, 1990.

Lie JT. Vascular involvement in Behçet's disease: arterial and venous and vessels of all sizes. J Rheumatol 19:341–343, 1992.

Waldherr R, Eberline-Gonska M, Noronha IL. Histopathological differentiation of systemic necrotizing vasculitides. APMIS Suppl 19:17–18, 1990.

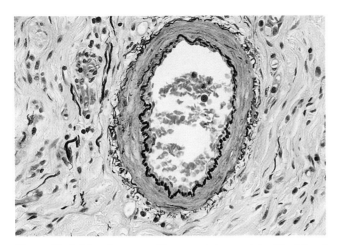

Figure 19–1. Muscular artery, Movat pentachrome stain. The internal and external elastic laminae are relatively discrete. Elastic tissue is stained black, and collagen is stained yellow.

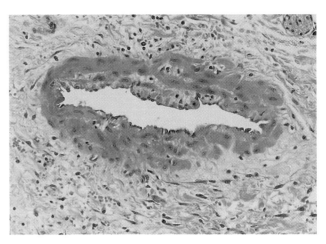

Figure 19–2. Muscular vein. The smooth muscle cells of the media are not as compact as those of arterial media and they are not parallel to one another.

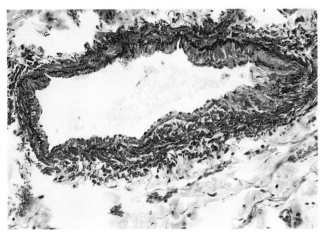

Figure 19–3. Muscular vein, Movat pentachrome stain. There is abundant elastic tissue. It is not arranged in two discrete layers, but is split into several interwoven strands, especially toward the adventitia.

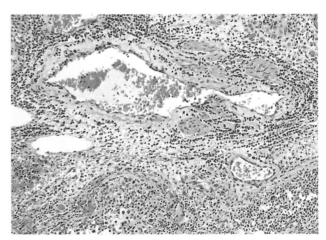

Figure 19–4. Testicular infarction. Acute and, later, chronic inflammatory cells typically infiltrate vessels of ischemic tissue and should not be taken as evidence of vasculitis. In this case, the infiltration of the vein wall is secondary to ischemia caused by torsion.

Figure 19–5. Margination. Acute margination of neutrophils occurs within minutes of surgical manipulation of tissues and should not be mistaken for vasculitis. This phenomenon, especially prominent on serosal surfaces, is especially well visualized in this photomicrograph.

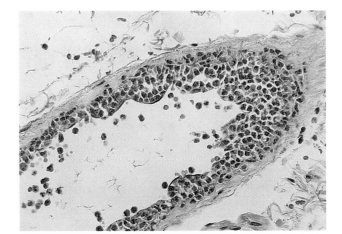

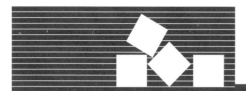

CHAPTER 20

Systemic Vasculitic Syndromes

Features of vasculitic syndromes are listed in Table 20–1.

POLYARTERITIS NODOSA

Polyarteritis nodosa is an idiopathic systemic syndrome characterized by inflammation of large and medium-sized muscular arteries.

Pathogenesis

- Circulating immune complexes are common, but deposits of complement and immunoglobulins are not consistently found within lesions
- Hepatitis B antigenemia is present in 8% to 40% of patients.
- Patients with microscopic polyarteritis and glomerulonephritis have a high incidence of antineutrophil cytoplasmic autoantibodies (ANCA).
- The significance of autoantibodies to endothelial cells is unclear.

Clinical Findings

- There is an incidence of 0.4 to 0.9 per 100,000 persons in the United States and United Kingdom.
- There is a constellation of symptoms and laboratory abnormalities.
- At least three of the following criteria must be met to make the diagnosis (Lightfoot et al, 1990):

  - Weight loss of more than 4 kg
  - Livedo reticularis
  - Testicular pain or tenderness
  - Myalgias, weakness, or leg tenderness
  - Mononeuropathy or polyneuropathy
  - Diastolic blood pressure of more than 90 mm Hg
  - Elevated blood urea nitrogen or creatinine level
  - Presence of hepatitis B surface antigenemia or antibody
  - Abnormal arteriogram showing idiopathic aneurysms or stenosis

  - Nondiagnostic biopsy demonstrating only suggestive features of polyarteritis (granulocytes or mononuclear leukocytes in arterial wall) or diagnostic biopsy with segmental fibrinoid necrosis

- Common sites of involvement include

  - Testis (testicular pain)
  - Bowel (acute abdomen/abdominal angina)
  - Lower extremities (pain, tenderness)
  - Skeletal muscle (pain)
  - Nerves (polyneuropathy, mononeuritis, mononeuritis multiplex)
  - Skin (cutaneous ulcers, scars, livedo reticularis)
  - Kidneys (elevated blood urea nitrogen and creatinine levels)
  - Liver (elevated transaminases)
  - Lungs (approximately 30% of cases)
  - Virtually any organ may be affected

- Prognosis is 63% survival at 5 years; poor prognosis is associated with age older than 50 years and gastrointestinal, renal, or cardiac involvement.

Pathologic Findings

- Muscular arteries and arterioles are involved and veins are spared.
- Segmental inflammation is typical, but may be concentric.
- The following lesions at different stages with segmental necrosis are characteristic:

  - Acute lesion: fibrinoid necrosis, neutrophils with mononuclear cells, aneurysms at branch points
  - Healing lesions: granulation tissue with segmental loss of media
  - Healed lesion: scarring with interruption of the elastic laminae; mild chronic inflammation

- Secondary changes include infarction and necrosis of the target organ.
- Complications include rupture, thrombosis of aneurysms, and fibrointimal proliferation with arterial occlusion.

Table 20–1
FEATURES OF VASCULITIC SYNDROMES

Type of Vasculitis	Clinical or Etiologic Factors	Vessels Involved	Pathologic Features
Polyarteritis nodosa	Hepatitis B (minority)	Muscular arteries	Segmental necrosis, healed lesions
Microscopic polyarteritis	ANCA	Arterioles, glomeruli, pulmonary capillaries	Necrotizing vasculitis
Wegener's granulomatosis	ANCA	Arteries, veins, glomeruli	Extravascular granulomas
Churg-Strauss vasculitis	Asthma, peripheral eosinophilia	Muscular arteries, veins	Necrotizing vasculitis, eosinophilic microabscesses
Giant cell arteritis	Polymyalgia rheumatica	Muscular and elastic arteries	Giant cell infiltrate of elastic laminae
Buerger's disease	Cigarette smoking	Muscular arteries, veins	Cellular thrombosis with luminal giant cells
Small cell vasculitis	Hypersensitivity, immune complexes	Venules, capillaries	Nuclear dust, lymphocytic infiltrate
Connective tissue vasculitis	Rheumatoid arthritis, SLE	Arteries, capillaries, pulmonary capillaritis	Necrotizing vasculitis, small vessel vasculitis
Behçet's disease	Immune complexes	Arteries, veins, capillaries	Aortitis, inflammatory aneurysms, thrombophlebitis
Takayasu's disease	Unknown	Aorta, arch vessels, pulmonary arteries	Stenoses, infrequently aneurysms
Kawasaki disease	Unknown; ANCA	Coronary arteries, other muscular arteries	Inflammatory aneurysms

ANCA, antineutrophil cytoplasmic autoantibody; SLE, systemic lupus erythematosus.

Microscopic Polyarteritis/Polyangiitis

- The term "microscopic polyarteritis" was originally applied to autopsied cases of systemic necrotizing vasculitis without gross aneurysms of classic polyarteritis nodosa.
- Later, the term was used for what is currently termed hypersensitivity, or small vessel vasculitis.
- Currently, it is most commonly used for arteritis of small to medium-sized arteries, especially of the skin, lungs, and kidneys.
- Unlike classic polyarteritis nodosa, patients are not typically hypertensive, lung involvement often causes clinical symptoms, and healed lesions are not often present histologically.
- The diagnosis is typically made in patients with immune complex–negative glomerulonephritis and pulmonary hemorrhage who have serologic evidence of ANCAs; there is overlap with Wegener's granulomatosis.

References

Guillevin L, Du LTH, Godeau P, Jais P, Wechsler B. Clinical findings and prognosis of polyarteritis nodosa and Churg-Strauss angiitis: a study of 165 patients. Br J Rheumatol 27:258–264, 1988.

Heptinstall RH. Polyarteritis (periarteritis) nodosa, Wegener's syndrome, and other forms of vasculitis. In Heptinstall RH (ed). *Pathology of the Kidney.* Boston, Little, Brown 1992, pp 1097–1162.

Lightfoot RW Jr, Michel BA, Bloch DA, et al. The American College of Rheumatology 1990 criteria for the classification of polyarteritis nodosa. Arthritis Rheum 33:1088–1093, 1990.

WEGENER'S GRANULOMATOSIS

Wegener's granulomatosis is a clinicopathologic syndrome of necrotizing granulomatous vasculitis of the upper and lower respiratory tract and glomerulonephritis.

Etiology

- The cause is unknown. There is an association with ANCA, which is used for diagnostic purposes and for monitoring disease:
  - C-ANCA: cytoplasmic staining (anti-proteinase 3)
  - C-ANCA most closely associated with Wegener's; present in more than 75% of patients
  - P-ANCA: perinuclear/nuclear staining (antimyeloperoxidase)
  - ANCA is commonly present in the sera of patients with microscopic polyarteritis and idiopathic crescentic glomerulonephritis.
  - ANCA has also been described in the sera of patients with classic polyarteritis nodosa, relapsing polychondritis, Kawasaki disease, and Churg-Strauss angiitis.

Clinical Findings

- There is an estimated incidence of 0.6 per 100,000 persons in the United Kingdom, inclusive of ANCA-positive microscopic polyarteritis/polyangiitis.
- Generalized symptoms include fever, weight loss, anorexia, malaise, arthralgias, and myalgias.
- Upper respiratory tract symptoms include sinusitis, epistaxis, rhinitis, nasal perforation, and subglottic stenosis.
- Lung manifestations include cough, hemoptysis, pleuritis, and presence of infiltrates.
- Renal manifestations include glomerulonephritis and renal mass.
- A variety of lesions, especially papulonecrotic eruption of extremities, occur on the skin.
- Nonspecific ulcers and granular gingivitis occur in the oral cavity.
- Conjunctivitis may occur.

■ Criteria for diagnosis include (Leavitt et al, 1990):

  • Nasal/oral inflammation (usually ulcers/purulent discharge)
  • Abnormal urinary sediment (microhematuria or red cell casts)
  • Chest radiograph showing nodules, geographic lesions, fixed infiltrates, or cavities
  • Hemoptysis

■ Unusual sites of involvement include the central nervous system, heart, genitourinary tract (prostatitis, cystitis, cervicitis, vaginitis), and gastrointestinal tract (necrotizing enteritis, perianal ulcers, Crohn-like manifestations).
■ Wegener's granulomatosis responds to cyclophosphamide and glucocorticoids.

Histopathologic Findings

■ Lung parenchyma shows necrotizing inflammation surrounded by palisading histiocytes. There are scattered giant cells, but well-formed sarcoid-like granulomas are absent.
■ Often inconspicuous, capillaritis (lung sections) is rarely the only manifestation. There is infiltrate of neutrophils in capillary walls with intra-alveolar hemorrhage.
■ Granulomatous vasculitis of arteries and veins is sometimes not prominent or even absent.
■ Mucosal biopsy shows mucosal ulceration (nonspecific), granulomatous inflammation, necrosis, and vasculitis.
■ Leukocytoclastic vasculitis and nonspecific ulcers occur on skin.
■ In the kidney, there are segmental necrotizing glomerulonephritis, glomerular thrombosis, and occasionally, granulomatous reaction to damaged glomeruli.
■ Peripheral arteries occasionally show changes indistinguishable from polyarteritis.

Differential Diagnosis

■ In the differential diagnosis are granulomatous infection, necrotizing sarcoid, lymphoma(toid granulomatosis), and Churg-Strauss angiitis.
■ In addition to Wegener's granulomatosis, ANCA-associated vasculitides include pulmonary capillaritis, microscopic polyarteritis, and nonimmune complex–related focal necrotizing glomerulonephritis with crescents (considered by some to be a vasculitis of glomerular capillaries). There is a trend among nephrologists to group these conditions together, especially because cytotoxic drugs, in addition to steroids, are indicated for treatment.
■ Pulmonary capillaritis (necrotizing alveolitis) can also be seen in patients with collagen vascular diseases, Goodpasture's syndrome, Henoch-Schönlein purpura, cryoglobulinemia, and toxic injury.

References

Bosch X, Font J, Mirapeix E et al. Antimyeloperoxidase autoantibody-associated necrotizing alveolar capillaritis. Am Rev Respir Dis 146:1326–1329, 1992.
Devaney KO, Travis WD, Hoffman G, Leavitt R, Lebovics R, Fauci AS. Interpretation of head and neck biopsies in Wegener's granulomatosis: a pathologic study of 126 biopsies in 70 patients. Am J Surg Pathol 14:555–564, 1990.
Fienberg R, Mark EJ, Goodman M, McCluskey RT, Niles JL. Correlation of antineutrophil cytoplasmic antibodies with the extrarenal histopathology of Wegener's (pathergic) granulomatosis and related forms of vasculitis. Hum Pathol 24:160–168, 1993.
Leavitt RY, Fauci AS, Bloch DA, et al. The American College of Rheumatology 1990 criteria for the classification of Wegener's granulomatosis. Arthritis Rheum 33:1101–1107, 1990.
Travis WD. Common and uncommon manifestations of Wegener's granulomatosis. Cardiovasc Pathol 3:217–225, 1994.
Velosa JA, Homburger HA, Holley KE. Prospective study of antineutrophil cytoplasmic autoantibody tests in the diagnosis of idiopathic necrotizing-crescentic glomerulonephritis and renal vasculitis. Mayo Clin Proc 68:561–565, 1993.

ALLERGIC ANGIITIS AND GRANULOMATOSIS OF CHURG-STRAUSS

Churg-Strauss angiitis is a systemic necrotizing vasculitis associated with severe asthma. It was originally considered a subset of polyarteritis nodosa.

Etiology

■ Unknown; may be a "malignant" expression of hypersensitivity with necrotizing arteritis
■ Antimyeloperoxidase antibodies often present (P-ANCA); antiproteinase-3 antibodies occasionally present (C-ANCA)

Clinical Findings

■ Young adults; no sex predominance
■ Prodromal phase:

  • Allergic rhinitis, sinusitis, allergic sinonasal polyps
  • Asthma, following or preceding rhinitis
  • Blood eosinophilia, moderate, rarely greater than 800/mm^2

■ Eosinophilic infiltrative disease:

  • Fleeting patchy irregular lung densities
  • Chronic eosinophilic pneumonia with fever and weight loss
  • Eosinophilic gastroenteritis with abdominal pain, diarrhea, bleeding, and obstruction

■ Vasculitic phase:

  • Fever, malaise, weight loss
  • Pulmonary infiltrates, fixed
  • Neuropathy, granulomatous myocarditis, coronary vasculitis

Histopathologic Findings

■ Eosinophilic infiltrates of arteries and veins, often with fibrinoid necrosis
■ Extravascular eosinophils, often with eosinophilic microabscesses
■ Medium-sized arteries and veins affected
■ The existence of localized forms controversial

Differential Diagnosis

- Similar findings may occur with drug reactions and visceral larva migrans.

References

Brill R, Churg J, Beaver PC. Allergic granulomatosis associated with visceral larva migrans. Am J Clin Pathol 23:1208, 1953.
Churg J. Systemic necrotizing vasculitis. Cardiovasc Pathol 3:197–204, 1994.
Churg J, Strauss L. Allergic granulomatosis, allergic angiitis and periarteritis nodosa. Am J Pathol 27:277–301, 1951.
Masi AT, Hunder GG, Michel BA, et al. The American College of Rheumatology 1990 criteria for the classification of Churg-Strauss syndrome (allergic granulomatosis and angiitis). Arthritis Rheum 33:1094–1100, 1990.

THROMBOANGIITIS OBLITERANS

Thromboangiitis obliterans is a nonatherosclerotic, inflammatory occlusive vascular disease that involves medium-sized arteries and veins, primarily in the distal extremities of young smokers; it is also called Buerger's disease.

Clinical Findings

- Most patients are young men; virtually all are cigarette smokers.
- Most cases regress with cessation of smoking, although there are exceptions.
- Cases of women with thromboangiitis obliterans are becoming more common with the increase in cigarette smoking in women.
- Obliteration of arm and leg arteries and veins may cause claudication and gangrene.
- Rarely, the temporal artery, mesenteric arteries, and veins may be affected, causing symptoms of temporal arteritis or ischemic bowel.

Histopathologic Findings

- Both arteries and veins are involved.
- Acute lesion consists of acute inflammation or microabscesses of media without fibrinoid necrosis or tissue reaction, and acute thrombosis.
- Chronic lesions demonstrate cellular thrombosis of arteries and veins, often with chronic inflammation, causing partial or complete obliteration of vessels.
- Giant cells within the organized thrombus is virtually pathognomonic for Buerger's disease.
- Elastic laminae of affected arteries are generally intact.

Differential Diagnosis

- In the absence of typical histologic lesions, proximal atherosclerosis and embolic diseases should be ruled out by angiography.
- Organizing thrombi usually lack the inflammation and giant cells typical of Buerger disease.
- Giant cell arteritis generally involves older patients, does not involve veins, and, histologically, there are giant cells within the media, not the lumen, of vessels.

References

Broide E, Scapa E, Peer A, Witz E, Abramowich D, Eschchar J. Buerger's disease presenting as acute small bowel ischemia. Gastroenterology 104;1192–1196, 1993.
Lie JT. Thromboangiitis obliterans (Buerger's disease) in women. Medicine (Baltimore) 66:65–72, 1987.
Mills JL, Porter JM. Buerger's disease (thromboangiitis obliterans). Ann Vasc Surg 5:570–572, 1991.

GIANT CELL ARTERITIS

Giant cell arteritis is a granulomatous inflammation of medium-sized arteries that usually affects cranial vessels in older individuals; it is often part of the syndrome of polymyalgia rheumatica.

Etiology

- Etiology is unknown; a cell-mediated T-cell regulated granulomatous reaction has been implicated in the pathogenesis.

Patient Characteristics

- There is a female predominance (female:male ratio 2–5:1).
- There is an incidence of 17 in 100,000 persons older than age 50 in the upper midwest of the United States with a large population of people of Northern European ancestry.
- The highest incidence is in Denmark (20 per 100,000 population).
- Giant cell arteritis is virtually unknown in the Orient.
- It is rare in blacks; only 40 biopsy-proven cases have been reported.
- It is rare in children and young adults; temporal arteritis in this group of patients may be a self-limiting disease not requiring steroid treatment.

Clinical Findings

- Three of the following five criteria should be met (Hunder et al, 1990):
  1. Age older than 50 years
  2. New onset of localized headache
  3. Tenderness of temporal artery or decreased temporal artery pulse
  4. Elevated Westergren erythrocyte sedimentation rate greater than 50 mm/h
  5. Biopsy of temporal artery demonstrating mononuclear cells with or without giant cells
- General symptoms include fatigue, fever, headaches, jaw claudication, vision loss, scalp tenderness, and polymyalgia rheumatica.
- Polymyalgia rheumatica occurs in 50% of patients late in the disease course; it is characterized by pain and stiffness in the shoulder and pelvic girdles, in the absence of atrophy or weakness, in association with other features of giant cell arteritis, such as elevated erythrocyte sedimentation rate (ESR), and a response to treatment with steroids.

- Polymyalgia rheumatica is more common than temporal arteritis; only a small fraction of patients with polymyalgia rheumatica develop temporal arteritis.
- ESR may be low in a small percentage of patients with temporal arteritis; these patients often have a history of polymyalgia rheumatica or steroid therapy. Even low-dose steroid therapy may lower ESR.

Histopathologic Findings

- The characteristic lesion is the destruction of the internal elastic laminae by a granulomatous infiltrate; giant cells are present in approximately 50% of cases.
- Lymphocytes and histiocytes are usually plentiful; eosinophils are sparse.
- Occasionally, an immunohistochemical stain for histiocytes may be helpful in identifying inflammatory cells within discontinuous areas of internal elastic laminae, supporting a diagnosis of giant cell arteritis.
- Fibrointimal proliferation is common in healed stages. Differential diagnosis is atherosclerosis and the intimal type of arterial dysplasia. In temporal arteritis, there is generally widespread destruction of elastic laminae.
- Inflammation of small branch vessels, usually lymphocytic, occurs commonly.
- Histologic changes often decrease after treatment, but there is little correlation between histologic stage and history of steroid therapy.

Role of Biopsy

- Between 25% and 50% of patients with presumed temporal arteritis have negative biopsy results.
- The response to steroid treatment is similar in patients with biopsy-proven versus biopsy-negative temporal arteritis.
- Patients with positive biopsy are more likely to have headaches, jaw claudication, and prior polymyalgia rheumatica than patients with negative biopsies.
- A negative biopsy may prompt the clinician to consider alternate diagnoses before instituting steroid therapy.

Differential Diagnosis, Giant Cell Arteritis of the Temporal Artery

- Age-related changes include mild to moderate fibrointimal proliferation and splitting (duplication) of the internal elastic laminae. However, if there is marked intimal proliferation resulting in more than 75% reduction of the luminal area or if there is significant loss of the internal elastic laminae, healed arteritis or atherosclerosis should be considered.
- Significant atherosclerosis is uncommon in the temporal artery. In atherosclerosis, the fibrointimal proliferation is usually eccentric, and there are generally one or more of the following: foam cells, cholesterol clefts, calcification, and a fibrous cap overlying pultaceous debris.
- Monckeberg's medial calcification may affect the temporal arteries; there is calcification of the media and/or elastic laminae, without inflammatory cells or luminal narrowing.

- Temporal arteritis is not always giant cell arteritis. Buerger's disease, polyarteritis nodosa, Wegener's granulomatosis, and the vasculitis of collagen vascular disease (e.g., rheumatoid arthritis) may affect the temporal artery.
- Epithelioid hemangioma may affect the temporal artery, resulting in a painful mass (see Chap. 25).
- The temporal artery may rarely be the site of arterial dysplasia, which may result in headaches, but usually with a normal sedimentation rate (see Chap. 20); additionally, traumatic aneurysms may affect the temporal artery (see Chap. 22).

Noncranial Giant Cell Arteritis

- Takayasu's disease and, occasionally, syphilis may have a giant cell component to the inflammatory infiltrate (see Chaps. 16 and 20).
- In a small percentage of patients with temporal arteritis, there is inflammation of the aorta, mesenteric arteries, and subclavian arteries that may result in aortic incompetence, intestinal ischemia, and claudication of the arm, respectively (see Chap. 16).
- Giant cell arteritis of the uterus and breast may be associated with temporal arteritis, or be an apparently isolated condition (see Chap. 21).
- Isolated giant cell/granulomatous arteritis has also been reported in the central nervous system (see Chap. 21), skin, lungs, and kidney.
- Visceral giant cell arteritis is rare, involving small arteries and arterioles of the internal organs, without extravisceral disease.

References

Achkar AA, Lie JT, Hunder GG, O'Fallon WM, Gabriel SE. How does previous corticosteroid treatment affect the biopsy findings in giant cell (temporal) arteritis? Ann Intern Med 120:987–992, 1994.

Chmelewski WL, McKnight KM, Agudelo CA, Wise CM. Presenting features and outcomes in patients undergoing temporal artery biopsy. A review of 98 patients. Arch Intern Med 152:1690–1695, 1992.

Costello JM Jr, Nicholson WJ. Severe aortic regurgitation as a late complication of temporal arteritis. Chest 98:875–877, 1990.

Hunder GG, Bloch DA, Michel BA, et al. The American College of Rheumatology 1990 criteria for the classification of giant cell arteritis. Arthritis Rheum 33:1122–1128, 1990.

Lie JT. Disseminated visceral giant cell arteritis: histopathologic description and differentiation from other granulomatous vasculitides. Am J Clin Pathol 69:299–305, 1978.

Ninet JP, Bachet P, Dumontet CM, Du Colombier PB, Stewart MD, Pasquier JH. Subclavian and axillary involvement in temporal arteritis and polymyalgia rheumatica. Am J Med 88:13–20, 1990.

Small P, Brisson ML. Wegener's granulomatosis presenting as temporal arteritis. Arthritis Rheum 34:220–223, 1991.

Tomlinson FH, Lie JT, Nienhuis BJ, Konzen KM, Groover RV. Juvenile temporal arteritis revisited. Mayo Clin Proc 69:445–447, 1994.

Wise CM, Agudelo CA, Chmelewski WL, McKnight KM. Temporal arteritis with low erythrocyte sedimentation rate: a review of five cases. Arthritis Rheum 34:1571–1574, 1991.

SMALL VESSEL VASCULITIS

Small vessel vasculitis is inflammation of arterioles, capillaries, and venules, presumably secondary to an allergic or hypersensitivity mechanism. Hypersensitivity vasculitis, hypersensitivity angiitis, and necrotizing venulitis are synonyms for small vessel vasculitis.

Clinical Findings

- Many patients have a history of recent drug ingestion and are older than 20 years of age.
- Skin is the most common site of involvement; occasionally, a systemic vasculitis occurs.
- Generally, there is a self-limited course.
- Three of the following five criteria should be met (Calabrese et al, 1990):

  1. Age older than 16 years
  2. History of medication use at onset of symptoms
  3. Palpable purpura
  4. Maculopapular rash
  5. Biopsy demonstrating neutrophils around arterioles or venules

Differential Diagnosis

- Patients with similar histopathologic findings may have underlying diseases, including the following:

  - Connective tissue disease
  - Malignancies
  - Henoch-Schönlein purpura
  - Mixed cryoglobulinemia
  - Hypocomplementemic urticarial vasculitis
  - Other vasculitides: polyarteritis nodosa, Churg-Strauss angiitis

Pathologic Features

- Involvement exclusively of arterioles, venules, and capillaries
- Cuffing of vessels with neutrophils, lymphocytes
- Karyorrhectic debris (leukocytoclastic vasculitis)
- Fibrinoid necrosis present in approximately 50% of cases
- Scattered eosinophils
- Lesions of the same age (i.e., no evidence of granulation tissue, scarring)
- Histiocytes with small granulomas occasionally present, but giant cells usually absent
- Deposition of immunoglobulins and complement shown with immunofluorescence

Additional Facts

- Small vessel vasculitis has been divided into a "lymphocytic" subset and "leukocytoclastic" subset. The presence of leukocytes, fibrinoid necrosis, and nuclear dust is variable, as this subclassification illustrates.
- Henoch-Schönlein purpura differs from hypersensitivity vasculitis in that patients are usually younger (mean 17 years vs. 47 years for hypersensitivity vasculitis); the gastrointestinal tract and kidneys are usually involved, as is the skin; the disease is chronic; IgA deposition in vessels with circulating IgA immune complexes are generally found.
- Cryoglobulinemic vasculitis is not associated with drug exposure. Many patients have elevated rheumatoid factor. Unlike typical hypersensitivity vasculitis, it is a chronic condition.
- Hypocomplementemic vasculitis is characterized by chronic urticaria of more than 6 months' duration, hypocomplementemia, small vessel vasculitis of the skin, arthralgias or arthritis, glomerulonephritis, and uveitis. There is significant overlap with SLE, but anti-DNA titers are generally low.

References

Calabrese LH, Michel BA, Bloch DA, et al. The American College of Rheumatology 1990 criteria for the classification of hypersensitivity vasculitis. Arthritis Rheum 33:1108–1113, 1990.

Imai H, Nakamoto Y, Hirokawa M, et al. Carbamazepine-induced granulomatous necrotizing angiitis with acute renal failure. Nephron 51:405, 1989.

Michel BA, Hunder GG, Bloch DA, Calabrese LH. Hypersensitivity vasculitis and Henoch-Schönlein purpura: a comparison between the 2 disorders. J Rheumatol 19:721–728, 1992.

VASCULITIS OF COLLAGEN VASCULAR DISEASE

Vasculitis of collagen vascular disease is vasculitis occurring in individuals with autoimmune connective tissue diseases characterized by inflammation of joints, serous membranes, and connective tissue. The term is primarily used for vasculitis of rheumatoid arthritis and diseases characterized by antinuclear autoantibodies.

Rheumatoid Vasculitis

- Annual incidence is 1.25 per 100,000 in the United Kingdom and is more common than polyarteritis nodosa or Wegener's granulomatosis.
- Rheumatoid vasculitis generally occurs in patients with long-standing disease (mean 10–13 years).
- Most patients have severe arthritis and high levels of rheumatoid factor.
- Clinically, the onset of vasculitis is characterized by fever, chills, and peripheral neuropathy, particularly mononeuritis multiplex (motor, sensory, or mixed deficits in the distribution of more than one peripheral nerve).
- Gangrene and leg ulcers may complicate peripheral vasculitis.
- Rare clinical manifestations include coronary vasculitis with myocardial infarction, mesenteric ischemia, or bowel perforation and cerebral infarcts.
- Biopsy for clinical confirmation is often obtained from the quadriceps or gastrocnemius muscles or the sural nerve.
- Histologically, there is a range of vasculitides, from a small vessel vasculitis to necrotizing arteritis similar to polyarteritis nodosa.
- Healed lesions demonstrate adventitial scarring and intimal proliferation.
- The syndrome of rheumatoid vasculitis may mimic polyarteritis nodosa, but renal involvement is rare.
- Polyarteritis-like vasculitis occurs less commonly, primarily in patients with severe disease and may affect any organ system.

- Digital vasculitis may occur and be relatively benign and localized, unlike disseminated rheumatoid vasculitis.

Systemic Lupus Erythematosus

- Incidence of vasculitis in SLE is lower than in rheumatoid arthritis.
- Digital arteritis with gangrene, similar to that seen in rheumatoid arthritis, responds to prednisone and may be localized.
- The most common cutaneous manifestation is small vessel vasculitis.
- Central nervous system symptoms occur in over 50% of patients with SLE, but the correlation with cerebral vasculitis is often unclear.
- Gastrointestinal vasculitis mimicking polyarteritis nodosa may affect the gastrointestinal tract, resulting in ischemia or bowel perforation.
- Coronary arteritis rarely results in myocardial infarction; histologically, a polyarteritis-like vasculitis is present.
- Pulmonary capillaritis may lead to massive pulmonary hemorrhage; histologically, it is identical to that seen in ANCA-associated conditions.
- Patients with antiphospholipid autoantibodies (lupus anticoagulant) may develop a thrombotic syndrome. Less commonly, there is a vasculitic syndrome. There is an overlap between the vasculitis of SLE and the vasculitis associated with antiphospholipid antibodies.

Miscellaneous Connective Tissue Diseases

- In scleroderma, the predominant vascular changes are obliterative with little inflammation, such as concentric intimal proliferation of renal or pulmonary or digital arteries. In the acute phase, there is hyaline necrosis of the arterial wall with little inflammation. Polyarteritis-like vasculitis is rare.
- In dermatomyositis, vasculitis is particularly common in the childhood variant.
- Vascular involvement in mixed connective tissue disease may be similar to that seen in SLE, scleroderma, or dermatomyositis.

References

Goldberger E, Elder RC, Schwartz RA, Phillips PE. Vasculitis in the antiphospholipid syndrome. A cause of ischemia responding to corticosteroids. Arthritis Rheum 35:569–572, 1992.

Sasamura H, Nakamota H, Ryuzaki M, et al. Repeated intestinal ulcerations in a patient with systemic lupus erythematosus and high serum antiphospholipid antibody levels. South Med J 84:515–517, 1991.

Schneider HA, Yonker RA, Katz P, et al. Rheumatoid vasculitis: experience with 13 patients and review of the literature. Semin Arthritis Rheum 14:280–286, 1985.

Watts RA, Carruthers DM, Symmons DPM, Scott DGI. The incidence of rheumatoid vasculitis in the Norwich Health Authority. Br J Rheumatol 33:832–833, 1994.

TAKAYASU'S DISEASE

- Aortic involvement, as well as arch vessel involvement, is invariably present (see Chap. 16).
- Takayasu's disease may involve coronary, renal, subclavian, left common carotid, mesenteric, and innominate arteries, and must be considered in the differential diagnosis of inflammatory aneurysms or constrictions in arteries of young adults, especially women.
- Pathologically, there is acute, granulomatous, necrotizing, or chronic inflammation with adventitial scarring and luminal fibrointimal thickening. Giant cells may be present. In the healed phase, fibrointimal proliferation and adventitial scarring are present with little inflammatory infiltrate.

KAWASAKI DISEASE

Kawasaki disease is an idiopathic, pediatric inflammatory disease characterized by fever, conjunctival congestion, oral erythema, rash, and lymphadenopathy. Although many infectious agents, including retroviruses, have been implicated, the cause is unknown. Synonyms include mucocutaneous lymph node syndrome and infantile polyarteritis nodosa.

Patient Characteristics

- Mean age at onset is 2.8 years (range 4 months to 14 years).
- There is a slight male predominance.
- There is a slight increased risk among blacks in the United States.
- Most cases are sporadic, although several American outbreaks have been described.
- Infantile polyarteritis nodosa, described in Western countries before Kawasaki's description of the epidemic disease in Japan, is thought to represent Kawasaki disease.

Acute Phase

- Fever of 1 to 2 weeks' duration (95%)
- Desquamation of fingertips (95%), nonvesicular rash, especially trunk (90%), edema of extremities with reddening of palms and soles (90%)
- Bilateral conjunctivitis (90%)
- Redness and fissuring of lips (90%), strawberry tongue (80%), oropharyngitis (90%)
- Cervical lymphadenopathy (75%)
- Cardiomegaly (20%)
- Fatal myocarditis (<2%)
- Serologic ANCA in 20% to 70% of patients

Latent Phase

- Inflammatory and necrotizing lesions occur in muscular arteries, especially coronary arteries.
- Coronary artery aneurysms are present in 15% to 30% of patients after the acute phase of illness.
- Aneurysms regress and disappear in 50% of patients; the remainder may partially regress or become obliterated, or result in arterial irregularities.
- Arterial lesions most commonly result in aneurysms but may result in sclerotic, obliterative, and thrombosed arteries.
- Virtually all muscular arteries may be involved.

- The aorta may demonstrate intimal thickening, but inflammation is rare.
- Serologic ANCA is found in 50% to 90% of patients.

Pathologic Findings

- Findings include fibrinoid necrosis, thrombosis, medial destruction, fibrointimal proliferation, and aneurysmal dilatation of muscular arteries.
- Vessels involved, in approximate order of frequency, are coronary, testicular, pulmonary, splenic, iliac, intercostal, mesenteric, renal, cerebral, axillary, pancreatic, and hepatic arteries.
- Inflammation may be at different stages, or there may a healed arteritis with little inflammation (fibrointimal proliferation with medial and adventitial scarring, and destruction of elastic laminae).
- Any arteritis in a child involving muscular arteries should raise the possibility of Kawasaki disease.

References

Bell DM, Brink EW, Nitzkin JL, et al. Kawasaki syndrome: description of two outbreaks in the United States. N Engl J Med 304:1568–1575, 1981.

Kawasaki T, Kosaki F, Okawa S, Shigematsu I, Yanagawa H. A new infantile acute febrile mucocutaneous lymph node syndrome (MLNS) prevailing in Japan. Pediatrics 54:271–276, 1974.

Landing BH, Larson EJ. Are infantile periarteritis nodosa with coronary artery involvement and fatal mucocutaneous lymph node syndrome the same? Comparison of 20 patients from North America with patients from Hawaii and Japan. Pediatrics 59:651–659, 1977.

Rider LG, Wener MH, French J, Sherry DD, Mendelman PM. Autoantibody production in Kawasaki syndrome. Clin Exp Rheumatol 11:445–449, 1993.

BEHÇET'S DISEASE

General

- Triad of relapsing iridocyclitis, recurrent oral ulcerations, and recurrent genital ulcerations of unknown cause
- Other manifestations: gastrointestinal ulcers, neuropathy, myopathy, and arthropathy

- Incidence: 190 in 100,000 in northern Turkey, 10 in 100,000 in Japan, 5 in 100,000 in Minnesota
- Association with HLA-B5 in Mediterranean and Japanese patients

Vasculopathy

- Vascular lesions occur in 25% to 35% of patients.
- Vessels of all sizes and types may be involved.

Arterial Lesions

- The aorta is involved most often (see Chap. 16), followed by pulmonary, femoral, popliteal, subclavian, and common carotid arteries.
- Approximately two thirds are aneurysms; one third are occlusive disease.
- Aneurysms may rupture, representing a leading cause of death.
- Nonspecific inflammatory lesions are seen histologically.

Venous Lesions

- Thirty percent to 40% of patients
- Deep thrombophlebitis (deep vein thrombosis of extremities, trunk, and intracranial venous sinus)
- Superficial thrombophlebitis
- Budd-Chiari syndrome

Small Vessel Vasculitis

- May be the cause of mucocutaneous lesions, genital ulcers, and other systemic manifestations
- May be the result of deposition of immune complexes
- Histologically, represented by the spectrum of lymphocytic and leukocytoclastic types

References

Koç Y, Gullu I, Akpek G, et al. Vascular involvement in Behçet's disease. J Rheumatol 19:402–410, 1992.

Lie JT. Vascular involvement in Behçet's disease: arterial and venous and vessels of all sizes. J Rheumatol 19:341–343, 1992.

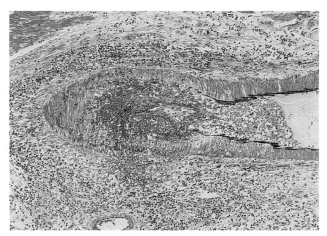

Figure 20–1. Polyarteritis nodosa, acute lesion, Movat pentachrome stain. There is segmental acute inflammation of the arterial wall with focal extension of the inflammatory infiltrate into the surrounding soft tissue.

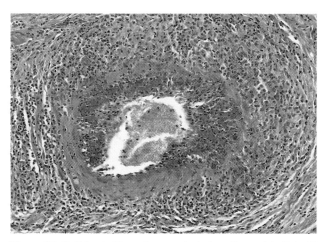

Figure 20–2. Polyarteritis nodosa, acute lesion. Segmental fibrinoid necrosis often accompanies the inflammatory infiltrate.

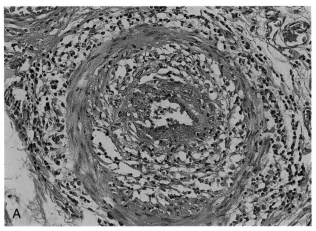 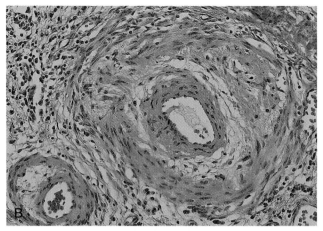

Figure 20–3. *A,* Polyarteritis nodosa, acute lesion. In this example, there is a circumferential ring of fibrinoid necrosis near the lumen, with inflammatory destruction of the outer portions of the intima, near the medial border. *B,* Polyarteritis nodosa, healed lesion. An artery adjacent to that shown in *A* demonstrates focal replacement of the media by loose connective tissue. This lesion is not diagnostic; in the absence of acute lesions, medial dysplasia or organized thrombus must be considered in the differential diagnosis.

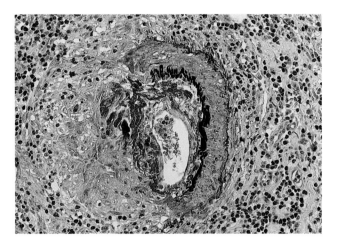 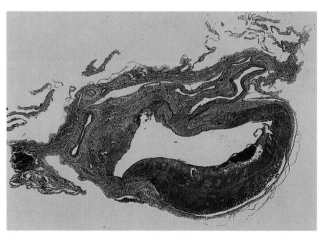

Figure 20–4. Polyarteritis nodosa, healing lesion, Movat pentachrome stain. There is granulation tissue replacement of a segment of arterial media.

Figure 20–5. Polyarteritis nodosa, aneurysm, Movat pentachrome stain. A common complication of the inflammatory lesions of polyarteritis is aneurysm formation. Note the focal dilatation of the involved artery.

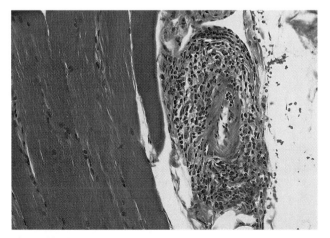 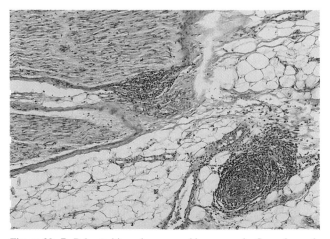

Figure 20–6. Polyarteritis nodosa, muscle biopsy sample. In biopsies performed to rule out systemic vasculitis, the muscles or nerves are often sampled. Because large vessels are not available, classic features are not always observed; note the perivascular mixed infiltrate in a patient with typical polyarteritis nodosa.

Figure 20–7. Polyarteritis nodosa, nerve biopsy sample. Several vessels demonstrate perivascular inflammation in this biopsy sample from a patient with suspected systemic vasculitis.

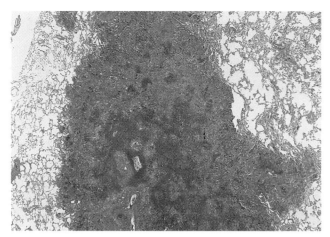

Figure 20–8. Wegener's granulomatosis. There is a well-demarcated parenchymal nodule of necrotizing granuloma. An infectious process must be considered in the differential diagnosis.

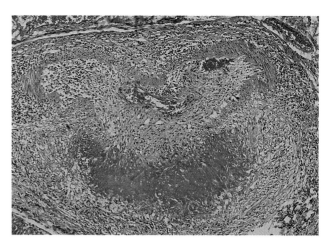

Figure 20–9. Wegener's granulomatosis. The vasculitic component of Wegener's granulomatosis may be relatively minor; in this case, there was a necrotizing granuloma partly destroying a muscular artery.

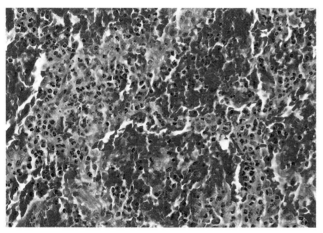

Figure 20–10. Pulmonary capillaritis. There is a neutrophilic infiltrate within the alveolar walls accompanied by alveolar hemorrhage. Pulmonary capillaritis may be present in antineutrophil cytoplasmic autoantibodies–associated vasculitis (Wegener's granulomatosis, microscopic polyarteritis) as well as in connective tissue vasculitis.

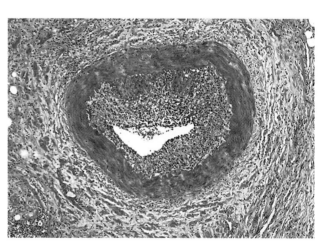

Figure 20–11. Churg-Strauss angiitis. There is a necrotizing vasculitis that resembles polyarteritis nodosa; the inflammatory infiltrate contains large numbers of eosinophils. The diagnosis of Churg-Strauss angiitis is made partly on a history of asthma and peripheral eosinophilia.

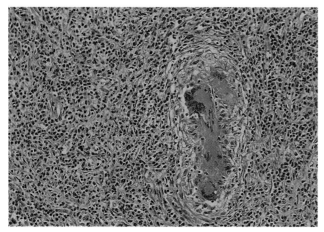

Figure 20–12. Churg-Strauss angiitis. In a different area of the lesion illustrated in Figure 20–11, there are extravascular granulomas with a pronounced eosinophilic infiltrate. These granulomas in the absence of vasculitis would suggest hypereosinophilic syndrome.

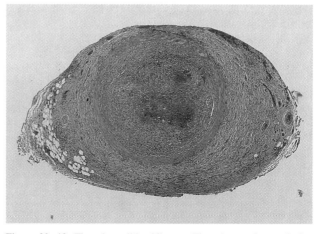

Figure 20–13. Thromboangiitis obliterans. There is complete occlusion of this muscular artery by an inflammatory process.

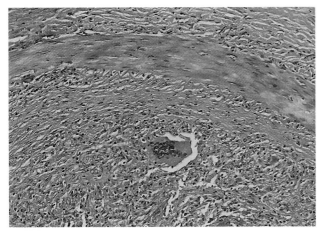

Figure 20–14. Thromboangiitis obliterans. A higher magnification of Figure 20–13 demonstrates a histiocytic giant cell within a cellular thrombus; this feature is pathognomonic of thromboangiitis obliterans.

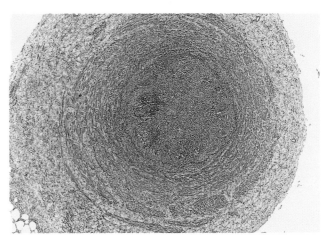

Figure 20–15. Thromboangiitis obliterans, Movat pentachrome stain. A muscular vein is completely occluded by cellular thrombus.

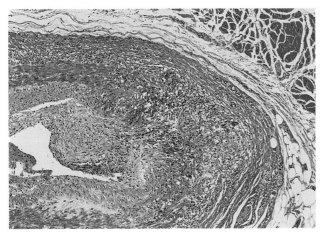

Figure 20–16. Giant cell arteritis, acute lesion. Temporal artery demonstrates granulomatous destruction of the vessel wall.

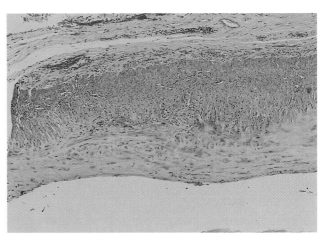

Figure 20–17. Giant cell arteritis, focal lesion. This section of temporal artery demonstrates a suggestion of giant cells lining the interface between the thickened intima and media.

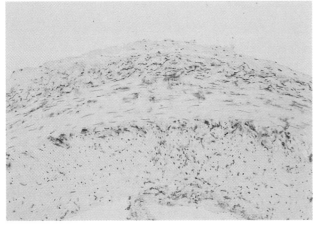

Figure 20–18. Giant cell arteritis. An immunohistochemical stain for histiocyte surface marker (KP-1) demonstrates a linear arrangement of KP-1–expressing cells along the area of the internal elastic laminae; this arrangement is typical of giant cell arteritis.

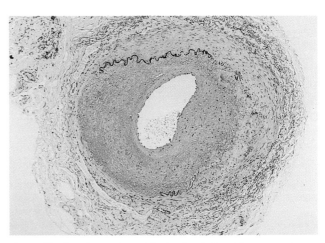

Figure 20–19. Giant cell arteritis, healing lesion, Movat pentachrome stain. At this magnification, all that is evident is fibrointimal proliferation with focal loss of elastic laminae. These features are nonspecific, but in the appropriate clinical setting, they are suggestive of giant cell arteritis. The differential diagnosis includes intimal arterial dysplasia (see Chap. 22), which is rare.

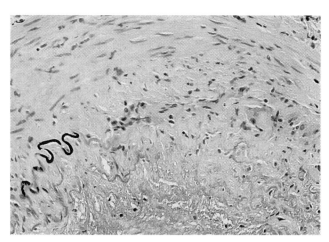

Figure 20–20. Giant cell arteritis, healing lesion, Movat pentachrome stain. A higher magnification of Figure 20–19 demonstrates a histiocytic reaction to degenerating elastic laminae, diagnostic of giant cell arteritis.

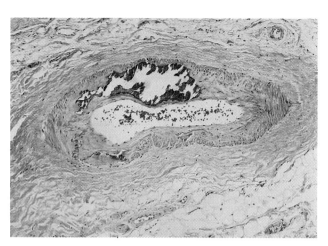

Figure 20–21. Mönckeberg's medial calcification. This degenerative, age-related process is characterized by medial calcification of arteries of the head, neck, and extremities. In contrast to healed giant cell arteritis, fibrointimal proliferation and luminal narrowing is usually absent.

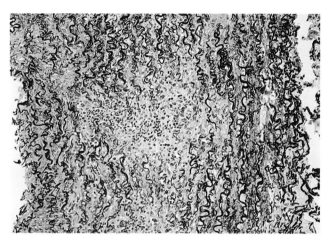

Figure 20–22. Noncranial giant cell arteritis, axillary artery, Movat pentachrome stain. The patient was a 64-year-old woman with claudication of the arm. Note the inflammation with destruction of elastic laminae. The differential diagnosis includes Takayasu's arteritis; the age of the patient and absence of intimal thickening weigh against this diagnosis.

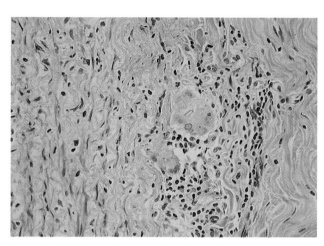

Figure 20–23. Noncranial giant cell arteritis, axillary artery. A routinely stained section of the artery shown in Figure 20–22 demonstrates giant cells.

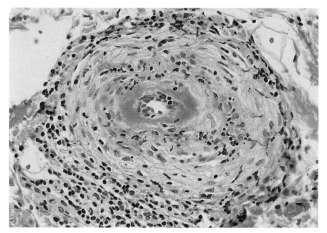

Figure 20–24. Small vessel vasculitis. Note the fibrinoid necrosis, nuclear dust, and perivascular lymphocytic infiltrate.

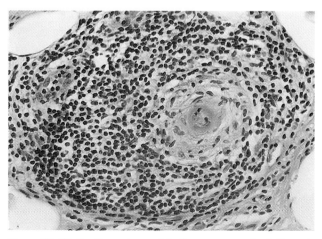

Figure 20–25. Small vessel vasculitis. In some cases, the infiltrate is predominantly lymphocytic, and little fibrinoid necrosis or leukocytoclastic debris is seen.

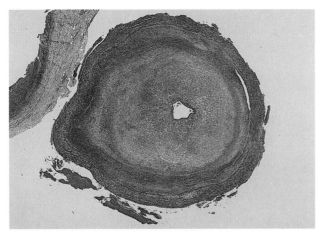

Figure 20–26. Takayasu's arteritis, Movat pentachrome stain. Takayasu's disease typically results in stenosis of arch vessels. A young woman presented with claudication of the upper extremity and focal narrowing of the subclavian artery. Surgery relieved the stenosis; angiography demonstrated aortic lesions consistent with Takayasu's disease. Note the marked intimal narrowing characteristic of Takayasu's disease.

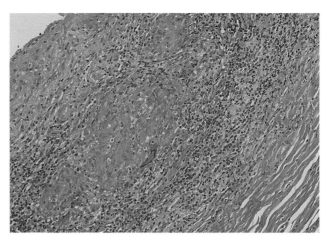

Figure 20–27. Takayasu's disease, hematoxylin and eosin stain. A higher magnification of the case illustrated in Figure 20–26 demonstrates a granulomatous infiltrate in the vessel wall.

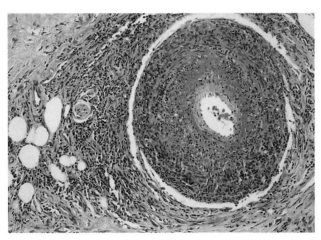

Figure 20–28. Rheumatoid vasculitis. This muscular artery is infiltrated by neutrophils and mononuclear cells, and there is fibrinoid necrosis of the wall. This histologic appearance is similar to that of polyarteritis nodosa.

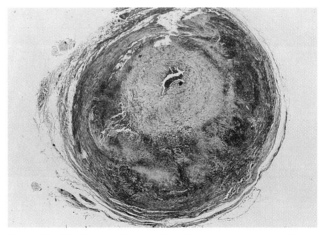

Figure 20–29. Rheumatoid vasculitis, Movat pentachrome stain. A young woman with a long history of rheumatoid arthritis developed temporal artery tenderness. Biopsy revealed marked inflammation, scarring, and fibrointimal proliferation.

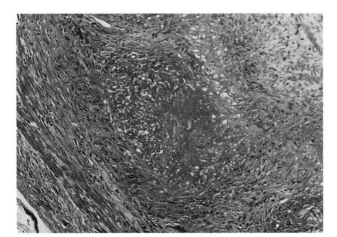

Figure 20–30. Rheumatoid vasculitis, hematoxylin and eosin stain. A higher magnification of Figure 20–29 demonstrates a necrobiotic nodule within the temporal arterial wall. Rheumatoid nodules are not usually found in rheumatoid vasculitis but are quite specific for the diagnosis.

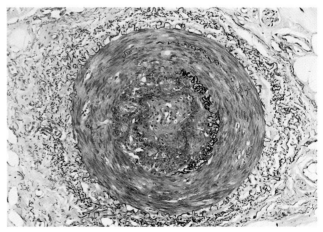

Figure 20–31. Scleroderma, peripheral artery. This muscular artery is occluded by fibrointimal proliferation and muscular hypertrophy. There is little inflammation. The vascular disease of scleroderma is often more sclerotic than inflammatory. The patient was a 64-year-old woman with gangrene of the tips of the middle and ring fingers of the right hand.

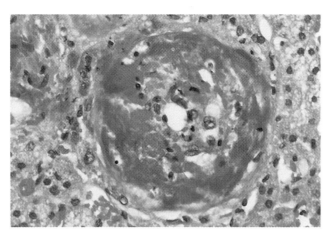

Figure 20–32. Scleroderma, adrenal artery. In this artery, there is hyaline necrosis of the vessel wall with little inflammation. These changes are characteristic of acute scleroderma, generally with progressive disease and renal failure. Similar arterial changes may occur in hypertension and diabetes mellitus.

CHAPTER 21

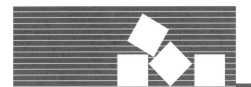

Vasculitis of Specific Organs and Localized Vasculitis

Patients with symptoms suggestive of systemic vasculitis may undergo biopsy to provide a tissue diagnosis. Sites of biopsy include the skin, skeletal muscle, nerve, and, less often, testis and gastrointestinal tract. In these cases, the presence or absence of vasculitis should be documented. Alternatively, vasculitis can occur in specific organs before there is a clinical suspicion of vasculitis. In these cases, a specific type of vasculitis should be diagnosed. The percentage of cases that later manifest as systemic disease is largely unknown but probably varies by histologic type.

CUTANEOUS VASCULITIS

Small Vessel Vasculitis

- Small vessel vasculitis is the most common cutaneous vasculitis.
- Synonyms include hypersensitivity vasculitis, small vessel necrotizing vasculitis, and necrotizing venulitis.
- It is believed to be secondary to circulating immune complexes in many cases.
- The hallmark clinical lesion is a palpable purpuric papule, often occurring in crops.
- Other dermatologic presentations are erythema elevatum diutinum and urticarial vasculitis.
- It is often a manifestation of systemic disease (see Chap 20), but, in more than 50% of cases, it remains apparently localized to the skin with a self-limited course.
- Other causes of vasculitis that histologically simulate small vessel vasculitis include septic emboli, cold injury, and adjacent ulcers.

Polyarteritis Nodosa

- Cutaneous involvement occurs in one fifth to one half of patients with systemic polyarteritis nodosa.
- Punctate cutaneous ulcers, digital gangrene, and livedo reticularis with ulcerating nodules are common clinical presentations.
- The most common histologic lesion is small vessel vasculitis. Typical lesions of muscular arteries are less common in the skin.
- "Benign cutaneous polyarteritis nodosa" is a localized form of polyarteritis characterized by painful, ulcerating nodules of the extremities. Systemic disease rarely develops in the first few years after diagnosis, but increased rates of late systemic involvement have been reported.

Churg-Strauss Angiitis

- Up to 70% of patients with Churg-Strauss vasculitis have cutaneous lesions, usually ulcers, and subcutaneous nodules.
- The histology is often a nonspecific small vessel vasculitis, and granulomas are uncommon.
- Isolated Churg-Strauss angiitis of the skin is essentially nonexistent.

Wegener's Granulomatosis

- Skin involvement in systemic Wegener's granulomatosis occurs in 10% of patients at presentation, and in up to 50% of all patients.
- Cutaneous Wegener's granulomatosis takes many forms, including perioral pyoderma gangrenosum and palpable purpura.
- The histology is nonspecific; disease isolated to skin has not been reported.

Miscellaneous Cutaneous Vasculitis

- In nodular vasculitis, arteritis is associated with panniculitis (erythema induratum).
- In "granulomatous" vasculitis, a granulomatous arteritis may occur in cutaneous lymphomas (lymphomatoid granulomatosis) or may be a component of cutaneous bacterial infection (syphilis, tuberculosis).

- Isolated granulomatous phlebitis of the skin is rare; histologically, there are necrotizing granulomas of vessel walls; clinically, there are recurrent subcutaneous nodules that may be painful.

References

Chen KR. Cutaneous polyarteritis nodosa: a clinical and histopathological study of 20 cases. J Dermatol 16:429–442, 1989.

Jorizzo JL. Classification of vasculitis. J Invest Derm 100:1065–1105, 1993.

VASCULITIS OF THE RESPIRATORY TRACT

Wegener's Granulomatosis

- Pulmonary lesions in patients with Wegener's granulomatosis occur in 50% of patients at presentation and up to 80% of patients during the course of disease.
- There is a subset of patients with Wegener's granulomatosis localized to the lung; these patients have a better prognosis.
- In upper airway involvement, biopsy demonstrates a polymorphous infiltrate with vasculitis, ischemic necrosis, and giant cells.
- Differential diagnosis of upper airway biopsies includes lymphoma and infectious processes.
- Diagnosis of Wegener's is often one of exclusion, and multiple biopsies may be necessary.

Polyarteritis Nodosa

- The lung is involved in about 30% of patients with classic polyarteritis nodosa, although reports suggest that up to 70% of cases have bronchial artery involvement.
- In addition to vasculitis, diffuse alveolar damage and interstitial fibrosis may occur.
- Vasculitic lesions are similar to polyarteritis involving other organs, without extravascular granulomas of Wegener's granulomatosis or Churg-Strauss angiitis.
- Pulmonary capillaritis is associated with microscopic polyarteritis (polyangiitis) and idiopathic crescentic glomerulonephritis (see Chap. 20).
- Polyarteritis nodosa isolated to the lung has not been described.

Churg-Strauss Angiitis

- Virtually all cases of Churg-Strauss angiitis involve the lung.
- Extrapulmonary manifestations are generally present, but a subset of patients have primarily pulmonary symptoms.
- Asthma and other allergic symptoms often precede a vasculitic phase.

Miscellaneous Pulmonary Vasculitis

- Hypersensitivity vasculitis is presumably immune complex mediated. Up to 25% of patients with hypersensitivity vasculitis have pulmonary symptoms.

- Histologically, there is a necrotizing small vessel vasculitis/venulitis.
- In Behçet's disease, thromboangiitis of pulmonary arteries with aneurysms may rupture as a secondary consequence of vasculitis of vasa vasorum.
- In pulmonary capillaritis, there is neutrophilic infiltration of capillaries with alveolar hemorrhage. It may complicate Wegener's granulomatosis and microscopic polyarteritis (antineutrophil cytoplasmic antibody–related), and a variety of other conditions (see Chap. 20).
- Systemic lupus erythematosus (SLE) may, like capillaritis, rarely result in a plexiform arteriopathy, which occasionally has a vasculitic component (see Chap 17).
- In rheumatoid arthritis, which is similar to SLE, there may be arteritis with pulmonary hypertension.
- Takayasu's arteritis involves elastic pulmonary arteries (demonstrated angiographically) in up to 50% of patients.

References

Carrington CB, Liebow A. Limited forms of angiitis and granulomatosis of Wegener's type. Am J Med 41:497–527, 1966.

Yousem SA, Colby TV, Carrington CB. Lung biopsy in rheumatoid arthritis. Am Rev Respir Dis 131:770–777, 1985.

VASCULITIS OF THE GASTROINTESTINAL TRACT AND ABDOMINAL VISCERA

Polyarteritis Nodosa

- Abdominal angina or bowel perforation occurs in approximately 25% of patients with polyarteritis nodosa. It is considered a surgical emergency and is often life threatening.
- Isolated polyarteritis nodosa of the gallbladder, pancreas, and small and large bowel has been reported. The incidence of development of systemic disease is unknown but is likely to be less than 25%.
- Isolated arteritis of the spleen may result in infarction and rupture. The splenic artery and its branches may be involved in patients with polyarteritis nodosa, lupus vasculitis, and antineutrophil cytoplasmic antibody–associated vasculitis.
- Vasculitis of the adrenal gland is a rare cause of isolated adrenal hemorrhage.

Connective Tissue Diseases

- SLE causes gastrointestinal symptoms in up to 50% of individuals, but vasculitis of the gut develops in only approximately 2% of patients. Acute abdomen may result in surgical bowel resection. SLE is histologically similar to polyarteritis in surgically resected cases; small vessel vasculitis also occurs.
- Rheumatoid arthritis causes a small vessel vasculitis in the rectum of up to 25% of individuals. Polyarteritis is less common but may result in mesenteric infarction similar to typical cases of polyarteritis nodosa.

Henoch-Schönlein Purpura

- Henoch-Schönlein purpura typically involves the bowel.
- It occurs primarily in children, after viral illness or ingestion of medication.
- Histologically, there is a small vessel vasculitis.
- Only rarely is surgical treatment required.

Intestinal Phlebitis

- Phlebitis is an uncommon disease of the bowel, not associated with collagen vascular disease, that affects primarily the right colon and omentum, although any location of the intestines may be involved.
- There are two types: giant cell phlebitis and lymphocytic phlebitis.
- Giant cell phlebitis typically presents as a mass lesion, perforation, or hemorrhage. Histologically, there is a mixed inflammatory infiltrate of large muscular veins, and there is a giant cell component.
- Lymphocytic phlebitis is associated with hypersensitivity to medications. Smaller veins are involved, and giant cells are not present.
- Intestinal phlebitis appears to have a relatively benign course, without development of a systemic illness.

Miscellaneous Gastrointestinal Vasculitis

- Churg-Strauss angiitis may rarely involve the bowel.
- Behçet's disease may result in bowel ulceration. The histology is that of small vessel vasculitis.
- Giant cell arteritis occasionally involves mesenteric arteries and may result in ischemia. There is usually aortic and cranial involvement. A rare form of visceral giant cell arteritis has been described (see Chap. 20).
- Buerger's disease occasionally involves mesenteric veins and arteries, resulting in ischemic bowel.

References

Adler RH, Norcross BM, Lockie LM. Arteritis and infarction of the intestine in rheumatoid arthritis. JAMA 180:922–926, 1962.

Burke AP, Sobin LH, Virmani R. Localized vasculitis of the gastrointestinal tract. Am J Surg Pathol 19:338–349, 1995.

Chen KT. Gallbladder vasculitis. J Clin Gastroenterol 11:537–540, 1989.

Fernandez-Nero A, Valdivielso P, Sanchez-Carrillo JJ, Donenech I, DeRamon E, Gonzalez-Santos P. Localized rheumatoid vasculitis presenting as acute alithiasic cholecystitis. Am J Med 91:90–92, 1991.

Helliwell TR, Flook D, Whitworth J, Day DW. Arteritis and venulitis in systemic lupus erythematosus resulting in massive lower intestinal haemorrhage. Histopathology 9:1103–1113, 1985.

Herrington JL, Grossman LA. Surgical lesions of the small and large intestine resulting from Buerger's disease. Ann Surg 168:1079–1087, 1968.

Ito M, Sano K, Inaba H, Hotchi M. Localized necrotizing arteritis. A report of two cases involving the gallbladder and pancreas. Arch Pathol Lab Med 114:780–783, 1991.

Powers BJ, Brown G, Williams RW, Speers W. Leukocytoclastic vasculitis, not associated with Henoch-Schönlein purpura, causing recurrent massive painless gastrointestinal hemorrhage. Am J Gastroenterol 87:1191–1193, 1992.

Saraga EP, Costa J. Idiopathic entero-colic lymphocytic phlebitis. A cause of ischemic intestinal necrosis. Am J Surg Pathol 13:303–308, 1989.

Stevens SM, Gue S, Finckh ES. Necrotizing and giant cell granulomatous phlebitis of caecum and ascending colon. Pathology 8:259–264, 1976.

Suen KC, Burton JD. The spectrum of eosinophilic infiltration of the gastrointestinal tract and its relationship to other disorders of angiitis and granulomatosis. Hum Pathol 10:31–43, 1979.

Sunder-Plassmann G, Geissler K, Penner E. Functional asplenia and vasculitis associated with antineutrophil cytoplasmic antibodies (letter). N Engl J Med 327:437, 1992.

Zizic TM, Shulman LE, Stevens MB. Colonic perforations in systemic lupus erythematosus. Medicine 54:411–426, 1975.

VASCULITIS OF THE NEUROMUSCULAR SYSTEM

Central Nervous System

Localized Primary Vasculitis of the Central Nervous System

- Localized vasculitis of the central nervous system is rare.
- The mean age at presentation is in the fifth decade.
- Clinically, patients with localized vasculitis of the central nervous system present with headache, focal deficits, visual disturbances, cognitive dysfunction, and altered consciousness.
- Unusual forms of presentation include brain tumor, chronic meningitis, abnormal pituitary function, spinal cord tumor, cerebellar dysfunction, and intracranial or subarachnoid hemorrhage.
- Unlike in giant cell arteritis, the erythrocyte sedimentation rate is normal.
- Histologically, both arteries and veins are involved, and any portion of the brain may be affected.
- The adventitia is preferentially inflamed with a lymphocytic or giant cell infiltrate.
- Neutrophils are sparse, and fibrinoid changes or aneurysmal dilatation is only occasionally present.
- The various histologic forms have been termed giant cell arteritis, necrotizing arteritis, and small vessel vasculitis.

Central Nervous System Involvement in Systemic Vasculitis

- Twenty percent to 40% of patients with polyarteritis nodosa demonstrate central nervous system abnormalities.
- Ten percent to 29% of patients with Behçet's disease have clinical central nervous system involvement; peripheral neuropathy and myopathy are rare.
- Up to 30% of patients with temporal arteritis have CNS symptoms, including syncope, confusion, stroke, hearing loss, ataxia, and visual disturbance.
- Intracerebral granulomas occur rarely in patients with Wegener's granulomatosis.

Peripheral Nervous System

- Polyarteritis nodosa involves the peripheral nerves as mononeuritis multiplex in up to 50% of patients. Nerve biopsy is often performed to confirm the diagnosis. Abnormal nerve conduction studies are helpful in determining the site of biopsy. Histologic appearance is generally that of small vessel necrotizing vasculitis of vasa vasorum. Nerve changes include axonal degeneration.
- Up to 75% of patients with Churg-Strauss angiitis have

peripheral neuropathy in the vasculitis phase. There are rare reports of vasculitis of vasa nervorum.

- Peripheral neuropathy occurs in almost 50% of patients with Wegener's granulomatosis. Vasculitis of peripheral nerves, muscle, and dorsal and ventral roots may occur.
- Rheumatoid arthritis can cause identical clinical findings (mononeuritis multiplex) and identical histologic findings as polyarteritis nodosa. Sometimes, histologic changes are less severe (mild inflammatory changes with intimal proliferation, absence of necrotizing vasculitis).

Vasculitis of Skeletal Muscles

- Polyarteritis localized in an extremity has been reported.
- Skeletal muscle involvement in patients with polyarteritis nodosa occurs in 35% of patients. Biopsy is often performed to confirm the diagnosis. Histologic findings include small vessel vasculitis, necrotizing arteritis, neurogenic muscular atrophy, and myositis.

References

Lie JT. Primary (granulomatous) angiitis of the central nervous system: a clinicopathologic analysis of 15 new cases and a review of the literature. Hum Pathol 23:164–171, 1992.

Wees SJ, Sunwoo IN, Oh SJ. Sural nerve biopsy in systemic necrotizing vasculitis. Am J Med 71:525–532, 1981.

VASCULITIS OF THE GENITOURINARY TRACT AND BREAST

Kidney

- Polyarteritis nodosa involves the kidney in 63% to 82% of cases. The classic type (vasculitis of small arteries without glomerulonephritis) is a less common cause of renal disease than the microscopic form (microscopic polyangiitis, see Chap. 20).
- Glomerulonephritis of polyarteritis is typically focal, segmental necrotizing glomerulonephritis with crescents. There is also a diffuse proliferative type.
- Wegener's granulomatosis involves the kidney in nearly all cases. Histologic features are similar to those of polyarteritis nodosa, although granulomatous glomerulonephritis is more common, and changes are usually more extensive and severe.
- Henoch-Schönlein purpura is caused by IgA immune complex deposition in small vessels.
- Churg-Strauss angiitis involves the kidney in only a minority of cases; glomerulonephritis similar to that seen in Wegener's granulomatosis has been reported, but the clinical outcome appears to be better.
- Rare cases of giant cell/granulomatous arteritis of the kidney have been reported. The relationship to hypersensitivity and classic giant cell arteritis is unknown.
- Hypersensitivity vasculitis of the kidney is rare, and the criteria for diagnosis are controversial.

Testis

- Approximately 20% of patients with clinically diagnosed polyarteritis nodosa have testicular pain. A biopsy of the testis is occasionally performed to provide a tissue diagnosis.
- Isolated polyarteritis of the testis and epididymis is a cause of testicular infarction and pain. A small (unknown) percentage of patients develop systemic polyarteritis.
- Isolated arteritis of the spermatic cord, often with giant cells, has been reported.

Urinary Tract

- Wegener's granulomatosis, in the form of necrotizing granulomas, rarely involves the prostate and bladder.
- Localized polyarteritis of the bladder and prostate occurs rarely.

Breast and Gynecologic Organs

- Giant cell arteritis of the breast occurs in elderly women with a history suggestive of polymyalgia rheumatica (50% of cases). It occurs as tender breast masses, accompanied by an elevated erythrocyte sedimentation rate.
- Giant cell arteritis of the uterus may precede temporal arteritis. There is an association with polymyalgia rheumatica. Prolapsed uterus may result.
- The finding of giant cell arteritis of the gynecologic organs should prompt an investigation for generalized giant cell arteritis.
- Systemic polyarteritis nodosa and systemic arteritis associated with connective tissue disease may involve the breast, uterus, and fallopian tubes, but symptomatic disease is rare.
- Localized polyarteritis of the breast may result in tender masses in younger women. The incidence of progression to systemic disease is unknown.
- Localized polyarteritis of the uterus, ovaries, and fallopian tubes occurs rarely. The incidence of progression to systemic disease is unknown.

References

Clement PB, Senges H, How AR. Giant cell arteritis of the breast: case report and literature review. Hum Pathol 18:1187–1189, 1987.

Heptinstall RH. Polyarteritis (periarteritis) nodosa, Wegener's syndrome, and other forms of vasculitis. In Heptinstall RH (ed). *Pathology of the Kidney.* Boston, Little, Brown, 1992, pp 1097–1162.

Jennette JC, Falk RJ. The pathology of vasculitis involving the kidney. Am J Kidney Dis 24:130–141, 1994.

Karnauchow PN, Steele AA. Isolated necrotizing granulomatous vasculitis of the spermatic cords. J Urol 141:379–381, 1989.

Levy A, Weinberger A, Mor C, Pinkhas J. Localized polyarteritis nodosa: cases involving the lower extremities and the breast. Rheumatol Int 6:43–44, 1986.

Nehra PC, Ramus DM, Peterson J. Giant-cell arteritis of the uterus with associated temporal arteritis: a case report. Obstet Gynecol 76:935–938, 1990.

Persellin ST, Menke DM. Isolated polyarteritis nodosa of the male reproductive system. J Rheumatol 19:985–988, 1992.

Shurbaji MS, Epstein JI. Testicular vasculitis: implications for systemic disease. Hum Pathol 19:186–189, 1988.

Susmano A, Roseman D, Haber MH. Giant cell arteritis of the breast. A unique syndrome. Arch Intern Med 150:900–904, 1990.

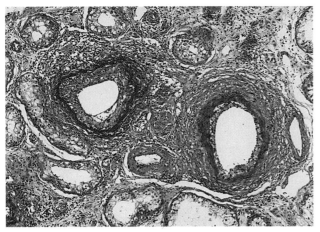

Figure 21–1. Polyarteritis, testis. Fibrinoid necrosis and acute inflammation are present in two arteries. Polyarteritis of the testis may occur as testicular pain or infarction, and it might not represent systemic illness.

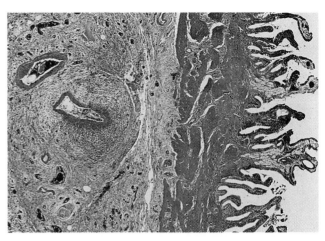

Figure 21–2. Polyarteritis, gallbladder. Isolated polyarteritis may occur in the gallbladder, resulting in alithiasic cholecystitis.

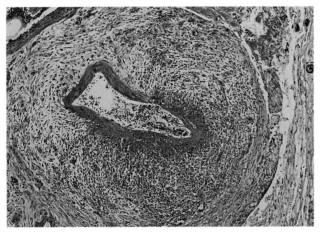

Figure 21–3. A higher magnification of Figure 21–2 demonstrating segmental necrosis and inflammation typical of polyarteritis nodosa.

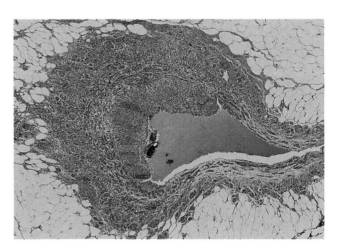

Figure 21–4. Giant cell phlebitis, right colon. Primary inflammation involving veins of the colon may result in infarction or masses of the bowel, especially the right colon and cecum. In this illustration, there is an inflammatory infiltrate involving a large segment of a muscular vein.

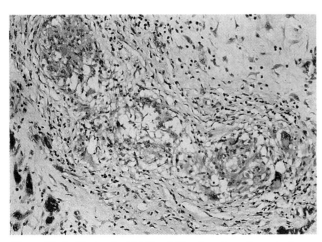

Figure 21–5. Giant cell phlebitis, right colon. A smaller vein from a different area of the section illustrated in Figure 21–4 demonstrates granulomatous inflammation with giant cells destroying a vessel, which on serial sections was seen as being a vein (not shown).

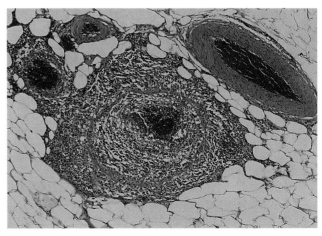

Figure 21–6. Phlebitis, colon. A vein accompanying a muscular artery is destroyed by a mononuclear infiltrate. Phlebitis without a granulomatous infiltrate may result in bowel symptoms and may be caused by a reaction to medications.

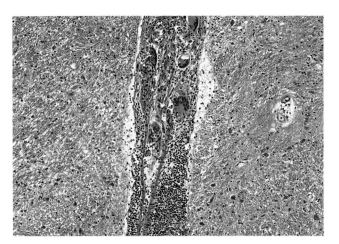

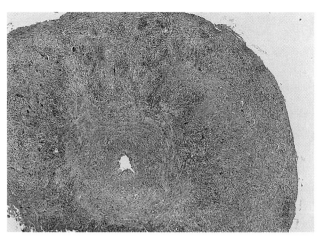

Figure 21–7. Giant cell arteritis, brain. Localized arteritis of the central nervous system may result in infarcts and localizing signs. In many cases, as in this illustration, giant cells are prominent. Unlike giant cell arteritis, the patients are not elderly and there is no evidence of polymyalgia rheumatica or elevated erythrocyte sedimentation rate.

Figure 21–8. Granulomatous phlebitis. One of multiple tender subcutaneous nodules was excised from a young woman with no clinical evidence of systemic vasculitis or connective tissue disease. Note the markedly thickened vein.

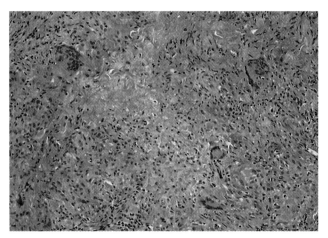

Figure 21–9. Granulomatous phlebitis. A higher magnification of Figure 21–8 demonstrates necrotizing granulomas.

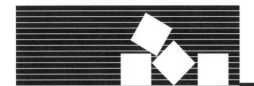

CHAPTER 22

Arterial Dysplasia, Aneurysms, and Dissections

FIBROMUSCULAR DYSPLASIA

Fibromuscular dysplasia (FMD) is a heterogeneous group of noninflammatory disorders characterized by disorganization of muscular arterial walls and resulting in arterial luminal narrowing and arterial aneurysms.

Clinical Findings

- Most patients are young white females.
- There is an association with estrogen exposure and pregnancy.
- The most common signs and symptoms are hypertension, stroke, and abdominal pain.
- The most frequent mode of inheritance is autosomal dominant with variable penetrance.
- Patients with neurofibromatosis are at increased risk for the development of dysplasia of various arteries. Stenotic arterial lesions in patients with neurofibromatosis are usually caused by FMD and, rarely, by compression by extrinsic neurofibroma.

Gross Pathologic Findings

- Segmental interrupted arterial narrowing of arteries results in an angiographic finding of a "string of beads."
- Complicated cases may show dissections or aneurysmal dilatation.

Microscopic Findings

- There is a multitude of findings, including fibrointimal proliferation (often segmental, alternating with normal areas), medial and adventitial scarring, and disorganization of elastic laminae.
- Secondary changes include dissections and aneurysmal dilatation.

- Histologically, FMD is classified into medial, intimal and adventitial types.
- Medial FMD accounts for 95% of cases and is further divided into medial fibroplasia, perimedial fibroplasia, and medial hyperplasia:

  - Medial fibroplasia is characterized by multifocal areas of close apposition of internal and external elastic laminae with intervening areas of smooth muscle cells, resulting in segmental narrowing and dilatation.
  - Perimedial hyperplasia denotes a predominance of fibrous tissue in the outer media.
  - Pure medial hyperplasia is rare; in this type of FMD, there is predominantly concentric hypertrophy of the medial wall with little fibrosis.

- Intimal FMD accounts for less than 5% of lesions. There is pure intimal proliferation of smooth muscle cells.
- In adventitial (periarterial) FMD, there is dense collagenous replacement of the adventitia and surrounding adipose tissue with normal media and intima.

Differential Diagnosis

- Atherosclerosis may mimic intimal FMD. In FMD, there is no lipid deposition or inflammatory cell infiltrate, and the internal elastic lamina is often preserved.
- Healed arteritis may be associated with intimal fibroplasia in muscular arteries that may mimic the histologic picture of intimal fibroplasia. In general, there is focal medial destruction with scarring and obliteration of the internal and/or external elastic laminae in healed arteritis.
- Dissections resulting from dysplasia must be distinguished from other causes of dissection (cystic medial change, iatrogenic dissections).
- Aneurysms resulting from dysplasia must be distin-

Table 22–1
PATHOLOGIC DIAGNOSES, SURGICALLY RESECTED NONAORTIC ANEURYSMS, AFIP* FILES 1970–1993

Diagnosis	Mean age	n	Mult	Diss	Site						
					Leg[1]	Viscera[2]	Face[3]	Arm[4]	Subcl	Carotid	Cor
Pseudoaneurysm	26	26	0	0	7	0	17	2	0	0	0
Noninflammatory**	43	19	3	2	4	8	0	5	1	1	0
FMD	42	17	4	4	5	4	2	0	2	4	0
Atherosclerotic	60	10	2	0	6	3	0	1	0	0	0
CMN	39	10	3	2	3	2	0	2†	1	1	1
Mycotic	53	4	0	0	1	3	0	0	0	0	0
Takayasu's disease	30	3	1	0	0	0	0	0	3	0	0
Kawasaki disease	2	2	0	0	0	0	0	1	0	0	1
Total	**40**	**91**	**13**	**8**	**26**	**20**	**19**	**11**	**7**	**6**	**2**

*Armed Forces Institute of Pathology.
**Not further classified; classification difficult due to inadequate sampling, secondary changes of dissection, or rupture.
†One patient had Ehlers-Danlos syndrome.
[1] 9 femoral, 8 iliac, 2 peroneal, 6 popliteal, 3 tibial artery aneurysms.
[2] 8 splenic, 3 celiac, 2 hepatic, 2 superior mesenteric, 4 renal aneurysms.
[3] 14 temporal, 2 preauricular, 2 lingual artery aneurysms.
[4] 3 axillary, 4 brachial, 2 ulnar, 2 radial artery aneurysms.
Mult, multiple; diss, dissecting; subcl, subclavian; cor, coronary; FMD, fibromuscular dysplasia; CMN, cystic medial necrosis (medial degeneration).

guished from other causes of aneurysms (vasculitis, atherosclerosis, aneurysms associated with medial degeneration).

Renal Vascular Dysplasia

- Renal vascular dysplasia accounts for 75% of cases of symptomatic FMD.
- It accounts for 25% of cases of renovascular hypertension and for approximately 2% of all cases of hypertension; angioplasty has been an effective treatment.
- Twenty-five percent of cases are associated with FMD of other arteries.
- The right renal artery is more often involved than the left.
- Bilateral renal FMD is associated with extrarenal FMD.
- The distal two thirds of the artery is typically involved by areas of narrowing and/or aneurysms, which may reach several centimeters in diameter.
- Renal vascular dysplasia may cause renal infarction, arterial dissection, embolization, and thrombosis.

Table 22–2
CHILDHOOD PERIPHERAL ARTERIAL
ANEURYSMS (SERIES OF 19 CASES)

Cause	n	Artery involved
Dysplasia	7	renal
Traumatic (pseudoaneursym)	6	ulnar (2), radial (2), popliteal (1), gastroepiploic (1)
Kawasaki disease	2	brachial, hepatic
Idiopathic	2	femoral, iliac
Neurofibromatosis	1	renal
Marfan syndrome	1	splenic

Data from Sarkar R, Coran AG, Cilley RE, Lindenauer SM, Stanley JC. Arterial aneurysms in children: clinicopathologic classification. J Vasc Surg 13:47–56, 1991.

- The arterial histologic changes in patients with neurofibromatosis and renal dysplasia (accounting for up to 25% of childhood renal FMD) are similar to those in patients without neurofibromatosis.

Fibromuscular Dysplasia of Aortic Arch Vessels

- FMD involves primarily the carotid, subclavian, and vertebral arteries, resulting in aneurysms and/or areas of segmental narrowing that are often asymptomatic.
- The internal carotid artery is typically involved at the level of C-1 and C-2 (distal to the most frequent site of atherosclerosis).
- Cerebrovascular FMD is associated with berry aneurysms of the intracranial internal carotid and middle cerebral artery.
- Symptoms occur if there is stenosis of major cephalic arteries, embolization from thrombosed areas of FMD, arterial dissections, or severe narrowing of the subclavian artery.
- Symptoms include transient ischemic attacks, strokes, subarachnoid hemorrhage from associated berry aneurysms of the circle of Willis, the subclavian steal syndrome, and weakness or claudication of the arms.
- Complications include arterial dissections and carotid–cavernous fistulas.

Visceral Fibromuscular Dysplasia and Fibromuscular Dysplasia of Other Arteries

- FMD of the extrarenal visceral arteries (celiac, mesenteric, hepatic, and splenic) is often asymptomatic, because abundant collaterals prevent the complication of ischemia.
- Rarely, patients with neurofibromatosis may develop

mesenteric artery dysplasia, resulting in ischemic bowel.

■ Occasionally, dissections and rupture with hemoperitoneum may result from visceral FMD.

■ FMD of the iliofemoral arteries, brachioaxillary arteries, coronary arteries, and aorta is less common than FMD of other sites and is often multifocal.

Cystic Adventitial Disease, Popliteal Artery

■ Cystic adventitial disease is an idiopathic accumulation of mucinous ground substance in the adventitia of the popliteal arterial wall, possibly related to trauma, ectopic ganglion cyst, or dysplasia.

■ It accounts for approximately 1 in 1200 cases of claudication.

■ There is a male predominance (male:female ratio 5–8:1).

■ The mean age at presentation is approximately 42 years (range 11–72 years).

■ The clinical differential diagnosis generally includes Buerger's disease and atherosclerosis.

■ Recurrence in an interposed vein graft has been reported.

■ Arteriography may show a smooth-walled narrowing or a nonspecific complete occlusion, or it may be normal.

■ Pathologically, there are mucus filled cysts of the adventitial layer of the popliteal artery and surrounding popliteal fossae, resulting from mucin-secreting synovial cells originating from the neighboring joint capsule or tendon sheath.

■ The lectin-binding pattern of cystic adventitial disease appears to be similar to the reactivity pattern of normal synovia.

■ Rarely, the media may be involved with the mucinous degeneration.

■ Rarely, there is involvement of other arteries in the extremities, and involvement of veins has been reported.

■ The gelatinous material may be easily evacuated without opening the arterial lumen.

■ Bypass of the lesion is necessary if there is luminal occlusion.

■ Angioplasty has not been successful in alleviating the stenoses.

References

Alimi Y, Mercier C, Pellissier JF, Piquet P, Tournigand P. Fibromuscular disease of the renal artery: a new histopathologic classification. Ann Vasc Surg 6:220–224, 1992.

Devaney K, Kapur SP, Patterson K, Chandra RS. Pediatric renal artery dysplasia: a morphologic study. Pediatr Pathol 11:609–621, 1991.

Finley JL, Dabbs DJ. Renal vascular smooth muscle proliferation in neurofibromatosis. Hum Pathol 19:107–110, 1988.

Insall RL, Chamberlain J, Loose HW. Fibromuscular dysplasia of visceral arteries. Eur J Vasc Surg 6:668–672, 1992.

Lie JT, Jensen PL, Smith RE. Adventitial cystic disease of the lesser saphenous vein. Arch Pathol Lab Med 115:946–948, 1991.

Luscher TF, Lie JT, Stanson AW, Houser OW, Hollier LH, Sheps SG. Arterial fibromuscular dysplasia. Mayo Clin Proc 62:931–952, 1987.

Sato S, Hata J. Fibromuscular dysplasia. Its occurrence with a dissecting aneurysm of the internal carotid artery. Arch Pathol Lab Med 106:332–335, 1982.

Schneider PA, LaBerge JM, Cunningham CG, Ehrenfeld WK. Isolated thigh claudication as a result of fibromuscular dysplasia of the deep femoral artery. J Vasc Surg 15:657–660, 1992.

Thevenet A, Latil JL, Albat B. Fibromuscular disease of the external iliac artery. Ann Vasc Surg 6:199–204, 1992.

ANEURYSMS, CLASSIFICATION, AND ETIOLOGY

Definitions

■ Aneurysms are often defined by their shape and size (e.g., saccular, small saccular [berry], fusiform, giant) and may be congenital or acquired. Types of aneurysms are listed in Tables 22–1 and 22–2.

■ Mycotic aneurysm is a term introduced by Osler before the microbiological distinction between fungi and bacteria was made; it signifies an underlying infection caused by bacteria or fungi.

■ Pseudoaneurysms are interruptions in the arterial wall and are focally lined by organized hematoma, scar, or granulation tissue; they are generally traumatic in origin.

Congenital Aneurysms

■ Intracranial berry aneurysms have a slight female predominance. Eighty percent to 85% occur in the anterior half of the circle of Willis. The most common location is the anterior cerebral artery. They are often considered to be congenital or may be secondary to a variety of conditions.

■ Sporadic congenital aneurysms may occur in virtually any arterial bed. The histologic changes are often nonspecific or show medial degeneration.

■ Aneurysms are associated with the following congenital syndromes:

• FMD may result in focal aneurysmal dilatation.

• Cerebral aneurysms may be associated with FMD of extracranial carotid arteries, aortic coarctation, and autosomal dominant polycystic kidney disease.

• Rarely, dysplasia of virtually any arterial bed develops in patients with neurofibromatosis. Although symptoms are generally related to arterial stenoses, aneurysms may result as well.

• Histologic features of Ehlers-Danlos syndrome (usually type IV) are not well documented.

• Marfan syndrome usually causes aneurysmal dilatation of the aorta. Occasionally, aneurysms with or without dissection of peripheral arteries occur. Cystic medial change is generally noted histopathologically.

Acquired Aneurysms

■ Traumatic (pseudo) aneurysms are usually present in superficial arteries. Typically, there is an abrupt interruption in the vessel wall, with granulation tissue or scar.

■ Atherosclerotic aneurysms are found in the abdominal aorta and popliteal, splenic, axillary, renal, iliac, femoral, and coronary arteries. Histologically, there may be an inflammatory infiltrate that is more marked than the infiltrate accompanying atherosclerosis in nonaneurysmal atherosclerotic vessels.

- Systemic hypertension may precipitate the formation of aneurysms of elastic and muscular arteries. Medial degeneration may be present histologically.
- Mycotic aneurysms are most commonly related to bacterial endocarditis and may be diagnosed years after endocarditis treatment. They affect, in descending order of frequency, the aorta and the superior mesenteric, splenic, coronary, posterior tibial, common iliac, popliteal, radial, ulnar, and renal arteries. The most frequent bacterial organisms are salmonella, staphylococci, and enterococci.
- Vasculitis (polyarteritis nodosa, Kawasaki disease, and Takayasu's disease) may cause inflammatory aneurysms in various arterial beds. Behçet's disease may cause aneurysmal arteriopathy of medium-sized arteries and pseudoaneurysms at angiographic puncture sites.
- Pregnancy is associated with aneurysms of the cerebral arteries, aorta, splenic artery, coronary artery, ovarian artery, carotid artery, and renal artery. More than 50% of ruptured aneurysms in women younger than 40 years of age are pregnancy-related.
- Histiocytosis X, embolic myxoma, and radiation therapy may result in aneurysms.

References

Faggioli GL, Gargiulo M, Bertoni F et al. Parietal inflammatory infiltrate in peripheral aneurysms of atherosclerotic origin. J Cardiovasc Surg (Torino) 33:331–336, 1992.

Freyrie A, Paragona O, Cenacchi G, et al. True and false aneurysms in Behçet's disease: case report with ultrastructural observations. J Vasc Surg 17:762–767, 1993.

Fukushige J, Nihill MR, McNamara DG. Spectrum of cardiovascular lesions in mucocutaneous lymph node syndrome: analysis of eight cases. Am J Cardiol 45:98–107, 1980.

Sarkar R, Coran AG, Cilley RE, Lindenauer SM, Stanley JC. Arterial aneurysms in children: clinicopathologic classification. J Vasc Surg 13:47–56, 1991.

ARTERIAL ANEURYSMS BY SITE

Visceral Aneurysms

- Splenic artery aneurysms are found most often in women in the distal artery and are associated with multiple pregnancies; 72% are calcified and 29% multiple. Causes include cystic medial change, other congenital (idiopathic) causes, and FMD.
- Renal artery aneurysms may be found incidentally. When found in women of childbearing age, in patients with FMD, or in patients with hypertension, surgery is indicated.
- Fifty percent of celiac/hepatic aneurysms are secondary to polyarteritis nodosa.
- Superior mesenteric artery aneurysms are frequently mycotic in patients with a history of bacterial endocarditis.
- Pancreatic, gastroduodenal, and pancreaticoduodenal artery aneurysms may be associated with adjacent pancreatitis (pseudoaneurysms).

Lower Extremity Artery Aneurysms

- There is a male predominance of lower extremity artery aneurysm. Most are atherosclerotic, and there is an association with hypertension.
- One third of iliac and femoral artery aneurysms are multiple.
- Popliteal aneurysms are generally considered atherosclerotic or degenerative; few may be secondary to entrapment of the artery.
- In younger patients, especially athletes, entrapment of the popliteal artery by anomalous or hypertrophied muscles or cystic adventitial disease may cause similar symptoms as popliteal aneurysms.

Aneurysms of Aortic Arch Arteries

- Inflammatory aneurysms in children are generally secondary to Kawasaki disease; in young adults, Takayasu's disease; in older adults, giant cell arteritis.
- Extracranial nondissecting carotid aneurysms are rare; they are usually located at or above the bifurcation and may result in dysphagia.
- Fusiform carotid aneurysms are more likely to be bilateral, atherosclerotic, and associated with hypertension, whereas saccular aneurysms are more likely to be congenital or idiopathic.
- Rare causes of carotid artery aneurysms include traumatic aneurysms from remote blunt trauma to the head and neck. Traumatic pseudoaneurysms are more common in distal vessels of the upper extremity.
- von Recklinghausen's neurofibromatosis may result in multiple aneurysms of the carotid, subclavian, and vertebral arteries.
- A congenitally aberrant right subclavian artery (arising distal to the left subclavian) is found in 0.5% of the population. Aneurysmal dilatation of its origin occurs rarely; these aneurysms may cause dyspnea, dysphagia, or sudden collapse from rupture. A mediastinal mass may be detected by roentgenography in asymptomatic patients.

References

Chiou AC, Josephs LG, Menzoian JO. Inferior pancreaticoduodenal artery aneurysm: report of a case and review of the literature. J Vasc Surg 17:784–789, 1993.

Holdsworth RJ, Gunn A. Ruptured splenic artery aneurysm in pregnancy. A review. Br J Obstet Gynaecol 99:595–597, 1992.

Kiernan PD, Dearani J, Byrne WD, et al. Aneurysm of an aberrant right subclavian artery: case report and review of the literature. Mayo Clin Proc 68:468–474, 1993.

McCready RA, Pairolero PC, Gilmore JC, et al. Isolated iliac artery aneurysms. Surgery 903:688–693, 1983.

Ramesh S, Michaels JA, Galland RB. Popliteal aneurysm: morphology and management. Br J Surg 80:1531–1533, 1993.

Rowe JG, Hosni AA. A common carotid artery aneurysm causing severe dysphagia. J Laryngol Otol 108:67–68, 1994.

Stehbens WE. Etiology of intracranial berry aneurysms. J Neurosurg 70:823–831, 1989.

Trastek VF, Pairolero PC, Joyce JW, et al. Splenic artery aneurysms. Surgery 91:694–699, 1982.

ARTERIAL DISSECTIONS

Arterial dissection is an accumulation of blood between planes of the arterial media or between the media and adventitia.

Etiology

■ There are varied underlying causes, including medial degeneration, trauma or instrumentation, medial dysplasia, and (rarely) vasculitis.

Clinical Findings

■ Spontaneous dissections occur in virtually all arterial beds, including renal, coronary, carotid, splanchnic (mesenteric, gastric, splenic), cerebral, vertebral, basilar, iliac, hepatic, femoral, and pulmonary arteries.
■ There is a slight male predominance. Most patients are 30 to 60 years of age; hypertension is present in up to 50% of cases.
■ Iatrogenic dissections occur during operative procedures or catheterizations. Carotid dissections have been reported with minimal trauma, such as with chiropractic manipulations.
■ The symptoms of arterial dissection relate to ischemia to the region of the body supplied (e.g., bowel infarct, stroke) or arterial rupture.
■ Pregnancy is associated with aneurysms and dissections of the splenic artery.
■ Arterial dissections of peripheral arteries may occur in clinical syndromes, specifically Marfan syndrome and Ehlers-Danlos type IV.

Pathologic Findings

■ In the earliest stages, there is a lining of platelets with or without fresh blood along the dissected planes.
■ In chronic dissections, the plane of dissection is lined by granulation tissue and fibrous tissue, distorting the media. A Movat pentachrome stain or other elastic stain is especially helpful in delineating intima, media, adventitia, and organized dissection.
■ There is formation of a false lumen, which may become the major channel of blood flow and which may compress the true lumen.
■ The false lumen may become distended and aneurysmal.
■ Aneurysmal dilatation is not a constant feature of arterial dissection; however, there may be an underlying aneurysm, especially in cases of cystic medial change.
■ Specific features of underlying causes of dissection (FMD, medial degeneration) should be sought.
■ Ulcerated atherosclerotic plaques, vasculitis (giant cell arteritis, Takayasu's arteritis, Behçet's disease), and segmental arterial mediolysis are rare causes of dissection.
■ Spontaneous dissections of the coronary arteries occur most often in women (left anterior descending coronary artery); they may be secondary to an inflammatory phenomenon, because, in most cases, there are abundant eosinophils.

References

Ast G, Woimant F, Georges B, Laurian C, Haguenau M. Spontaneous dissection of the internal carotid artery in 68 patients. Eur J Med 2:466–472, 1993.

Bahar S, Coban O, Gurvit IH, Akman-Demir G, Gokyigit A. Spontaneous dissection of the extracranial vertebral artery with spinal subarachnoid haemorrhage in a patient with Behçet's disease. Neuroradiology 35:352–354, 1993.

Declemy S, Kreitmann P, Popoff G, Diaz F. Spontaneous dissecting aneurysm of the common iliac artery. Ann Vasc Surg 5:549–551, 1991.

Merrel SW, Gloviczki P. Splenic artery dissection: a case report and review of the literature. J Vasc Surg 15:221–225, 1992.

Sasaki O, Ogawa H, Koike T, Koizumi T, Tanaka R. A clinicopathological study of dissecting aneurysm of the intracranial vertebral artery. J Neurosurg 75:874–882, 1991.

Schievink WI, Mokri B, Piepgras DG. Angiographic frequency of saccular intracranial aneurysms in patients with spontaneous cervical artery dissection. J Neurosurg 76:62–66, 1992.

Slavin RE, Cafferty L, Cartwright J Jr. Segmental mediolytic arteritis. A clinicopathologic and ultrastructural study of two cases. Am J Surg Pathol 13:558–568, 1989.

Vignati PV, Welch JP, Ellison L, Cohen JL. Acute mesenteric ischemia caused by isolated superior mesenteric artery dissection. J Vasc Surg 16:109–112, 1992.

Witte JT, Hasson JE, Harms BA, Corrigan TE, Love RB, Fatal gastric artery dissection and rupture occurring as a paraesophageal mass: a case report and literature review. Surgery 107:590–594, 1990.

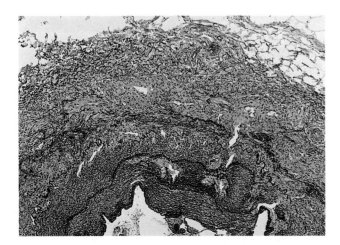

Figure 22–1. Arterial dysplasia, elastic van Gieson's stain. There were multiple aneurysms in the arteries of the lower extremities in a young man. The section demonstrates irregular, haphazard layers of the arterial wall.

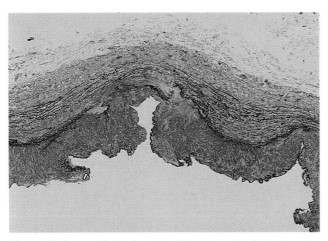

Figure 22–2. Arterial dysplasia, medial type. A longitudinal section shows the renal artery in a young woman with hypertension.

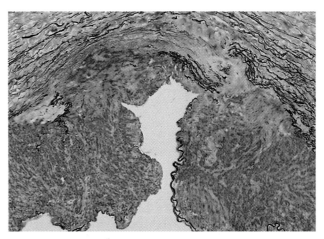

Figure 22–3. Arterial dysplasia, medial type. A higher magnification of Figure 22–2 demonstrates a gap in the arterial media. A succession of such defects results in the string-of-beads appearance on angiogram.

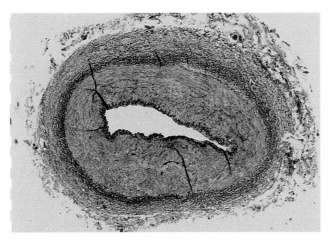

Figure 22–4. Arterial dysplasia, medial type. A section of renal artery demonstrates marked thickening of the medial wall.

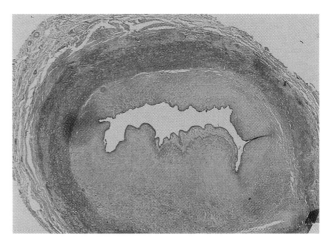

Figure 22–5. Arterial dysplasia, intimal type. The medial wall is of normal thickness; there is marked fibrointimal proliferation. In contrast to atherosclerosis, foam cells, cholesterol clefts, and calcification are absent.

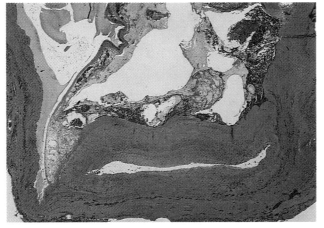

Figure 22–6. Adventitial cystic disease, popliteal artery. Note the large cystic area adjacent to the arterial adventitia; the cyst had caused compression of the lumen and symptoms of claudication in a 47-year-old woman.

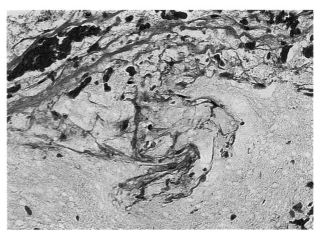

Figure 22–7. Adventitial cystic disease, popliteal artery. A higher magnification of Figure 22–6 demonstrates mucoid material with occasional spindled cells.

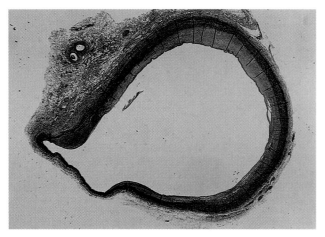

Figure 22–8. Carotid aneurysm, Movat pentachrome stain. The patient was a young woman with a palpable bruit in the neck. The section demonstrates the carotid artery, which was partially excised. There is focal thinning and aneurysm formation of the arterial wall.

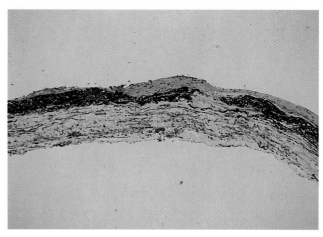

Figure 22–9. Carotid aneurysm, Movat pentachrome stain. There is nearly complete absence of media in the thinned area seen in Figure 22–8, suggesting arterial medial dysplasia.

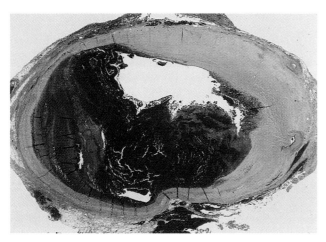

Figure 22–10. Traumatic pseudoaneurysm, Movat pentachrome stain. The patient was a young man with a history of head trauma and pulsatile mass over the temporal artery. The illustration demonstrates a massively dilated structure lined by fibrous tissue (pseudoaneurysm). The arterial lumen is barely visible at the right side of the photograph.

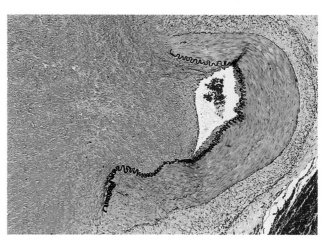

Figure 22–11. Traumatic pseudoaneurysm, Movat pentachrome stain. A higher magnification of Figure 22–10 demonstrates sharp transition between normal artery and aneurysm.

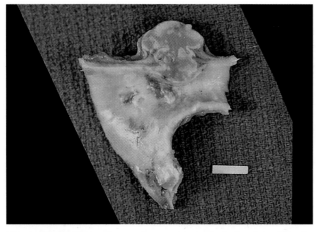

Figure 22–12. Traumatic pseudoaneurysm, innominate artery. Note the focal outpouching of the arterial wall with organized thrombus. The aneurysm was discovered incidentally at autopsy; the patient had a remote history of vehicular trauma.

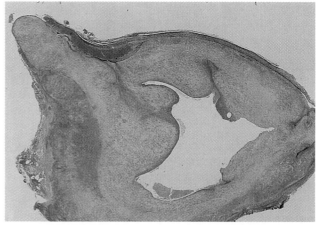

Figure 22–13. Ulnar artery aneurysm, Movat pentachrome stain. This photograph illustrates a dilated, thick-walled artery from a young boy with a pulsatile mass in the arm.

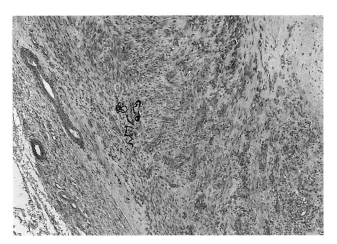

Figure 22–14. Ulnar artery aneurysm. A higher magnification of the vessel wall shown in Figure 22–13 demonstrates destruction of the elastic laminae and replacement by granulation tissue. These features suggest a healed arteritis; in the pediatric age range, healed Kawasaki disease is the most likely diagnosis.

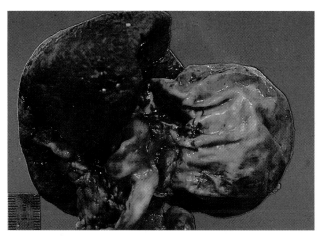

Figure 22–15. Splenic artery aneurysm. The gross photograph demonstrates a massively dilated structure adjacent to the spleen. Histologic features of most splenic artery aneurysms are nonspecific, and most splenic artery aneurysms are therefore considered idiopathic, although there is an association with pregnancy. There may be secondary atherosclerotic changes that are likely not causatory.

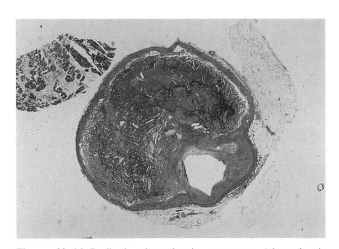

Figure 22–16. Popliteal atherosclerotic aneurysm. Atherosclerotic aneurysms affect the aorta and peripheral vessels, such as the popliteal artery shown here. Although severe atherosclerosis is present, there is likely an additional genetic predisposition to aneurysm formation.

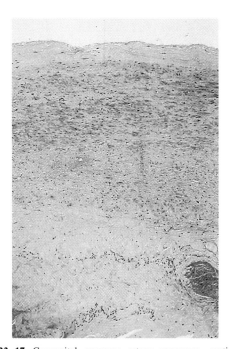

Figure 22–17. Congenital coronary artery aneurysm, cystic medial change, Movat pentachrome stain. The patient was a 45-year-old man with palpitations and angiographically detected massive aneurysms of the left anterior descending and left circumflex coronary arteries. The aneurysms were surgically resected. The wall of the vessel shows lack of inflammation, loss of elastic lamellae, and medial changes that are discernible as bluish areas.

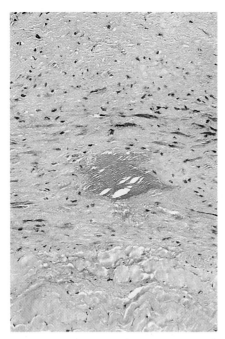

Figure 22–18. Coronary artery aneurysm, cystic medial change, Movat pentachrome stain. A higher magnification of Figure 22–17 shows the proteoglycan deposits in the media and loss of elastic lamellae.

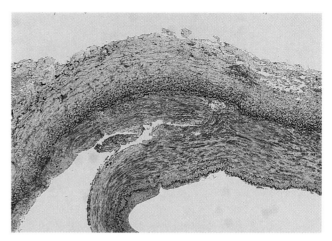

Figure 22–19. Spontaneous dissection, renal artery. Note the cleft within the outer portion of the media. The cause of the dissection in this case was not obvious, although disorganization in the medial layer suggested dysplasia.

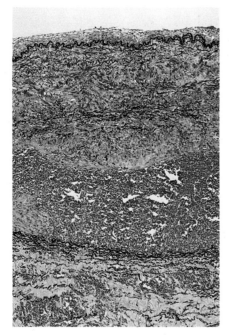

Figure 22–20. Spontaneous dissection, renal artery. A higher magnification of the artery illustrated in Figure 22–19 from a different field demonstrates blood between medial layers.

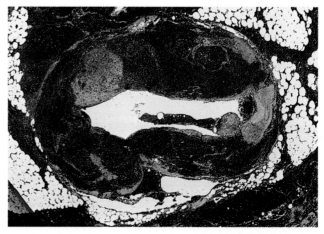

Figure 22–21. Spontaneous dissection, mesenteric artery. Note the large accumulation of blood between the adventitia and media of the vessel and focal replacement of the vessel wall with blood. This pattern of dissection is suggestive of so-called segmental arteriolytic mediolysis.

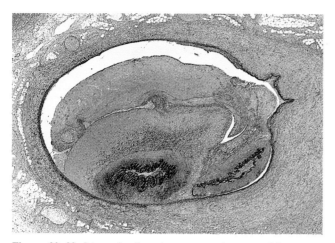

Figure 22–22. Iatrogenic dissection, mesenteric artery, Movat pentachrome stain. The patient suffered from abdominal angina and had recently undergone exploratory surgery for an unrelated condition. Note the huge expansion of dissected space (false lumen) with compression of true lumen (two small cavities).

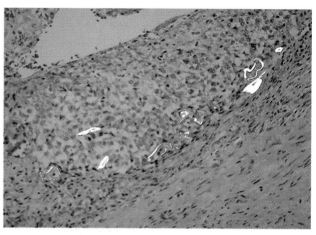

Figure 22–23. Iatrogenic dissection, mesenteric artery. Note the refringent material within the dissected area in a higher magnification of Figure 22–22, viewed with polarized light.

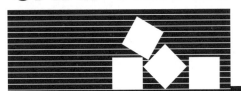

CHAPTER 23

Atherosclerosis

MORPHOLOGIC CHARACTERISTICS OF NATIVE ATHEROSCLEROSIS

Fatty Streak

- Earliest lesion of atherosclerosis
- Flat or slightly raised yellow intimal lesion
- Intimal foam cells and extracellular lipids, mainly cholesterol and its esters

Fibrous Plaque

- Proliferative lesion
- Amorphous central lipid core of acellular debris (pultaceous debris), cholesterol and its esters, and foam cells
- Fibrous cap of smooth muscle cells in collagen and proteoglycan matrix, surrounding central lipid core

Complicated Plaque

- Calcification
- Hemorrhage into plaque
- Ulceration and/or fissure of fibrous cap
- Plaque rupture
- Luminal thrombosis

CLINICOPATHOLOGIC CORRELATES

Stable Angina

- Sixty percent of patients have fibrous plaque with lipid core.
- Forty percent of patients have pure fibrous plaque.
- Lumen is concentric (28%) or eccentric (72%); hemorrhage into plaque may be present.
- Plaque ulceration and thrombosis are generally absent, but recanalized thrombi are common.

Unstable Angina

- Plaques are usually complicated (64% hemorrhage into plaque, 36% plaque rupture, 29% thrombus).

- Most plaques are eccentric.
- Organized thrombi are nearly always present.

Acute Myocardial Infarction

- Acute thrombus is almost always present.
- There is underlying plaque hemorrhage, fissure, or ulceration in 90% of cases.

PATHOLOGY OF CORONARY ATHERECTOMY

Percutaneous directional atherectomy uses a transluminal approach to remove strips of atherosclerotic plaque and thrombus from stenotic vessels.

De Novo Lesions

- In previously noninstrumented coronary arteries, plaque morphology is that of native atherosclerosis.

Restenosis Lesions

- Approximately 40% of coronary artery lesions dilated by balloon angioplasty or atherectomy become reoccluded (restenosis lesion).
- Restenosis results from the proliferation and migration of smooth muscle cells within a proteoglycan matrix.
- Smooth muscle cells change their phenotypic expression from synthetic, in early lesions, to contractile smooth muscle cells in late lesions of restenosis.
- Synthetic smooth muscle cells are generally polyhedral, muscle-specific actin-positive, smooth muscle actin-negative, and rich in endoplasmic reticulum.
- Contractile smooth muscle cells are more spindled, smooth muscle actin–positive, and aligned parallel to the lumen.

Pathologic Reporting of Atherectomy Specimens

- The following items should be noted in the pathologic reporting of atherectomy specimens:

- Arterial media, as identified by elastic stains (media is present in 60% of cases)
- Adventitia, present in 30% of cases
- Intimal hyperplasia (smooth muscle proliferation in proteoglycan matrix), present in 42% of de novo lesions and 91% of restenosis lesions
- Acute (fibrin/platelet–rich) or organized thrombi
- Plaque hemorrhage and inflammation
- Foam cells, chronic inflammation, cholesterol clefts, and calcium
- Active lesions, defined as thrombus, hemorrhage, and abundant and disorganized smooth muscle cells in a loose connective tissue proteoglycan matrix

Clinical Correlates, Atherectomy Reporting

- There is no adverse clinical outcome with recovery of media or adventitia on restenosis; recovery of adventitia is associated with a higher incidence of pseudoaneurysm formation (ectasia) by angiography in approximately 13% of cases.
- Thrombi and foam cells are more commonly seen in saphenous vein graft atherectomy.
- Mural thrombi and plaque hemorrhage are more common in unstable angina than in stable angina (22% vs 2%).
- Active lesions are more common in unstable angina (56%) or restenosis (50%) patients than in patients with stable angina (<5%).
- Some studies have reported that the rate of smooth muscle cell proliferation, determined by cell proliferation studies (e.g., proliferative cell nuclear antigen [PCNA] immunostaining), is higher in restenosis lesions than in de novo lesions.
- The presence of transforming growth factor-β messenger RNA in atherectomy specimens has been correlated with a higher restenosis rate.

References

DiSciascio G, Cowley MJ, Goudreau E, Vetrovec GW, Johnson DE. Histopathologic correlates of unstable ischemic syndromes in patients undergoing directional coronary atherectomy: in vivo evidence of thrombosis, ulceration, and inflammation. Am Heart J 128:419–426, 1994.

Escaned J, van Suylen RJ, MacLeod DC, et al. Histologic characteristics of tissue excised during directional coronary atherectomy in stable and unstable angina pectoris. Am J Cardiol 71:1442–1447, 1993.

Flugelman MY, Virmani R, Correa R, et al. Smooth muscle cell abundance and fibroblast growth factors in coronary lesions of patients with non-fatal unstable angina: a clue to the mechanism of transformation from stable to the unstable clinical state. Circulation 88:2493–2500, 1993.

Garratt KN, Edwards WD, Kaufmann UP, Vlietstra RE, Holmes DR Jr. Differential histopathology of primary atherosclerotic and saphenous vein bypass grafts: analysis of tissue obtained from 73 patients by directional atherectomy. J Am Coll Cardiol 17:442–448, 1991.

Hofling B, Welsch U, Heimerl J, Gonschior P, Bauriedel G. Analysis of atherectomy specimens. Am J Cardiol 72:96E–107E, 1993.

Nobuyoshi M, Kimura T, Ohishi H, et al. Restenosis after percutaneous transluminal coronary angioplasty. Pathologic observations in 20 patients. J Am Coll Cardiol 17:433–439, 1991.

Ueda M, Becker AE, Tsukada T, Numano F, Fujimoto T. Fibrocellular tissue response after percutaneous transluminal coronary angioplasty. An immunocytochemical analysis of the cellular composition. Circulation 83:1327–1332, 1991.

Umans VA, Robert A, Foley D, et al. Clinical, histologic and quantitative angiographic predictors of restenosis after directional coronary atherectomy: a multivariate analysis of the renarrowing process and late outcome. J Am Coll Cardiol 23:49–58, 1994.

Virmani R, Farb A, Burke AP. Coronary angioplasty from the perspective of atherosclerotic plaque; Morphologic predictors of immediate success and restenosis. Am Heart J 127:163–179, 1994.

Waller BF, Johnson DE, Schnitt SJ, Pinkerton CA, Simpson JB, Baim DS. Histologic analysis of directional coronary atherectomy samples. A review of findings and their clinical relevance. Am J Cardiol 72:80E–87E, 1993.

PERIPHERAL ATHERECTOMY

Clinical Findings

- Atherectomy performed for peripheral occlusive disease results in angiographic success in 87% of cases.
- Dissection is the most common complication and occurs in 2.2% of treated lesions.

De Novo Lesions

- Primary (de novo) stenoses are composed of atherosclerotic plaque (88%), fibrous intimal thickening overlying internal elastic laminae (9%), or organizing thrombus (3%).
- Atherosclerotic plaques have variable morphology: 80% are complex, 60% show thrombus formation, 50% show calcification, 40% show hemorrhage, and 30% show ulceration.

Restenosis Lesions

- Restenosis may complicate peripheral atherectomy or angioplasty, similar to coronary artery instrumentation.
- Thrombus is present in 30% of postangioplasty restenoses and in 10% of postatherectomy restenoses.
- There is hyperplasia in 90% of postangioplasty restenoses and in 70% of postatherectomy restenoses.
- In approximately 25% of cases, only atherosclerotic plaque is present.

Reference

Johnson DE, Hinohara T, Selmon MR, Braden LJ, Simpson JB. Primary peripheral arterial stenoses and restenoses excised by transluminal atherectomy: a histopathologic study. J Am Coll Cardiol 15:419–425, 1990.

CORONARY ENDARTERECTOMY

Coronary endarterectomy is the intraoperative removal of atherosclerotic plaque, usually at the time of bypass graft surgery, enabling diffusely diseased, inoperable arteries to be grafted.

Clinical Findings

- The mortality rate is higher in patients with left coronary endarterectomy compared with those with right coronary endarterectomy.
- Perioperative myocardial infarction is highest in pa-

tients undergoing multiple endarterectomies (13%) versus those requiring single endarterectomy (7%) or no endarterectomy (6%).

■ Early graft patency rates are similar in patients with or without endarterectomy (90%).

■ Late graft patency (>1 year) is higher in vessels without endarterectomy (76%) than in those requiring endarterectomy (71%).

■ Five-year survival is reduced in patients requiring endarterectomy compared with those requiring bypass surgery only.

Pathologic Findings

■ Pathologic findings of endarterectomy specimens vary according to clinical syndrome.

■ The presence of media, which is generally avoided in surgical endarterectomy, should be reported.

■ Endarterectomy sites heal by fibrin platelet mural thrombus, which organizes, becomes replaced by fibrointimal proliferation of smooth muscle cells in a proteoglycan matrix, and eventually is replaced by fibrosis.

Reference

Walley VM, Byard RW, Kean WJ. A study of the sequential morphologic changes after manual coronary endarterectomy. J Thorac Cardiovasc Surg 102:890–894, 1991.

CAROTID ENDARTERECTOMY

Clinical Background

■ Correlation between carotid artery disease and stroke was made as early as 1856 by Savory.

■ Cerebral emboli originating from carotid artery plaques were first identified as a cause of stroke by Hiari in 1905.

■ Symptomatic carotid artery disease is usually located at the carotid sinus and at the origin of the internal carotid artery.

Primary Carotid Endarterectomy

■ Primary carotid endarterectomy is performed in symptomatic patients (history of transient ischemic attacks) and in asymptomatic patients with severe stenosis.

■ The surgeon attempts to remove plaque in a single piece, but occasionally, fragmented plaque is obtained.

■ Plaque should be cross-sectioned at 1- to 2-mm intervals to determine the presence of calcification, hemor-

rhage into plaque, plaque rupture, ulceration, and thrombosis.

■ The incidence of ulceration is 46%, thrombosis 9%, necrotic atheroma 12%, and smooth intimal surface 34%.

Clinical Correlates

■ Asymptomatic patients with more than 75% stenosis and morphologically soft plaques are at the greatest risk of transient ischemic attack or stroke.

■ Asymptomatic patients with less than 75% stenosis and calcified plaques are at the lowest risk of transient ischemic attacks or stroke.

■ The presence of plaque hemorrhage is more frequent in symptomatic (35%) than in asymptomatic (20%) patients.

■ Plaque hemorrhage shows a significant correlation with severity of plaque stenosis.

Recurrent Carotid Disease

■ Plaque morphology of recurrent carotid disease is dependent on the time interval between primary and reoperative endarterectomy.

■ Early recurrent lesions (<36 months) have a significantly greater content of smooth muscle cells in a proteoglycan matrix than late recurrent lesions (>36 months).

■ Late recurrent lesions have the features of disorganized atherosclerosis (foam cells, cholesterol clefts, dense collagen, calcification) with pultaceous debris without a fibrous cap.

■ The incidence of intralesional thrombus and surface thrombi is high in both early (100%) and late (75%) recurrences.

■ Neovascularization is more prominent in late lesions than in early recurrent lesions.

References

Bornstein NM, Krajewski A, Lewis AJ, Norris JW. Clinical significance of carotid plaque hemorrhage. Arch Neurol 47:958–959, 1990.

Clagett GP, Robinowitz M, Youkey JR, et al. Morphogenesis and clinicopathologic characteristics of recurrent carotid disease. J Vasc Surg 3:10–23, 1986.

Imparato AM, Riles TS, Mintzer R, Baumann FG. The importance of hemorrhage in the relationship between gross morphologic characteristics and cerebral symptoms in 376 carotid artery plaques. Ann Surg 197:195–203, 1983.

Lusby RJ, Ferrell LD, Ehrenfeld WK, Stoney RJ, Wylie EJ. Carotid plaque hemorrhage. Its role in the production of cerebral ischemia. Arch Surg 117:1479–1487, 1982.

O'Holleran LW, Kennelly MM, McClurken M, Johnson JM. Natural history of asymptomatic carotid plaque. Five year follow-up study. Am J Surg 154:659–662, 1987.

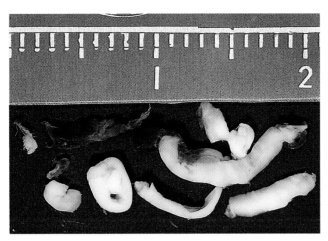

Figure 23–1. Atherectomy specimen, gross appearance. Note the multiple small pieces of plaque; the specimen was removed from the femoral artery in a patient with claudication.

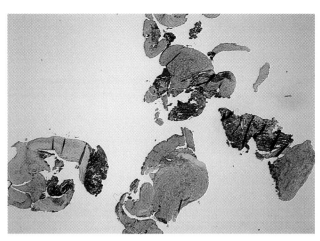

Figure 23–2. Coronary atherectomy, Movat pentachrome stain. Note the multiple pieces of plaque consisting of fibrous cap (yellow), fibrointimal proliferation (green), and necrotic core and fibrin thrombus (dark).

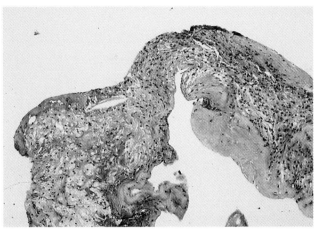

Figure 23–3. Atherectomy, foam cell–rich lesion, Movat pentachrome stain. There are foam cells and inflammatory cells within a fibrous cap.

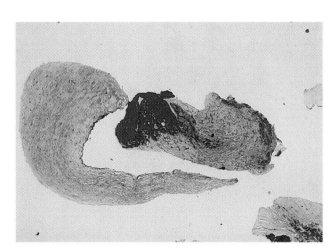

Figure 23–4. Atherectomy thrombus. This specimen was removed from a patient with unstable angina. Note the presence of organizing thrombus and underlying smooth muscle cell–rich plaque.

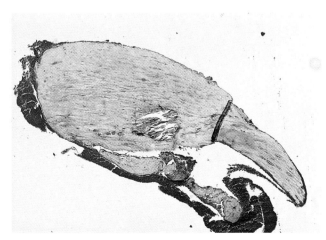

Figure 23–5. Atherectomy, calcification, Movat pentachrome stain. There is a small focus of calcification in the center of this fibrous plaque. Extensive calcification is infrequently seen in coronary atherectomy specimens.

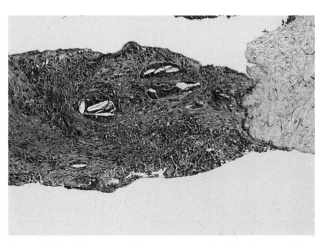

Figure 23–6. Atherectomy, inflammatory reaction. Note the chronic inflammation with cholesterol clefts and surrounding giant cells. This degree of inflammation is rarely seen in atherosclerotic disease.

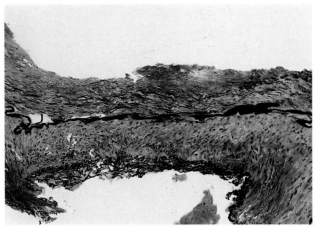

Figure 23–7. Atherectomy with excision of media and adventitia, Movat pentachrome stain. Internal and external elastic laminae and fibrous adventitia (upper half) are highlighted.

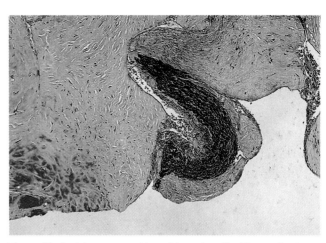

Figure 23–8. Atherectomy with excision of media. The proximal portion of the left main coronary artery is an elastic artery; therefore, media obtained at atherectomy of the left main coronary artery may demonstrate layers of elastic laminae, without discrete internal and external elastic laminae.

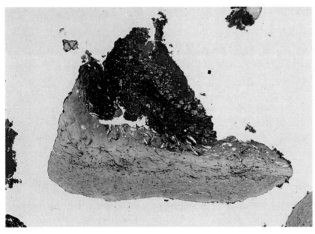

Figure 23–9. Atherectomy, saphenous vein graft. There is hemorrhagic plaque with scattered foam cells, cholesterol clefts, and an underlying thin layer of fibrous tissue.

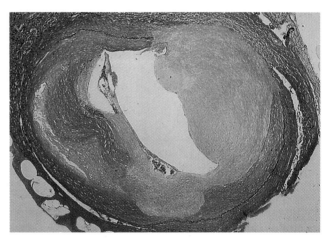

Figure 23–10. Restenosis lesion, elastic van Gieson's stain. Coronary artery section from a patient who had undergone atherectomy 3 months prior to death. Note the abrupt replacement of the coronary wall by fibrointimal proliferative tissue in areas where a previous atherectomy procedure had been performed. (Courtesy of Dr. William D. Edwards.)

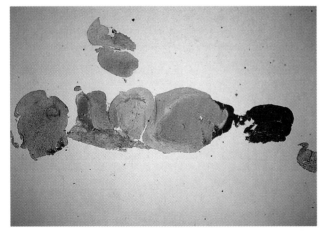

Figure 23–11. Atherectomy, restenosis lesion, Movat pentachrome stain. The patient had undergone balloon angioplasty 6 months earlier and developed restenosis at the same site. Note the alternating fibrous plaque with areas rich in proteoglycan matrix (green).

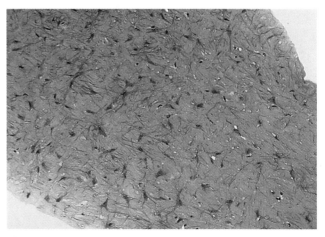

Figure 23–12. Atherectomy, restenosis lesion, Movat pentachrome stain. A higher magnification of Figure 23–11 showing marked smooth muscle cell proliferation in a proteoglycan matrix, typical of restenosis.

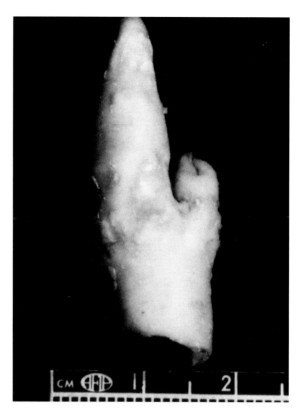

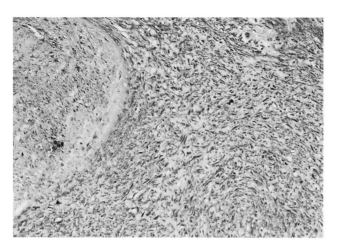

Figure 23–13. Atherectomy, restenosis lesion *(right of field)*. Immunohistochemical stain for smooth muscle actin demonstrates a large number of immunoreactive cells.

Figure 23–14. Carotid endarterectomy. External view of carotid plaque.

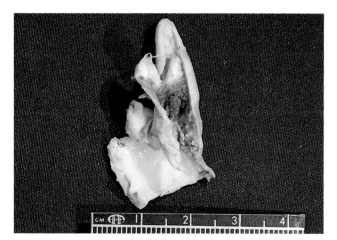

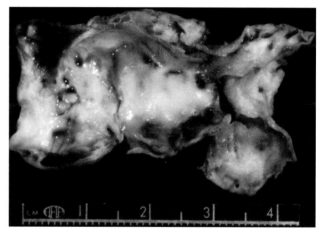

Figure 23–15. Carotid endarterectomy. The lumen has been opened and a thrombus is identified.

Figure 23–16. Carotid endarterectomy. The intima is exposed. Note the focal hemorrhage *(dark areas)* within the plaque.

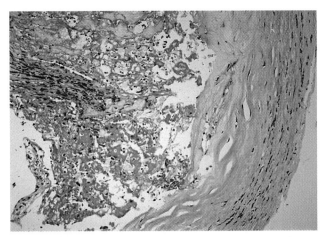

Figure 23–17. Carotid endarterectomy. Note the large necrotic core with overlying fibrous plaque. The necrotic core is rich in foam cells.

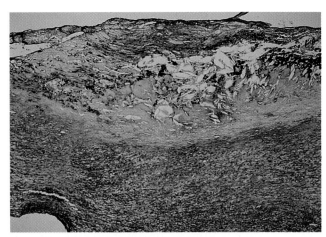

Figure 23–18. Carotid endarterectomy, recurrent stenosis. The patient had undergone carotid endarterectomy 40 months earlier. Note an underlying plaque rich in smooth muscle cells and an overlying atherosclerotic necrotic core with cholesterol clefts and hemorrhage. The fibrous cap is extremely thin and friable.

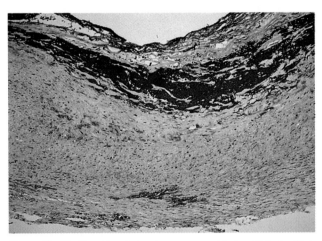

Figure 23–19. Carotid endarterectomy, recurrent lesion. Note the fibrin thrombus within the wall of the plaque. This plaque was removed from a patient with previous endarterectomy and late recurrence.

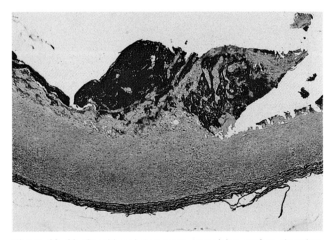

Figure 23–20. Carotid endarterectomy, organizing surface thrombus. The surface is covered with thrombus, which is attached to a fibrointimal lesion. Carotid endarterectomy had been performed 30 months earlier.

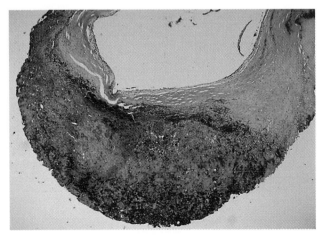

Figure 23–21. Carotid endarterectomy, organizing thrombus. Note the organizing thrombus in a recurrent carotid atherosclerotic plaque. The lesion is rich in granulation tissue.

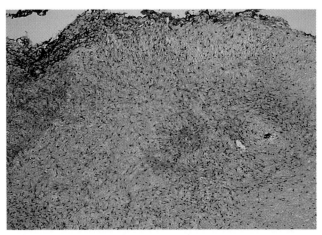

Figure 23–22. Carotid endarterectomy, early recurrent lesion. Note the fibrointimal lesion rich in smooth muscle cells in a proteoglycan matrix. There is some neovascularization. There is a portion of medial wall in the upper left corner of the illustration.

CHAPTER 24

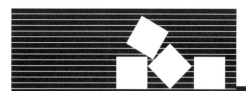

Metabolic, Thrombotic, and Embolic Diseases

METABOLIC DISEASES OF BLOOD VESSELS

- Metabolic diseases involving blood vessels are rarely encountered by the surgical pathologist.
- Acquired diseases are more common than primary, congenital metabolic diseases of vessels.
- The criteria for what defines a metabolic disease are sometimes vague and there is no standard classification.
- For a detailed pathologic review that discusses biochemical defects and pathways, refer to *The pathology of blood vessels in metabolic disorders* by R. Subramanian, R. Virmani, and V. Ferrans in *Vascular Pathology,* W.E. Stehbens and J.T. Lie (eds), London, Chapman & Hall Medical, 1995, pp 129–174.

Classification of Selected Metabolic Diseases Affecting Blood Vessels

Diseases of Carbohydrate Metabolism

- Mucopolysaccharidoses
  - Type I (Hurler-Scheie)
- Mucolipidoses
- Hyperoxalurias
  - Primary oxalurias
  - Secondary oxalosis
  - Diabetes mellitus

Diseases of Lipid Metabolism

- Lysosomal storage diseases
- Fabry's disease
- Farber disease
- Hyperlipoproteinemias/atherosclerosis

Diseases of Amino Acid Metabolism

- Ochronosis
- Homocystinuria

Diseases of Connective Tissue Synthesis

- Marfan syndrome
- Cutis laxa
- Pseudoxanthoma elasticum
- Ehlers-Danlos syndrome

Diseases of Carbohydrate Metabolism

- Mucopolysaccharidoses may result in thickened arteries, with vacuolated cells.
- The most common mucopolysaccharidosis to involve vessels is type I (Hurler-Scheie). Histologic findings include concentric fibrous plaques and occasional Hurler cells (connective tissue cells filled with membrane-bound vacuoles).
- Mucolipidoses may occasionally result in arterial thickening.
- Hyperoxalurias either are of the rare primary types or are secondary to renal failure, oxalic ingestion, xylitol feeding, small bowel resections, or pyridoxine deficiency.
- Histologic findings in hyperoxalurias include oxalate crystals or calcification of muscular arteries and, less often, elastic arteries.
- Oxalate crystals are bluish-gray or yellow-brown with hematoxylin and eosin stain and are birefringent with polarized light.
- Diabetes mellitus causes a microangiopathy with concentric hyaline thickening and capillary basement membrane thickening of arterioles of the retina, kidney, and peripheral nerves.

Diseases of Lipid Metabolism

- Fabry's disease may result in ectasia of small blood vessels, cystic medial necrosis of the aorta, and smooth muscle vacuolization of media of pulmonary arteries and other arteries.
- An ultrastructural finding in Fabry's disease is the presence of myelin figures with alternating light and dark bands.

■ Fabry's disease may result in yellow plaques in the pulmonary arteries, coronary arteries, and aorta.

■ Hyperlipoproteinemias of many types may result in accelerated atherosclerosis.

Diseases of Amino Acid Metabolism

■ Ochronosis results in chronic alkaptonuria and is secondary to a deficiency of homogentisic acid oxidase.

■ Vascular lesions of ochronosis include brown-black pigment in heart valves, endocardium, aortae, coronary arteries, muscular arteries, veins, and capillaries.

■ Cardiovascular symptoms in ochronosis may result from the deposition of pigment and calcification in the aortic valve, resulting in aortic stenosis.

■ Homocystinuria may result in peripheral arterial occlusions, premature atherosclerosis, and venous thromboses.

■ Homocystinuria results histologically in fragmentation of elastic fibers, especially internal elastic laminae, fibromuscular intimal thickening, medial fibrosis, and luminal narrowing.

Diseases of Connective Tissue Synthesis

Marfan Syndrome

■ Marfan syndrome is an autosomal dominant disease resulting from a deficiency of the microfibril component of elastic fibers, specifically fibrillin-1, related to mutations of the fibrillin gene (located on chromosome 15).

■ Cardiovascular pathology of Marfan syndrome is manifest in four ways:

1. Fusiform ascending aortic aneurysms (39%) (see Chap 15)
2. Aortic dissections (36%) (see Chap 15)
3. Mitral regurgitation without other cardiovascular involvement (21%)
4. Miscellaneous cardiovascular pathology (4%)

■ The clinical syndrome exhibits considerable overlap with annuloaortic ectasia (see Chap 15), mitral valve prolapse syndrome, and familial dissecting aortic aneurysms.

■ The term "MASS" phenotype, from *M*itral valve, *A*ortic, *S*keletal, and *S*kin involvement, has been used for patients who have some, but not all, features of Marfan syndrome.

■ The histologic hallmark of Marfan syndrome is aortic medial degeneration (cystic medial change); this change is quantitative, rather than qualitative, and is seen in other degenerative conditions.

Cutis Laxa

■ Cutis laxa may be acquired or congenital.

■ Cutis laxa results grossly in loose skin and dilatation of the ascending and thoracic aortae.

■ Cutis laxa results histologically in a decrease in elastic fibers; it may resemble Marfan syndrome.

Pseudoxanthoma Elasticum

■ Pseudoxanthoma elasticum results in premature atherosclerosis.

■ Pseudoxanthoma elasticum histologically is typified by the degeneration and calcification of elastic fibers in the endocardium and arterial circulation (especially femoral, radial, and ulnar arteries); in contrast to cutis laxa or Marfan syndrome, elastic fibers are large and fragmented.

■ Aneurysms of the ascending aorta may occur.

■ A cardiomyopathy (restrictive or dilated) may rarely occur (see Chap 2).

Ehlers-Danlos Syndrome

■ Ehlers-Danlos syndrome embraces at least 12 related syndromes, the histopathologic changes of which are not well documented.

■ Gross pathologic changes in Ehlers-Danlos syndrome include dissection of aortae, peripheral or coronary artery aneurysms, tortuous arteries, multiple arterial dissections, and sinus of Valsalva aneurysms, most commonly seen in Ehlers-Danlos type IV (deficiency of type III collagen).

Osteogenesis Imperfecta

■ Osteogenesis imperfecta is a generalized disorder of connective tissue, possibly caused by a defect in alpha-1 and alpha-2 type collagen.

■ Cardiovascular complications are unusual, but nonprogressive aortic root dilatation has been observed in a few patients, with a familial pattern.

References

Haust MD. Arterial involvement in genetic diseases. Am J Cardiovasc Pathol 1:231–285, 1987.

Subramanian R, Virmani R, Ferrans V. The pathology of blood vessels in metabolic disorders. In Stehbens WE, Lie JT (eds). *Vascular Pathology.* London, Chapman & Hall Medical, 1995.

THROMBOTIC DISEASE OF BLOOD VESSELS

Hypercoagulable States

■ Antiphospholipid syndrome
■ Protein C deficiency
■ Protein S deficiency
■ Decreased factor XII
■ Antithrombin III deficiency
■ Heparin-induced thrombopathy
■ Myeloproliferative syndromes
■ Cancer

Deep Venous Thrombosis

Clinical Findings

■ Clinical findings vary by site of vessel.

■ Clinical presentations include extremity pain, swelling, and tenderness, and intestinal pain if there is mesenteric thrombosis.

■ Pulmonary embolism is the most important complication of deep venous thrombosis of the lower extremities.

■ Predisposing factors include hypercoagulable states, postoperative state, sedentary lifestyle, increased systemic venous pressure, and malignancy. (Thrombosis may precede the clinical detection of malignancy.)

Pathologic Findings

- Acute and organizing thrombi occur in veins of affected vessels.

Superficial Thrombophlebitis

- Superficial thrombophlebitis may be classified as migratory, nonmigratory (often associated with varicosity), Mondor's disease (limited to chest wall), and traumatic (associated with intravenous lines).
- Risk factors for superficial thrombophlebitis include hypercoagulable state, malignancy, Behçet's disease, inflammatory bowel disease, secondary syphilis, and Buerger's disease. Many cases are idiopathic.
- Histologically, there are organizing thrombi in superficial veins.

Arterial Thrombosis

- Arterial thrombosis may involve virtually any artery, including the aorta.
- Risk factors in normal arteries include hypercoagulable states, malignancy, polycythemia vera, estrogen use, and heparin-induced thrombopathy.
- Pathologic vascular conditions predisposing the patient to arterial thrombosis include atherosclerosis, arterial dysplasia, and vasculitis (Behçet's disease, Buerger's disease, giant cell arteritis).

References

Lesher JL Jr. Superficial migratory thrombophlebitis. Cutis 177:80, 1991.
Nachman RL, Silverstein R. Hypercoagulable states. Ann Intern Med 119:819–827, 1993.
Rosove MH, Brewer PM. Antiphospholipid thrombosis: clinical course after the first thrombotic event in 70 patients. Ann Intern Med 117:303–308, 1992.
Shibata S, Harpel PC, Gharavi A, Rand J, Fillit H. Autoantibodies to heparin from patients with antiphospholipid antibody syndrome inhibit formation of antithrombin II–thrombin complexes. Blood 83:2532–2540, 1994.
Visentin GP, Ford SE, Scott JP, Aster RH. Antibodies from patients with heparin-induced thrombocytopenia/thrombosis are specific for platelet factor 4 complexed with heparin or bound to endothelial cells. J Clin Invest 93:81–88, 1994.

EMBOLIC DISEASES

Thromboemboli

- Sources of thromboemboli to the pulmonary circulation include mural thrombi in the right atrium or ventricle, marantic vegetations of the tricuspid valve, and deep venous thrombosis.
- Thromboemboli of the systemic circulation include marantic (nonbacterial thrombotic) and infectious vegetations of the mitral or aortic valves and mural thrombi in the left ventricle or atrium.

Atheroemboli

- Atheroemboli are essentially limited to the systemic circulation.
- They may be spontaneous in patients with ulcerative aortic atherosclerosis, or they may result from catheterization, surgery, or other manipulations of the aorta.
- Symptoms result from ischemic complications.
- Atheroembolic syndrome is characterized by focal bluish discoloration of toes with intact pedal pulses and painful bilateral foot ulcers.
- Renal failure and visceral infarction may occur.
- Clinically, the diagnosis may be suspected by elevated erythrocyte sedimentation rate, transient amaurosis fugax, cholesterol emboli in the ocular fundi, angiographic demonstration of irregular aortic plaques, and acral skin ulcers.
- Histopathologic diagnosis may be made on the basis of surgically excised intestine, mucosal biopsy, skin biopsy, or renal biopsy.
- Histologic findings are the presence of cholesterol clefts in small arteries.
- Cholesterol clefts are surrounded by fibrin, foreign body giant cells, and organizing thrombus.

Tumor Emboli

- Tumor emboli of the systemic arterial circulation are usually papillary fibroelastoma or cardiac myxoma (see Chap. 11); more rarely, they are aortic intimal sarcomas.
- Tumor emboli of the pulmonary circulation are usually from right-sided atrial myxomas or are from diverse sites, including carcinomas, often adenocarcinomas, or choriocarcinoma.

Nontumorous Tissue Emboli

- Nontumorous tissue emboli are generally fat emboli and are present in the pulmonary arterial circulation (see Chap. 17).

Foreign Body Emboli

- Foreign body emboli are most often present in the pulmonary circulation, but they may enter the systemic circulation in cases of patent foramen ovale and pulmonary hypertension.
- They may be a result of instrumentation, cardiopulmonary bypass, or intravenous drug abuse.
- Histologically, birefringent particles are found in arterioles with a foreign body reaction.
- Materials in emboli of intravenous drug addicts include

  - Polyethyleneglycol
  - Tragacanth
  - Magnesium stearate
  - Magnesium trisilicate (talc)
  - Cotton fibers
  - Cornstarch

- Vegetable emboli may occur in systemic arteries in patients with aortoesophageal fistulas.

References

Kaufman JL, Stark K, Brolin RE. Disseminated atheroembolism from extensive degenerative atherosclerosis of the aorta. Surgery 102:63–70, 1987.
McGowan JA, Greenberg A. Cholesterol atheroembolic renal disease. Report of 3 cases with emphasis on diagnosis by skin biopsy and extended survival. Am J Nephrol 6:135–139, 1986.
O'Brian DS, Jeffers M, Kay EW, Hourihane DO. Bleeding due to colorectal atheroembolism. Diagnosis by biopsy of adenomatous polyps or of ischemic ulcer. Am J Surg Pathol 15:1078–1082, 1991.

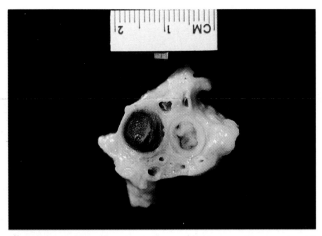

Figure 24–1. Venous and arterial thrombosis. An elderly man with metastatic colonic adenocarcinoma developed gangrene of the lower extremities. A section of popliteal artery and vein demonstrates thrombotic occlusion of both vessels.

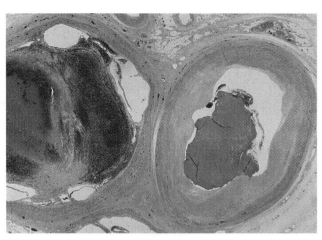

Figure 24–2. Venous and arterial thrombus. A histologic section of Figure 24–1 demonstrates organizing thrombus (note the hemorrhagic appearance in Figure 24–1) within the vein and fibrin platelet thrombus within the artery (note the creamy white appearance in Figure 24–1).

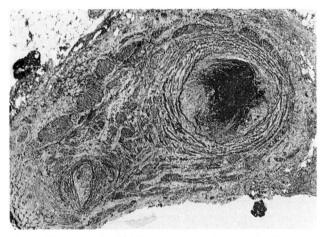

Figure 24–3. Thrombophlebitis, Movat pentachrome stain. Note organizing thrombus within the vein.

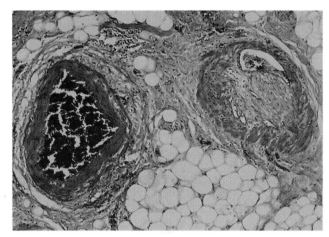

Figure 24–4. Mesenteric thrombosis. Most cases of mesenteric thrombosis are caused by venous obstruction. Note the organized eccentric thrombus within a vein; the accompanying artery is not involved.

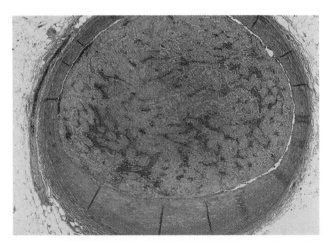

Figure 24–5. Coronary artery (left main) thrombosis, acute. The patient was a young female smoker who used birth control pills. Death occurred before a coagulation workup could be performed. Note the occlusive thrombus in the absence of atherosclerosis.

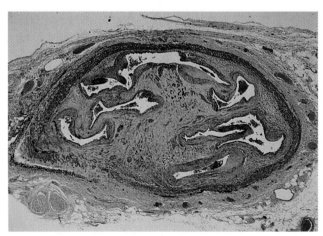

Figure 24–6. Coronary artery (left anterior descending) thrombosis, organized, Movat pentachrome stain. Recanalization of a thrombus may result in channels lined by smooth muscle cells.

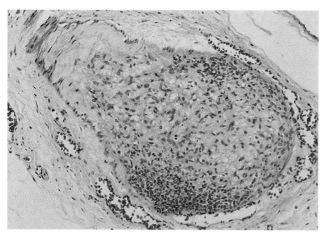

Figure 24–7. Organized thrombus, myxoid change. There may be deposition of proteoglycans within an organized thrombus, similar to restenosis lesions (see Chap. 23). Unlike in myxoma, myxoma cells are absent.

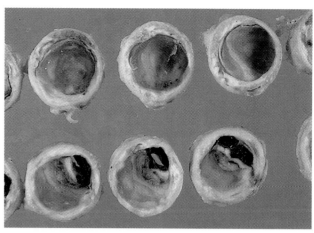

Figure 24–8. Aortic thrombosis. Thromboses in patients with hypercoagulable syndromes are not restricted to muscular arteries. The patient was a middle-aged woman who was given heparin for suspected pulmonary embolism. Thrombocytopenia with multiple arterial thrombi, including aortic thrombosis, occurred in response to antiheparin antibodies. Note the multiple sections of aorta with acute thrombosis.

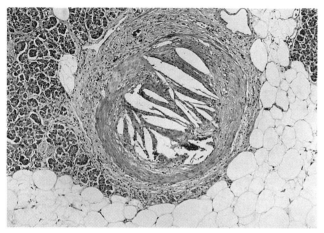

Figure 24–9. Atheroembolism. The patient was a 56-year-old man with congestive heart failure and severe peripheral vascular disease. He developed the atheroembolism syndrome after cardiac catheterization. Note the characteristic cholesterol crystals within the arterial lumen.

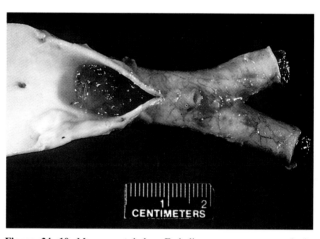

Figure 24–10. Myxoma embolus. Embolic myxoma may result in Leriche's syndrome from obstruction at the iliac bifurcation.

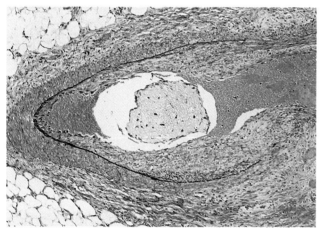

Figure 24–11. Myxoma embolus, Movat pentachrome stain. Histologically, detached fragments of myxoma, often with accompanying thrombus, are seen.

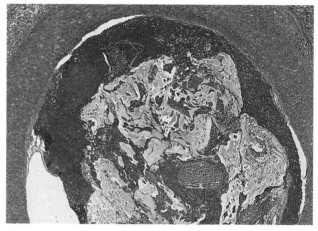

Figure 24–12. Foreign body embolus. The patient was a middle-aged man with irradiated esophageal carcinoma and presumed aortoesophageal fistula who developed ischemia of the upper extremity. Amputation revealed vegetable matter within the thrombosed lumen of the brachial artery.

CHAPTER 25

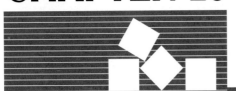

Tumors and Tumor-like Proliferations of Peripheral Blood Vessels

- The true nature of many vascular proliferations of blood vessels is unclear; it is often unknown whether many of these proliferations, especially those tumors designated "hemangiomas," are true neoplasms, hamartomas, or reactive processes.
- Lesions loosely classified as hemangiomas include capillary hemangioma, pyogenic granuloma, cavernous hemangioma, arteriovenous malformation, venous hemangioma, and intramuscular hemangioma.
- Conditions of blood vessels that are often considered reactive include intravascular fasciitis, papillary endothelial hyperplasia, and epithelioid hemangioma.
- Proliferations that are considered low-grade neoplasms are epithelioid hemangioendothelioma, spindle cell hemangioma, and Dabska tumor.
- Kaposi's sarcoma and bacillary hemangiomatosis are seen primarily in immunocompromised individuals. The former is probably a neoplasm, although an infectious cause has not been completely excluded; the latter is a reactive proliferation to a known bacterial agent.
- Malignant or high-grade neoplasms of blood vessels are generally classified as angiosarcomas.

CAPILLARY HEMANGIOMA

Capillary hemangiomas are benign vascular neoplasms composed of capillary-like vessels. Synonyms include infantile hemangioendothelioma, juvenile hemangioma, and cellular capillary hemangioma.

Clinical Findings

- Capillary hemangioma, or "strawberry" nevus, is the most frequent tumor of infancy.

- It occurs on the skin or subcutis of the head and neck.
- Kasabach-Merritt syndrome was reported initially in a patient with capillary hemangioma (platelet trapping and thrombocytopenia).
- Gradual regression and involution is the rule for infantile cutaneous hemangioma.
- Rare life-threatening or disfiguring tumors respond to selective embolization, laser treatment, and interferon alpha-2A.

Histologic Findings

- In the proliferative phase, there are lobules of endothelial cells, pericytes, and fibroblasts, and few capillary lumens. Mitotic activity is common.
- At maturation, patent lumens form at the periphery of lobules.

Differential Diagnosis

- Macular stains (nevus flammeus, port wine stains) are not proliferations but are telangiectases that, on histologic evaluation, demonstrate nearly normal skin.
- "Acquired tufted angioma," or progressive capillary hemangioma, is a rare tumor characterized by progressive skin lesions that stabilize after years. Lesions occur on the trunk and neck, and "cannonballs" of capillary hemangioma are separated by bands of collagen within the dermis. These lesions rarely regress or involute, but do not metastasize.
- "Glomeruloid hemangioma" is a multifocal vascular tumor of skin associated with the POEMS syndrome (polyneuropathy, organomegaly, endocrinopathy, monoclonal protein, skin lesions); the lobular collections of capillaries in the skin lesions occur within larger vessels, such as occurs in the renal glomerulus.

References

Chan JKC, Fletcher CDM, Hicklin GA et al. Glomeruloid hemangioma, a distinctive cutaneous lesion of multicentric Castleman's disease associated with POEMS syndrome. Am J Surg Pathol 14:1036–1046, 1990.

Padilla RS, Orkin M, Rosai J. Acquired tufted angioma (progressive capillary hemangioma), a distinctive clinicopathologic entity related to lobular capillary hemangioma. Am J Dermatopathol 9:292–300, 1987.

PYOGENIC GRANULOMA

Pyogenic granuloma is a lobular proliferation of capillary-like vessels; possibly an exuberant reactive type of granulation tissue or a lobular variant of capillary hemangioma.

Clinical Findings

- Involved tissues include mucosa, skin, subcutaneous tissue, or blood vessels.
- The most common sites of involvement are gingiva, fingers, lips, face, and tongue.
- In persons younger than 18 years of age, there is a male predilection.
- In persons aged 19 to 40 years, there is a female predilection, with tumors occurring in the oral and nasal mucosa.
- There is a history of trauma in one third of cases.
- There is occasional local recurrence.
- Tumors occur in 1% of women in their first trimester of pregnancy, usually in the oral mucosa.

Gross Pathologic Findings

- Generally solitary
- Sessile, polypoid, or pedunculated
- Rapid onset growth
- Lesions as large as to 2 to 3 cm

Histologic Findings

- Well-marginated
- Capillary-sized vessels
- Multilobular
- Mitotic activity common

Differential Diagnosis

- Bacillary angiomatosis
- Angiosarcoma
- Nodular Kaposi's sarcoma

Reference

Mills SE, Cooper PH, Fechner RE. Lobular capillary hemangioma: the underlying lesion of pyogenic granuloma: a study of 73 cases from the oral and nasal mucous membranes. Am J Surg Pathol 4:471–479, 1980.

CAVERNOUS HEMANGIOMA

Cavernous hemangiomas are benign vascular tumors composed of dilated thin-walled vessels.

Clinical Findings

- Cavernous hemangiomas occur in children and adults.
- For dermal cases, the upper half of the body is more frequently involved.
- Lesions do not regress.
- They may occur in deep soft tissues and viscera.
- They may cause Kasabach-Merritt consumptive coagulopathy syndrome.
- In the central nervous system (CNS), they are less likely to bleed than arteriovenous malformation. Feeder vessels are not shown on angiogram, and they are only 50% visible by magnetic resonance imaging. Cavernous hemangiomas are 5 to 10 times less common than arteriovenous malformations.
- Cavernous hemangiomas lack arteriovenous connections and do not predispose the patient to congestive heart failure.

Gross Pathologic Findings

- Lesions are soft, elevated, dark blue or purplish masses.

Histologic Findings

- Lobulated or marginated engorged thin-walled vessels are lined with flattened endothelium.
- Pericytes, smooth muscle cells, and fibroblasts are less conspicuous than in capillary hemangiomas.
- Overlap with capillary hemangioma is not uncommon.
- In Maffucci's syndrome, there are dyschondroplasia and hemangiomas. Extensive enchondromatosis may give rise to chondrosarcoma.
- In blue rubber bleb nevus syndrome, multiple small dome-shaped vascular lesions involve the skin; it is associated with gastrointestinal lesions and anemia.

VENOUS HEMANGIOMAS

Venous hemangiomas are deep benign vascular tumors formed of thick-walled vein-like vascular channels; they are sometimes considered a type of cavernous hemangioma, but the latter have thinner walls.

Clinical Findings

- Venous hemangiomas are rare.
- Adults are affected more frequently than children.
- Sites of occurrence include skeletal muscle, bones, mediastinum, joint spaces, hollow viscera, spinal cord, and CNS.
- Venous hemangiomas are poorly visualized by arteriography; venography is more sensitive for radiologic diagnosis.
- Venous hemangiomas may be less likely to cause hemorrhage in the CNS than cavernous hemangiomas; many classifications of CNS vascular lesions do not separate these from cavernous hemangiomas.

Histologic Features

- Blood-filled, vein-like channels have prominent muscular walls.

■ Secondary changes, such as papillary endothelial hyperplasia, are common.

Reference

Jones WP, Keller FS, Odrezin GT, et al. Venous hemangioma of the gallbladder. Gastrointest Radiol 12:319–321, 1987.

ARTERIOVENOUS MALFORMATION

Arteriovenous malformations are acquired (posttraumatic) or congenital benign vascular tumors with arteriovenous anastomoses. Synonyms include cirsoid/racemose aneurysms.

Clinical Findings

■ Traumatic tumors are solitary tumors, usually subcutaneous (arteriovenous fistula). Typical causes are low-velocity fragment trauma, skull fracture, and surgery. Clinical signs include varicose veins, cardiac dilatation, aneurysm, and thrombosis. The lower extremities are most commonly involved.
■ Congenital tumors are often multiple and have a female predominance.
■ Sites of involvement include deep soft tissues of the extremities, head, and neck; stomach mucosa (Dieulafoy aneurysm); and the CNS.
■ Clinical signs include swelling of the extremity, superficial varicosities, bruits, high output cardiac failure, and hemorrhage.
■ In Klippel-Trenaunay syndrome, signs include a lower extremity port wine stain, varicose veins, and skeletal and soft-tissue hypertrophy of the affected site, with lengthening of the limb.
■ In Parkes Weber (Klippel-Trenauney-Weber) syndrome, there are unilateral arteriovenous malformations, often with congestive heart failure.
■ Diagnosis by arteriography is as important as histopathologic diagnosis.
■ "Acral arteriovenous tumor" of the perioral region and the extremities of adults manifests as small papules in the dermis of the skin or submucosa of the lip.
■ CNS lesions are most prevalent in the central cerebral hemispheres and are characterized on angiogram by large feeding vessels. The rate of bleeding is approximately 4% per year.

Histologic Findings

■ Malformed arteries and veins
■ "Arterialized" veins with fibrointimal hyperplasia, medial muscular hypertrophy, and prominent internal elastic laminae, reflecting increased luminal pressure secondary to anastomosis

References

Adams RD, Victor M. Cerebrovascular diseases. In Adams RD, Victor M (eds). Principles of Neurology. New York, McGraw-Hill, 1993, pp 729–743.
Linder F. Acquired arterio-venous fistulas. Report of 223 operated cases. Ann Chir Gynaecol 74:1–5, 1985.

INTRAMUSCULAR HEMANGIOMA

Intramuscular hemangiomas are benign vascular tumors that are poorly circumscribed and occur within skeletal muscle. The histologic appearance ranges from capillary/cavernous hemangiomas to arteriovenous malformations. The presence of fat in many lesions suggests that they may be hamartomas (infiltrating angiolipomas).

Clinical Findings

■ Most patients are younger than 30 years old.
■ Lower extremities (especially the quadriceps femoris muscle) are the most commonly affected.
■ Arteriography is frequently diagnostic.
■ Incomplete excision may occur because of infiltrative growth.
■ Recurrence is not uncommon after incomplete excision.

Histologic Features

■ Capillary, cavernous, arteriovenous hemangiomas
■ Fat
■ Ossification (occasionally), especially in lesions that resemble arteriovenous hemangiomas

Differential Diagnosis

■ Angiosarcoma (rare in muscle)
■ Liposarcoma

Reference

Allen PW, Enzinger FM. Hemangiomas of skeletal muscle: an analysis of 89 cases. Cancer 29:8–23, 1972.

ANGIOMATOSIS

Angiomatosis is a benign vascular proliferation growing contiguously in multiple tissue planes or extensively in tissues of the same type (e.g., apposed muscles).

Clinical Findings

■ There is a female predominance (female:male ratio 3:2).
■ Mean age is second to third decades.
■ Persistent diffuse swelling, pain, and tenderness occur. There is infrequent limb hypertrophy.
■ Superficial discoloration and signs of arteriovenous shunting are usually absent.
■ The lower extremity, including the buttock, is the most frequently affected site, followed by the trunk and the upper extremity. Less commonly, the head and neck, back, pelvis, and retroperitoneum are involved.
■ The process involves the deep subcutaneous tissue and muscles, although more superficial tissues or underlying bone may also be involved.
■ There is a strong propensity for local recurrence.

Histologic Findings

■ An admixture of large irregular venous segments with disorganized muscular walls, cavernous vessels, and capillary channels are scattered diffusely throughout tissue planes and are often associated with large amounts of adipose tissue.

- Arteries and lymphatic channels may also be noted, but they are typically not seen in direct communication with the former.
- Capillary-sized vessels proliferate adjacent to, and within the walls of, the disorganized venous segments.

Differential Diagnosis

- Intramuscular hemangioma is generally more localized.
- Diffuse arteriovenous malformation is more likely to be associated with edema, phlebectasia, and arteriographic features of shunting; histologically, there is a predominance of thick-walled arteries and "arterialized" veins.

Reference

Rao VK, Weiss SW. Angiomatosis of soft tissue: an analysis of the histologic features and clinical outcome in 51 cases. Am J Surg Pathol 16:764–771, 1992.

INTRAVASCULAR FASCIITIS

Intravascular fasciitis is a growth that is histologically similar to nodular fasciitis and occurs in intimate association with vessels, usually veins.

Clinical Findings

- Intravascular fasciitis occurs at any age, but usually in children and young adults.
- The head and neck region is affected.
- The lesion may be fast-growing.

Gross Pathologic Findings

- The circumscribed or infiltrative mass may be multiple, but its association with a vessel is often not appreciated.
- Masses are usually smaller than 3 cm.

Microscopic Findings

- Findings are similar to those of nodular fasciitis.
- "Feathery" growth of myofibroblasts occurs within the vessel wall and adventitia.
- The mass may grow into surrounding soft tissue.
- Osteoclast-like giant cells, cystic degeneration, and keloid-like collagen are occasionally present.

Differential Diagnosis

- Sarcoma is considered in the differential diagnosis. Intravascular fasciitis may have abundant mitoses and cellularity.
- Dense fascicular growth of leiomyoma is usually absent in intravascular fasciitis.

Reference

Patchevsky AS, Enzinger FM. Intravascular fasciitis. A report of 17 cases. Am J Surg Pathol 5:29–32, 1981.

PAPILLARY ENDOTHELIAL HYPERPLASIA

Papillary endothelial hyperplasia is a reactive, unusually exuberant form of organizing thrombus (Masson's vegetant intravascular hemangioendothelioma, intravascular angiomatosis).

Clinical Findings

- In the "pure" form, there is a subcutaneous mass, often of fingers, head, neck, or hemorrhoidal vessels.
- In most cases, papillary endothelial hyperplasia is a component of an organizing thrombus or other vascular tumor; clinical findings pertain to the specific process.

Gross Pathologic Findings

- In the pure form, a bluish mass is usually well circumscribed and less than 1 cm.

Microscopic Findings

- There is a proliferation of endothelial cells.
- Papillary fronds contain a core of fibrin (early stage) or hyalinized collagen (later stage).
- There is no significant atypia, and mitotic activity is low.
- Fronds may appear to be "free-floating" within the vessel lumen.

Differential Diagnosis

- In comparison with angiosarcoma, papillary endothelial hyperplasia is usually confined to the lumen, lacks pleomorphism, has a single layer of cells, has a low mitotic rate, and demonstrates little necrosis.

References

Kuo T, Sayers PM, Rosai J. Masson's "vegetant intravascular hemangioendothelioma": a lesion often mistaken for angiosarcoma. Study of seventeen cases located in the skin and soft tissues. Cancer 38:1227–1236, 1976.

Pins MR, Rosenthal DI, Springfield DS, et al. Florid extravascular papillary endothelial hyperplasia (Masson's pseudoangiosarcoma) presenting as a soft-tissue sarcoma. Arch Pathol Lab Med 117:259–263, 1993.

Stern Y, Braslavsky D, Segal K, Shpitzer T, Abraham A. Intravascular papillary endothelial hyperplasia in the maxillary sinus. A benign lesion that may be mistaken for angiosarcoma. Arch Otolaryngol Head Neck Surg 117:1182–1184, 1991.

EPITHELIOID HEMANGIOMA (ANGIOLYMPHOID HYPERPLASIA WITH EOSINOPHILIA)

Epithelioid hemangioma is a benign vascular proliferation, most likely reactive, with epithelioid endothelial cells and often eosinophils. Histiocytoid hemangioma is a related term that likely includes other entities. Kimura's disease is a related but probably separate entity.

Clinical Findings

- Subcutaneous tissues or dermis of the head and neck are affected.
- Lymphadenopathy and peripheral eosinophilia are less common than in Kimura's disease.
- There is no Asian predilection.
- There is local recurrence in up to one third of patients.

Histologic Findings

- The proliferation is composed primarily of uncanalized capillaries.
- There are epithelioid (histiocytoid) endothelial cells.
- The process is often centered about a medium-sized artery or vein.
- The lesion is usually well circumscribed and often bordered by lymphoid follicles.
- Eosinophils may be plentiful but are occasionally rare or absent.
- Dermal (superficial) lesions are less well marginated, more often mature (canalized), and not generally associated with a vessel or lymphoid follicles.

References

Allen PW, Ramakrishna B, MacCormac LB. The histiocytoid hemangiomas and other controversies. Pathol Annu 27:51–87, 1992.

Olsen TG, Helwig EB. Angiolymphoid hyperplasia with eosinophilia: a clinicopathologic study of 116 patients. J Am Acad Dermatol 12:781–796, 1985.

SPINDLE CELL HEMANGIOENDOTHELIOMA

Spindle cell hemangioendothelioma is a vascular tumor of indeterminate biologic potential that was originally considered to be a low-grade neoplasm and is currently believed by some to be a reactive proliferation.

Clinical Findings

- Spindle cell hemangioendothelioma is a superficial, slow-growing, painless mass.
- The hands and feet are affected in more than 50% of cases.
- Lesions are usually less than 2 cm.
- There is a predilection for the third and fourth decades.
- Local recurrence is common. Metastasis is rare or nonexistent.

Histologic Findings

- Well circumscribed
- Cavernous hemangioma with spindle cell proliferation
- Epithelioid endothelial cells (occasionally)

Differential Diagnosis

- Kaposi's sarcoma

References

Ding J, Hashimoto H, Imayama S, et al. Spindle cell hemangioendothelioma: probably a benign vascular lesion not a low grade angiosar-

coma. Virchows Archiv A Pathol Anat Histopathol 420:77–85, 1992.

Imayama S, Murakami Y, Hashimoto H, Hori Y. Spindle cell hemangioendothelioma exhibits the ultrastructural features of reactive vascular proliferation rather than of angiosarcoma. Am J Clin Pathol 97:279–287, 1992.

Perkins PL, Weiss SW. Spindle cell hemangioendothelioma: a clinicopathologic analysis of 77 cases. Mod Pathol 7:9A, 1994.

Weiss SW, Enzinger FM. Spindle cell hemangioendothelioma: a low grade angiosarcoma resembling a cavernous hemangioma and Kaposi's sarcoma. Am J Surg Pathol 10:521–530, 1986.

ENDOVASCULAR PAPILLARY ANGIOENDOTHELIOMA (DABSKA TUMOR)

Clinical Findings

- Exceedingly rare
- Limited potential for aggressive behavior
- Affects all ages

Gross Pathologic Findings

- Superficial skin lesions
- May grow into underlying structures, including muscle and bone

Histologic Features

- Hemangioma containing characteristic papillary tufts with a central avascular hyaline core
- Possible epithelioid appearance of endothelial cells

Differential Diagnosis

- Other epithelioid hemangiomas (spindle cell hemangioendothelioma, epithelioid hemangioendothelioma, epithelioid hemangioma)

References

Dabska M. Malignant endovascular papillary angioendothelioma of the skin in childhood. Clinicopathologic study of six cases. Cancer 24:503–510, 1969.

Morgan J, Robinson MF, Rosen LB, et al. Malignant endovascular papillary angioendothelioma (Dabska tumor). A case report and review of the literature. Am J Dermatopathol 11:64–68, 1989.

EPITHELIOID HEMANGIOENDOTHELIOMA

Epithelioid hemangioendothelioma is a malignant vascular tumor composed of epithelioid endothelial cells. The clinical course is more favorable than that of angiosarcoma. "Intravascular sclerosing bronchoalveolar tumor" is the term used for epithelioid hemangioendothelioma of the lung.

Clinical Findings

- Epithelioid hemangioendothelioma occurs at any age, but is rare in childhood.
- Affected sites include soft tissue of the extremities, lungs, liver, and bones.

TUMORS AND TUMOR-LIKE PROLIFERATIONS OF PERIPHERAL BLOOD VESSELS ▪ 211

- More than 50% of cases are associated with a medium-sized or larger vessel, usually a vein.
- Metastases occur in 31% of cases, and tumor-related death occurs in 13% of patients (mean follow-up period 48 months).
- Aggressive histologic features include mitotic activity greater than 1 mitosis per 10 high-power fields, spindled tumor cell morphology, and the presence of necrosis.

Gross Pathologic Findings

- Marginated nodules with rubbery consistency

Microscopic Findings

- Epithelioid (histiocytoid) endothelial cells
- Spindle or dendritic cells in cord-like arrangements within a chondromyxoid or myxohyaline matrix
- Prominent cytoplasmic vacuoles within neoplastic cells
- Positivity for endothelial markers shown by immunohistochemistry; helpful in distinction from carcinoma

Differential Diagnosis

- Epithelioid hemangioma
- Epithelioid sarcoma
- Metastatic carcinoma
- Chondrosarcoma

References

Weiss SW, Enzinger FM. Epithelioid hemangioendothelioma: a vascular tumor often mistaken for a carcinoma. Cancer 50:970–981, 1982.
Weldon-Linne CM, Victor TA, Christ ML, et al. Angiogenic nature of the "intravascular bronchoalveolar tumor" of the lung: an electron microscopic study. Arch Pathol Lab Med 105:174–179, 1981.

BACILLARY ANGIOMATOSIS

Bacillary angiomatosis is a nonneoplastic vascular proliferation found usually in immunocompromised individuals, caused by bacterial species (*Rochalimaea henselae,* Bartonella sp., and similar gram-negative bacteria).

Clinical Findings

- Bacillary angiomatosis most often affects patients with acquired immunodeficiency syndrome.
- Cutaneous lesions are the usual initial manifestation; a systemic infection may follow that may involve virtually any organ.
- Treatment consists of therapy with erythromycin, rifampin, or doxycycline over a 4- to 6-week course.

Gross Pathologic Findings

- Multiple cutaneous lesions are present.
- Bacillary angiomatosis must be differentiated from Kaposi's sarcoma.

Microscopic Findings

- There is lobulated proliferation of capillary-sized vessels.

- The endothelium lining the vessels may be mildly atypical.
- Neutrophils and leukocytoclastic debris are present.
- Clumps of small curved rods appear approximately 0.5 to 1.0 μm in length with the Warthin Starry stain, pH 4.0.

Differential Diagnosis

- In comparison with pyogenic granuloma, bacillary angiomatosis contains atypical vessels and inflammatory foci in the absence of surface ulceration.
- In comparison with Kaposi's sarcoma, bacillary angiomatosis demonstrates a well-formed, lobulated vascular pattern, and it has a polymorphonuclear, rather than lymphoplasmacytic, inflammatory reaction.
- Demonstration of organisms, which are usually numerous, is pathognomonic of bacillary angiomatosis.

References

Chan JKC, Lewin KJ, Lombard CM, et al. Histopathology of bacillary angiomatosis of lymph nodes. Am J Surg Pathol 15:430–437, 1991.
Schwartzman WA. Infections due to *Rochalimaea:* the expanding clinical spectrum. Clin Infect Dis 15:893–902, 1992.

KAPOSI'S SARCOMA

Kaposi's sarcoma is a multifocal neoplasm of spindled and endothelial cells, which is associated in most cases with immunosuppression.

Clinical Findings

- In nonimmunosuppressed patients, there is a marked predominance in men aged 50 to 80 years, especially those of Mediterranean descent. Skin of the lower extremities is primarily affected.
- The spectrum of lesions spans coalescent macules, papules, and plaques; early lesions resemble petechiae or papulonodules; later stage lesions are nodules, often ulcerating.
- In disseminated disease, mucosal surfaces, lymph nodes, salivary glands, and viscera are affected.

Histologic Findings

- In early lesions, there are prominent periadnexal capillaries with chronic inflammation and focal endothelial atypia.
- Nodular lesions have spindle and endothelial cells, which are often cellular; occasionally, epithelioid areas are present.
- There are hemosiderin deposits throughout the lesion; globules that are positive on periodic acid–Schiff are characteristic features.

Differential Diagnosis

- Granulation tissue (early lesion) and leiomyosarcoma (cellular nodular lesion) are in the differential diagnosis.
- Infantile kaposiform hemangioendothelioma is a rare vascular tumor of infants that is deep seated and ag-

gressive, resulting in jaundice or intestinal obstruction. The histologic appearance is that of cellular capillary hemangioma with focal slit-like areas that resemble Kaposi's sarcoma. Unlike Kaposi's sarcoma, however, the tumor is lobulated, lacks inflammatory cells and hemosiderin deposits, and is not associated with immunosuppression.

References

Chor PJ, Santa Cruz DJ. Kaposi's sarcoma: a clinicopathologic review and differential diagnosis. J Cutan Pathol 19:6–20, 1992.

Fukunaga M, Silverberg S. Hyaline globules in Kaposi's sarcoma: a light microscopic and immunohistochemical study. Mod Pathol 4:187–190, 1991.

Tsang WYW, Chang JKC. Kaposi-like infantile hemangioendothelioma: a distinctive vascular neoplasm of the retroperitoneum. Am J Surg Pathol 15:982–989, 1991.

ANGIOSARCOMA

Angiosarcoma is a malignant neoplasm derived from and composed of endothelial cells of blood vessel or lymph vessel origin.

Clinical Findings

■ Cutaneous and subcutaneous angiosarcomas occur in the head and neck of elderly individuals, and in the breast and upper extremity of postmastectomy patients (lymphedema or Stewart-Treves syndrome).
■ Angiosarcomas of the breast have rarely been reported in patients with lumpectomy and radiation therapy.
■ Angiosarcomas of the deep soft tissue are relatively rare and may appear at any age; they may be associated with thrombocytopenia.
■ Sites of deep angiosarcomas include the heart and pericardium (see Chaps. 12 and 14), adrenal gland, thyroid gland, retroperitoneum, uterus, CNS, and extremities.

■ Treatment of cutaneous tumors is complete excision; grading is not prognostically helpful.
■ The clinical course of deep angiosarcoma is probably aggressive, although there are no large series to date.
■ Treatment of deep angiosarcoma remains to be determined; complete surgical extirpation is recommended.

Histologic Appearance

■ Cutaneous tumors are multicentric, well-formed vascular channels.
■ Deep tumors are often epithelioid, spindled, or histiocytoid; they are poorly differentiated with sheets of cells.
■ Extensive sampling may be necessary to identify areas of endothelial cell differentiation.
■ Factor VIII–related antigen, *Ulex europaeus* lectin, and CD34 antigen are expressed in well-differentiated angiosarcomas.
■ Epithelioid angiosarcoma may also stain strongly for keratin; however, other epithelial markers are generally negative.

Differential Diagnosis

■ Epithelioid hemangioma
■ Papillary endothelial hyperplasia
■ Spindle cell hemangioendothelioma
■ Kaposi's sarcoma

References

Mark RJ, Tran LM, Sercarz J, Fu YS, Calcaterra TC, Juillard GF. Angiosarcoma of the head and neck. The UCLA experience 1955 through 1990. Arch Otolaryngol Head Neck Surg 119:973–978, 1993.

Mena H, Ribas JL, Enzinger FM, Parisi JE. Primary angiosarcoma of the central nervous system. Study of eight cases and review of the literature. J Neurosurg 75:73–76, 1991.

Stokkel MP, Peterse HL. Angiosarcoma of the breast after lumpectomy and radiation therapy for adenocarcinoma. Cancer 69:2965–2968, 1992.

Wolov RB, Sato N, Azumi N, Lack EE. Intra-abdominal angiosarcomatosis report of two cases after pelvic irradiation. Cancer 67:2275–2279, 1991.

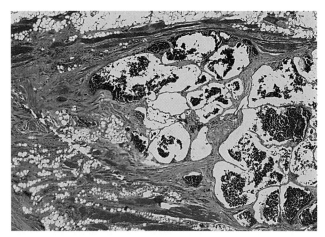

Figure 25–1. Intramuscular hemangioma. Note the cavernous spaces typical of hemangioma. There is also a proliferation of fat within the skeletal muscle, a typical feature of intramuscular hemangioma.

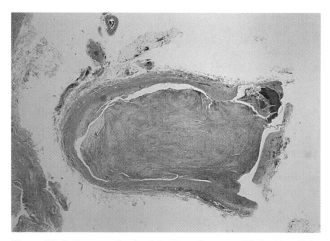

Figure 25–2. Intravascular fasciitis. Note the artery filled with cellular proliferation.

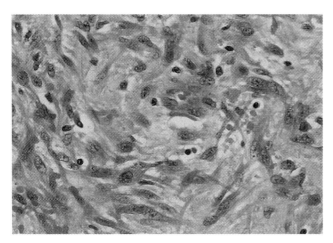

Figure 25–3. Intravascular fasciitis. A high magnification of Figure 25–2 demonstrates cellular features similar to nodular fasciitis of soft tissue, with a characteristic tissue culture appearance to the fibroblasts.

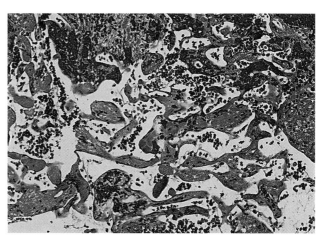

Figure 25–4. Papillary endothelial hyperplasia. There are anastomosing channels lined with endothelial cells and organizing fibrin, and there is an absence of endothelial atypia.

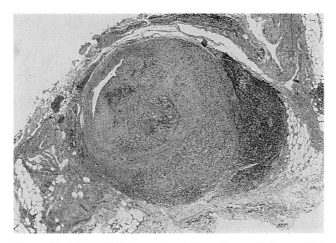

Figure 25–5. Epithelioid hemangioma. There is a well-circumscribed proliferation with focal lymphoid reaction involving a medium-sized artery.

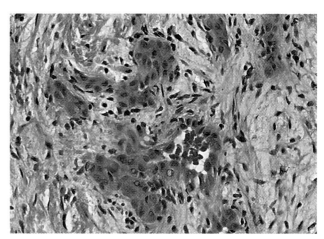

Figure 25–6. Epithelioid hemangioma. The proliferating endothelial cells are plump, with an epithelioid appearance, and there is a myxoid background.

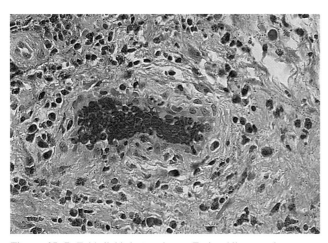

Figure 25–7. Epithelioid hemangioma. Eosinophils may be present within the walls of the proliferating vessels.

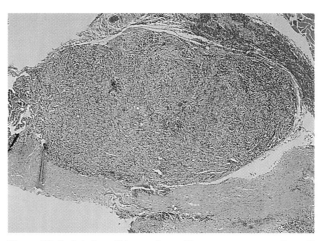

Figure 25–8. Spindle cell hemangioma. These tumors are usually well circumscribed, as are most benign vascular tumors.

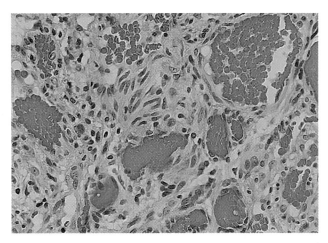

Figure 25–9. Spindle cell hemangioma. Spindle cells are interspersed among benign-appearing cavernous channels; this juxtaposition is not present in Kaposi's sarcoma.

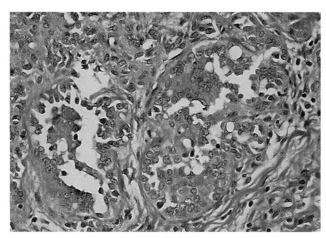

Figure 25–10. Dabska tumor (endovascular papillary angioendothelioma). The endothelial cells have a papillary, epithelial appearance.

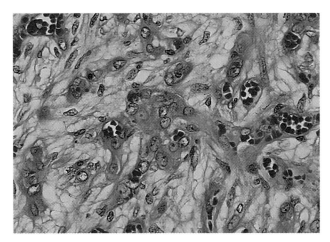

Figure 25–11. Epithelioid hemangioendothelioma. Typical features are cords and anastomosing bands of epithelioid cells. Despite their distinctly epithelioid appearance, vacuoles containing red blood cells are present. These are not present in carcinoma.

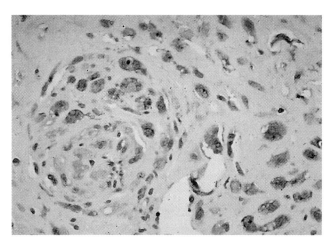

Figure 25–12. Epithelioid hemangioendothelioma. Immunohistochemical stain for CD34 demonstrates cytoplasmic positivity for this endothelial marker.

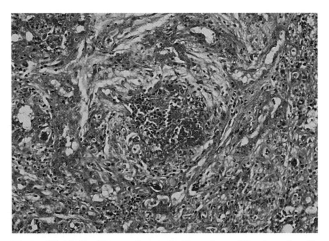

Figure 25–13. Bacillary angiomatosis. Note the proliferation of capillary-type vessels and the focal abscess.

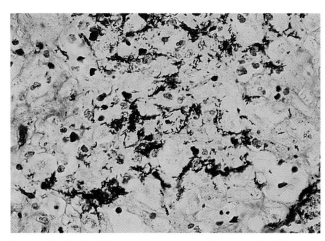

Figure 25–14. Bacillary angiomatosis. A silver stain highlights the bacilli, which are numerous and enlarged by silver impregnation.

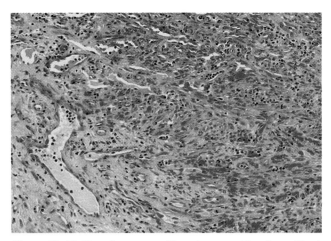

Figure 25–15. Kaposi's sarcoma. There is a transition from dilated, mildly atypical vascular channels to a cellular, atypical proliferation diagnostic of Kaposi's sarcoma.

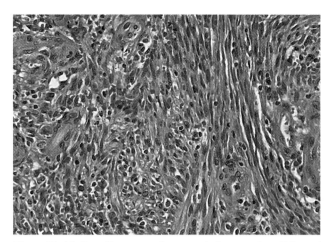

Figure 25–16. Kaposi's sarcoma. Late-stage lesions may be cellular and fascicular and may resemble leiomyosarcoma.

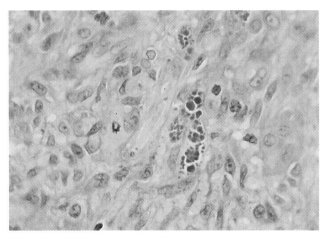

Figure 25–17. Kaposi's sarcoma. Globules that are positive for periodic acid–Schiff and that are diastase resistant are often present. Although not specific, they are, like hemosiderin deposits, a helpful feature in the differential diagnosis.

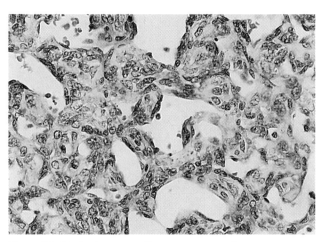

Figure 25–18. Angiosarcoma. There are anastomosing structures composed of and lined by atypical endothelial cells.

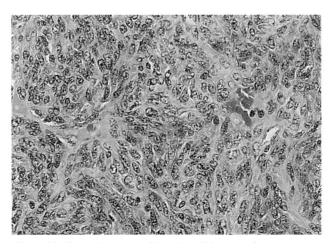

Figure 25–19. Angiosarcoma. The endothelial nature of the tumor may not be evident in cellular areas of the tumor.

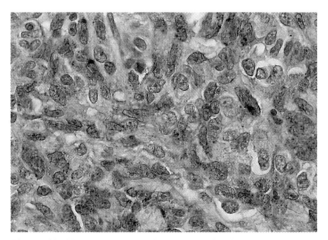

Figure 25–20. Angiosarcoma, factor VIII–related antigen. In many cases of angiosarcoma, expression of factor VIII–related antigen is demonstrated by immunohistochemical techniques. The positivity is generally cytoplasmic and diffusely punctate; this photomicrograph illustrates the same tumor shown in Figure 25–19.

INDEX

Note: Page numbers in *italics* refer to illustrations;
page numbers followed by t refer to tables.

217